Geriatric Residential Care

Geriatric Residential Care

Edited by

Robert D. Hill, PhD
Brian L. Thorn, PhD
John Bowling, PhD
Anthony Morrison, PhD
University of Utah

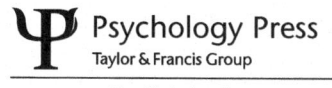 Psychology Press
Taylor & Francis Group

New York   London

First pubished by

Lawrence Erlbaum Associates, Inc., Publishers
10 Industrial Avenue
Mahwah, NJ 07430

This edition published 2012 by Psychology Press

Psychology   Psychology
Taylor & Francis Group   Taylor & Francis Group
711 Third Avenue   27 Church Road, Hove
New York, NY 10017   East Sussex BN3 2FA

Cover design by Kathryn Houghtaling Lacey

Library of Congress Cataloging-in-Publication Data

Geriatric residential care / Robert D. Hill ...[et al.].
        p. cm.
Includes bibliographical references and index.
ISBN 0-8058-3846-5 (cloth : alk. paper)
ISBN 0-8058-3847-3 (pbk. : alk. paper)
1. Old age homes. 2. Aged—Institutional care. 3. Geriatrics. I. Hill,
    Robert D.
HV1454 .G47 2001
362.6'1—dc21   2001023994
                                                      CIP

Contents

Preface

It is well-known that adults are living longer than ever before. For the first time in U.S. history, the Census Bureau has created a three-digit space for age in recognition of the more than 70,000 centenarians who are living into the 21st Century. With this increase in average life expectancy as well as the greater numbers of adults who are living into very old age, it is becoming more critical to address the care needs of the frail elderly. In recent history, this has been accomplished primarily through nursing home facilities that have operated exclusively within the medical model of care. In fact, in the 1980s there was a 29% increase in the number of frail older adults residing in nursing homes.

As greater numbers of people find themselves in need of nonmedical assistance with basic activities of daily living, more options must become available for long-term care. It is not surprising; therefore, that residential care is currently a "top-growth" industry in the United States and will likely be one of the more important resources for addressing the needs of the frail elderly throughout the 21st century.

Residential care has been difficult to define because it has encompassed such a wide range of living options including family care, board and care homes, and assisted living environments. Thus, there is a rapidly growing need to develop models of residential care that can fully address the contemporary issues of the frail elderly. A major goal of this book; therefore, is to examine the concept of residential care from a psychological perspective. The chapter authors of this text espouse a psychological approach to long-term residential care, and throughout the text an effort is made to present a model of care that encompasses the whole individual. Given that psychologists are being increasingly asked to provide consultation to long-term residential care facilities, the need for psychologically based care models has become apparent. This text offers assistance in developing and maintaining residential care environments that maximize quality of life and personal well-being in the presence of declining physical and emotional resources that are associated with the vicissitudes of living into advanced aging.

This text is divided into four parts. Part I addresses psychological and social issues facing the frail elderly who are candidates for, or are living in, residential care settings. The three chapters in Part I highlight the wide range of individual differences among the frail elderly. Conceptualizing the needs of this very heterogeneous population involves balancing the need for autonomy and individual respect in the presence of age-related deterioration of basic capabilities for self-care. Several models were presented highlighting the progress society has made to maximize individual choice within such closed communities. A critical theme that runs through Part I is the notion that the highest quality of care can only be obtained through establishing a strong sense of continuity with the individual's previous social and psychological contexts.

Part II addresses issues in the assessment of individuals in residential care. The chapters in this part cover psychological and neuropsychological assessment strategies, as well as the acknowledgement that medical problems and psychological state are highly interconnected. One goal of Part II is to build a conceptual framework to allow for the assessment of the effectiveness of multidisciplinary interventions designed to improve quality of life in residential care.

Part III highlights the design and execution of intervention strategies in residential care. Case studies and empirical research are presented to develop a set of tailored intervention approaches to some of the more common issues facing individuals in this context. Such strategies encompass behavioral management and pharmacological strategies.

Part IV, the final section of this text, addresses how organizational aspects of residential care contexts can optimize the quality and meaningfulness of care. For example, strategies for training staff and altering the basic living environment are described with respect to the optimization of care. The final chapter highlights future directions in residential care and how these assisted-living communities will look in the 21st century.

We express appreciation to the following family members who supported us while we developed this text. These are Debra K. Hill, Lynette Thorn, Debra Morrison, and Judith Bowling. Special thanks to the creativity and support provided by Loren Shook, CEO, and Steve Winner, Chief of Culture at Silverado Senior Living. Special thanks from R. D. Hill to his Great Aunt, C. Belle Grischow who is 92 years old and aging optimally.

I

General Concepts in Residential Care

1

Older Adults in Residential Care: A Population at Risk

Robert D. Hill and Chuck Gregg
University of Utah

INTRODUCTION

It is well documented that the population of the United States is progressively aging. In 1990, 12.7% of the U.S. population was over age 65, and by 2020 this will increase to 18% (American Association of Retired Persons [AARP], 1991). Although the majority of older adults can expect to live healthy and independent lives, a substantial minority will require long-term care to compensate for age-related functional impairment. For the purpose of this chapter, residential-based care is the mechanism by which many of these needs are met. Hawes (1999) has defined residential care as a closed community-based living arrangement that houses two or more unrelated adults and provides assistance with instrumental activities of daily living such as laundry, meals, household upkeep, medication supervision, organized activities, and transportation. This type of care has been commonly characterized by many names including board and care homes, residential living centers, assisted living homes, congregate living facilities, personal care homes, homes for the aged, shelter care homes, adult care homes, and family care homes, to name just a few (see Hawes, 1999). Because residential care is a somewhat elusive term, its definition in this chapter encompasses all forms of residential-based services, including nursing home care. Specifically, residential care involves a range of services that exist along a continuum of care with the endpoints defined as housing and social support for the least impaired endpoint, to the provision of housing, professional services, and 24-hour medical care at the more severe endpoint. With respect to the more severe residents, these individuals would be considered incapable of performing even the most basic self-care functions including toileting, feeding, moving from one place to another, and dressing without assistance. They would also need 24-hour medical supervision to deal with progressive disease or other health-related problems. In other words, it is likely that an individual with such significant care needs would not survive independently without the receipt of this level of care. Chapter 2 explores this definition of residential care in more depth; however, the goal of this chapter is to characterize individuals who are most likely to need residential care services and to describe two theoretical models of aging that can be extended to residential care.

It has been estimated that between 1980 and 1990 the annual rate of growth in residential care facilities has been between 15% and 20% (Assisted Living Facilities of America, 1993; AARP, 1993). Individuals who are in need of residential care have traditionally been identified as the frail elderly, and they possess three distinguishing characteristics that differentiate them from older adults who are able to live independently in their own home or outside of an institutional environment: advanced age, disability, and diminished resources to live independently. As highlighted throughout this chapter, the concept of residential care in this regard includes the provision of assistance to the frail elderly across a wide variety of formal and informal settings.

The Very Old

As our society progresses through the 21st century, it is clear that there will be an unprecedented increased in the oldest old (Suzman, Manton & Willis 1992). Although this subgroup of very old adults has been traditionally defined as those 85 years of age and older, recent population estimates have moved this arbitrary cut off point to 90 years, and there is a growing literature highlighting centenarians who have unique care needs (Taueber & Rosenwaike, 1992). It is noteworthy that for the first time in our history, the U.S. Census Bureau's census forms have added a 3-digit column for "age," highlighting the approximately 70,000 centenarians in the United States (Koplan & Fleming, 2000). There are a number of predictable issues that face the very old including the need for supportive services to meet the growing physical and psychological dependency that is associated with very advanced age.

With respect to demographics, population estimates have noted that for those individuals who live to be 85 years or older, the ratio of women to men is in excess of 3 to 1 (Taueber & Rosenwaike, 1992). In addition, it is fairly well documented that the oldest-old have less formal education than younger aged cohorts, although recent population projections have estimated that this educational disadvantage will diminish as younger age-groups move into more advanced age. The extant literature has indicated that lower levels of education are predictive of cognitive problems and among the predominant number of individuals with dementia of the Alzheimer's type, many report completing fewer years of formal education (Mortimer & Graves, 1993).

Although much research and clinical data has been presented to characterize the oldest old who are living independently in the community from those who are at risk for institutionalized care, there are a number of issues common to this high-risk group when compared with older adults who are relatively unimpaired. These common characteristics include (a) the need to remain independent and somewhat self-sufficient, (b) a desire to be recognized and treated with respect within the social system, and (c) the need to feel connected to others in a meaningful way. In many ways the concept of independence must include aspects of functional independence, namely activities of daily living (ADL) and instrumental activities of daily living (IADL), but also a sense that one is capable of engaging with others to achieve personal gains. In some respects, it might appear that placement in a long-term care facility would indicate a subjugation of this need; however, research argues to the contrary. In fact, maintaining functional independence within a residential care context may become even more pronounced as one moves into very late life. Thus, a critical need that the very old face is the desire to be recognized and supported by various systems within ones living environment. This includes the family and the community at large. This point is evidenced in the following case scenario:

> When his wife died several years ago Charles, age 82, continued to reside in the family home. However, the surrounding neighborhood had changed considerably over the years and was now dominated by younger couples with school aged children. Charles found himself increasingly socially isolated with few friends or visitors. As a result he began to experience periodic bouts of depression and feelings of uselessness and helplessness. After considerable discussion his family convinced him that he likely would fare better in a residential living center for older adults. Following his initial adjustment to this new living situation, Charles did indeed begin to establish friendships with the other residents of the center and participate in numerous activities and outings. His symptoms of depression gradually subsided and he began to speak more optimistically of his life and his future.

This vignette highlights the notion that very old adults, by virtue of age-related developmental processes, disengage from work and community-related activities and are defined as a group of adults who are dependent with respect to social systems. However, they are also an extension of our social network inasmuch as they represent a normative end-state through which all individuals in society must pass. Thus, dealing with the problems of advanced aging and the care of those with predictable disability that occurs as one moves into very old age is an issue that not only characterizes this group of older adults, but ultimately affects all members of society who will likely live into advanced age.

Disability in Old Age

One of the more distinguishing features of older adults who are in need of residential care is age-related disability. The nature of disability is complex and interacts in part with increased mortality risks associated with old age. Manton and Saldo (1992) highlighted this complexity by suggesting that a selection bias (through death) may mediate the presence and the various forms of disability in a given individual within the overall population. Nonetheless, it is clear that disability increases as a function of advanced aging, although it is not necessarily the case that disability is only present in the very old. For example, data from the 1970s and 1980s documented that although older Americans were living longer, the level of disability increased (see Crimmons, Saito, Ingegneri, 1989). In other words, an increase in population life expectancy has the effect of increasing the presence of health problems and disability across all age groupings of older adults. Lubitz, Beebe, and Baker (1995) have suggested that health care expenditures by the individual and society (including various forms of institutionalized care for older adults) depends in part on a number of factors, including the absolute number of older adults with respect to the total population and their health status. The term active life expectancy has emerged to define this issue and denotes the interaction of disability and age in predicting relative functioning in a given population. Using active life expectancy as a gauge of disability in the United States, the highest proportion of disabled adults varies across geographical regions but are usually between the ages of 70 and 90. Interestingly, for those who live beyond 90, relative disability remains stable (or in some cases declines) given the high morbidity that is a normative process in very old age. In other words, there is an increased likelihood in very old age that those who experience disability succumb to death in contrast to those who, by virtue of genetic propensity, live beyond 90 years of age in good health. As noted earlier, centenarians are a good example of those who are very old but are able to manage their chronic conditions outside of institutional settings.

Thus, in addition to age, chronic illness is a source of disability. In this chapter, chronic illness is defined as a disease or dysfunction that lasts an extended period of time, involves remission and exacerbation of symptoms, and increases the likelihood of functional impairment. There is large individual variation with respect to chronic illness, although it is noteworthy that 80% of those over 65 years of age will have at least one chronic health condition. Multiple chronic illnesses are common for those who live to be 75 and older (AARP, 1998) and increases the likelihood of disability and the need for professional services in order for the individual to maintain functional independence. It can also create strong discontinuities that foster social stereotypes making it more difficult for the individual to live in the community (e.g., we must keep our impaired family member out of the public eye; Luborsky, 1994). Some of the more common chronic illnesses facing adults 65 and older are arthritis (50%), hypertension (36%), hearing impairment (32%), heart disease (29%), cataracts (17%), orthopedic impairment (16%), and diabetes (10%). There are a number of factors that influence at what point and to what degree a person will experience disability associated with chronic health conditions (AARP, 1998). These include genetics, lifestyle behaviors, and the social environment. These factors also play a role in the timing of the need for long-term care services such as those found in residential care settings.

Disability due to cognitive impairment deserves special consideration as a risk factor for placement in residential care. Individuals who experience significant deficits in memory, language, abstract thinking, and judgement have great difficulty maintaining functional independence with respect to activities of daily living or instrumental activities of daily living. Chronic disease states that are associated with cognitive impairment generally involve some form of dementia. The traditional long-term care option for dementia patients has been nursing home care (Davis, et al., 2000). However, in the past few years there has been an increase in the number of special care units that have as their focus the care and management of individuals with cognitive impairments such as dementia of the Alzheimer's type (Davis et al., 2000; Zimmerman & Sloane, 1999). Although residential care facilities have, as yet, an unproven track record for housing and caring of individuals with dementia, Zimmerman and Sloane (1999) have highlighted a number of potential strengths that residential care facilities offer, particularly with respect to helping an individual to maintain limited autonomy as well as continuity within a long-term care setting.

In summary, physical and cognitive disability, as they emerge in later life are important determinants of the need for residential care. Although disability and old age are not the same, there are significant overlaps given that age is associated with both physical and cognitive decline. It appears, however, that the age range in which disability is the greatest and most likely to precipitate placement in residential care is between 70 and 90 years. In very old age, disability loses its prominence as a predictor of long-term care needs due, in part, to selective morbidity and mortality in favor of those who can function independently in old age even in the presence of disease.

Loss of Resources

A good number of older adults live in their home, which is true of those who have less disability but are simply in advanced age. This previous vignette is indicative of the phenomenon that as living conditions change (e.g., moving in with members of one's extended family), the risk of long-term care in contexts that are residential increases. The choice of where and how to live is affected by multiple factors including whether the individual is living with a partner, one's relative ability to engage in everyday living activities, and the nature of formal and informal support resources. Research also suggests that older adults who live without a partner are at the highest risk to need informal and formal care-related services. At its most fundamental level, being old and living alone magnifies the risk for loss of functional independence. Population estimates indicate that more than one third of adults 85 years of age and older live with a family member (see Atchley, 2000).

Although the majority of older adults in the United States prefer to live independently, financial status, functional status, and physical health may dictate consideration of alternative housing options that provide a more protective and supportive environment. For example, one of the most difficult issues facing aging individuals is the loss of their social support system through death of loved ones, and this is especially true when the loss involves close family members including parents and spouse. Loneliness, despair, and isolation are often associated with such losses, and these can lead to intractable psychiatric conditions such as depression (Ingebretsen & Solem, 1998), increasing the need for residential care services. Several studies have highlighted the fact that emotional conditions such as loneliness and depression can predispose an individual for care, and one treatment option for such conditions may involve the creation of a community where social support is more readily available. In addition to loss of one's support system, changes in financial state, loss of employment through retirement, and changes in ones living environment (moving away from one's home of origin) can all play a role in creating vulnerabilities that would predispose a person for residential care services. Unlike the nursing home, the concept espoused within the residential care field is the term "aging in place." (Hawes, 1999). This concept highlights the notion that the provision of health care should be provided, even to the most impaired and disabled person, in the least restrictive and most home-like environment as possible. This notion of aging in place is in contrast to nursing home care that has been molded and shaped by the medical model to focus intervention efforts on the presenting problem through strategies and techniques that are driven by specific diagnostic categories.

In summary, this section has highlighted characteristics of individuals who have the highest likelihood for placement in residential care. These characteristics include being very old, disabled, and having insufficient personal resources to maintain oneself independently in the community. The next section explores models of adult development and aging that may be useful in understanding how residential care can be made maximally effective.

EXTENDING THEORIES OF ADULT DEVELOPMENT TO THE CARE OF THE VERY OLD

Most of the research and professional literature in long-term care is atheoretical in nature. This, in part, has highlighted the trend to view long-term care as a pragmatic problem facing the frail elderly. However, in the past 10 years there has been rapid growth in developmental theories of adulthood and aging that could be used to guide research and planning in long-term care. Thus, integrating contemporary developmental models would seem critical if one were interested in optimally addressing the needs of the very old. Two prominent theories of aging are summarized in this section: SOC (selectivity, optimization, and compensation; see Baltes, Staudinger, & Lindenberger, 1999) and continuity theory (see

Atchley, 1989, 2000). Both of these theories have been described with respect to enhancing counseling interventions in the old and very old (see Hill, Thorn, & Packard, 2000), and in a similar way their linkage to issues of residential care are highlighted. It should be noted that one of the unique features of this book is the integration of these two models of adult development within several of the chapters. A major purpose of this chapter, therefore, is to provide the reader with an introductory description of these theories and to describe how they might apply to older adults in residential care.

(SOC) Theory

SOC as a theoretical construct has received significant attention in the scientific literature for more than two decades. It is part of a broad meta-theory of individual development from conception to old age. In this regard, its basic premise is that development involves not only acquisition and maturation, but also decomposition and attrition of life processes. Old age highlights these latter two forces. The complexity of SOC is beyond the scope of this chapter; however, there are aspects of this theory that can be used to inform and guide the structure and function of residential care. The first principle of SOC highlights the notion that with increased age the need for culture to offset age-related losses increases. For example, consider what has happened to life expectancy (which has increased dramatically) and educational status (such as reading skills) in the past five years. Although the fundamental genetic make-up of the population has changed very little in the past 100 years, more advanced levels of culture (including technology) have emerged to allow people to maintain functional independence into very old age that was not possible 100 years ago. For example, the advent of glasses, and more recently laser surgery for cataracts, in addition to multiple mediums through which to obtain information (e.g., radio, television, interactive computer displays, the internet) have allowed people to function for longer intervals of time in the presence of declining sensory capability. Thus, culture creates opportunities to facilitate function in the presence of eventual biological decline through degenerative processes associated with aging (e.g., declining health, vision loss, and increased disability). In other words, extended care (or assisted living) has its genesis in cultural efforts to offset the loss of independent functioning in very old age. As noted earlier, residential care promotes the concept of aging in place to highlight the increasing sophistication of this form of long-term care to address the unique preferences and needs of older individuals receiving care. Thus, the goal of residential care is both to extend the length of life and to create a care environment that facilitates active life expectancy in the presence of age-related cognitive impairment, physical impairment, or both. Thus, residential care can be theoretically construed as a culture-initiated compensatory force to promote functioning in the presence of degenerative physiological processes and death. The assumption underlying residential care is not to prevent death or remediate degenerative disease per se, but to maintain active life expectancy for as long as is possible.

A second component of SOC that is highlighted throughout the chapters in this text involves how the individual takes advantage of culture; the three relevant factors are selectivity, optimization, and compensation. Briefly, *selection* involves reducing the number of options available so as to focus one's skills and abilities on obtainable outcomes. It is well known that aging decreases objective levels of social support. In many cases such a decrease can be viewed as positive inasmuch as the individual begins to select only those relationships that are the most meaningful to her or him. In doing so, the individual can focus on these while letting go of other relationships which are not as important for continued life adjustment (e.g., former colleagues at work). *Optimization* involves a functional response to loss by focusing on abilities that are still intact. For example, if an older adult is becoming disoriented at night, it might be possible to optimize what capabilities still remain in the person's visual system by increasing the amount of ambient light in the bathroom at night. *Compensation*, the final component of SOC, involves developing new strategies to compensate for loss. In the case of long-term care, the use of asbsorptive pads when one is incontinent is a form of compensation. Because continence is lost and there is no way to regain this capability, developing compensatory strategies, such as the use of absorptive pads, is a compensatory alternative to deal with this issue. A powerful manifestation of this theory is the notion of wisdom, where although there is declining cognitive and physical ability in old age, the interaction of SOC can produce a form of knowledge in terms of mobilizing past experience and learning that, in a practical sense, can exceed the intellectual capability possessed by younger age groups. Baltes & Baltes (1990) highlighted this example of SOC in normal aging as follows:

> When the concert pianist Arthur Rubinstein, as an 80-year-old was asked in a television interview how he managed to maintain such a high level of expert piano playing, he hinted at the coordination of three strategies. First, he played fewer pieces (selection); he practiced these pieces more often (optimization); and to counteract his loss in mechanical speed he now used a kind of impression management, such as playing more slowly before fast segments to make the latter appear faster (compensation). (p. 22)

The above example provides a conceptual framework for SOC. The example of SOC that follows demonstrates the potential of using these three individual mechanisms to maximize functional adaptation in a residential care setting.

> Steve had a number of issues related to his behavior in a local residential care facility. The staff felt that part of the problem was that Steve became overstimulated when he

was in a large group of people, especially, those he was not familiar with. Thus, to assist Steve, a small support group of other residents was created of those with similar cognitive functioning and background by the on-site recreational therapist (selection). Activities were developed that Steve was comfortable with and could still gain information from, for example, he enjoyed having some of the members of the group read the newspaper to him (optimization). Because Steve had a tendency to wander, even though he enjoyed the group, one of the nurses aids was directed to gently encourage him to stay seated while the group was in session and the time of the group was shortened to better meet his attentional needs (compensation).

Although Steve is highlighted as the primary beneficiary of this intervention, it had a positive impact on others in the group as well.

Continuity Theory

Continuity theory was first proposed by Robert Atchley (1989) as a way to describe psychological adaptation in old and very old age. Although continuity theory was originally proposed to describe normal aging, it can easily be extended to older adults dealing with issues of advanced aging in residential care settings. The basic premise of continuity theory is that in making adaptive choices, older adults attempt to preserve and maintain existing internal and external psychological structures; that is, an older adult will draw from her or his central identity to solve current and future problems of living. Thus, continuity theory asserts that older individuals are integrally connected to the past to guide them in future decision-making. Within this framework, Atchley proposed two types of continuity: internal and external.

Internal continuity is defined by the individual in relation to a remembered inner structure, such as the persistence of temperament, affect, experiences, preferences, dispositions, and skills. It is noteworthy that even in individuals who experience profound deficits in cognitive functioning, basic internal structures associated with one's identity remain intact. As a specific example, consider an individual who maintains his or her identity through social interaction with others. This person (in the absence of a psychiatric condition such as depression) will gravitate toward this behavior even if he or she is significantly cognitively or physically impaired and in a new living situation. If allowed to continue, the individual will shape her or his living environment so that it facilitates the creation of opportunities for social interaction. In other words, a popular person will remain popular even when he or she is placed in a long-term care facility. This notion of internal continuity is a major factor underlying individual differences between residents in long-term care. To assume that all older adults are the same and do not vary with regard to internal psychological structures and capacities to shape their environment is to make an assumption that is counter to continuity theory and that will create a more difficult living environment for the individual. In the case described earlier, contexts that promote isolation will not help this person cope with an environmental change such as placement in a residential care facility.

External continuity involves stability of the structure of physical and social environments. This is inclusive of roles, relationships, and specific activities. Perceptions of external continuity occur when a person is in a familiar environment, practices familiar skills, and interacts with familiar people. Thus, there are everyday locations in social and physical space that are uniquely typical of the individual (e.g., this is Grandpa's favorite chair). Continuity theory predicts that reinstating these physical structures will facilitate adaptation. As noted in the example earlier, both internal and external continuity often interact; that is, individuals create and shape their own environment so that it is more amenable to one's internal sense of self. Finding ways to reinstate a sense of external continuity may work to facilitate adaptation. Chapters 9 and 13 highlight innovative environmental interventions that work to enhance external continuity in residential care settings.

Discontinuity involves change that is perceived by the individual as diminishing her or his capacity for coherence with respect to some aspect of external or internal continuity. A predicted manifestation of continuity theory is an individual's attempt to manipulate the external environment to address continuity needs (e.g., "I have always listened to the radio while I sleep, and I can't understand why I am not able to do this now"). When this effort is blocked, significant discontinuity ensues along with negative psychological sequale. It is this aspect of continuity theory that has important meaning for issues of long-term care. The vignette that follows highlights how one residential care setting used continuity theory to address a troublesome behavior of an individual resident who made frequent expensive calls from the center's telephone:

Bob, a 79 year old White male, was admitted to a residential care facility by his son who complained that changes in Bob's memory and cognitive functioning had become so severe that he was unable to maintain him in his home. Bob had a very close relationship with his father, and one particularly troubling behavior was Bob's frequent calls to his son at work, and this continued after Bob had been placed in the facility. The director of the facility suggested that the phone be removed from Bob's room so that he would be unable to make the calls. An attempt to do this caused Bob to withdraw and experience what appeared to be a depressive episode. The loss of the phone represented a significant discontinuity. The consulting psychologist suggested that the care center reinstate the phone, but disconnect it or rewire the connection so that it dialed the nursing staff. The latter option was chosen and Bob's phone was returned with a rewired connection. Soon, Bob's mood improved and he frequently called the nursing staff to ask how his son was doing at work. When they reassured him that things were well, Bob's mood and behavior improved. He had now made a successful transition to the residential care environment.

It is not surprising that older adults, even in the presence of cognitive or physical disability, tend to feel that it is very important to maintain themselves in familiar contexts despite the apparent risks to health and safety. This issue was highlighted in a national survey that queried whether older adults would be willing to consider nursing home placement. In this report, 30% of older adults surveyed indicated that they would rather "die" than be placed in a nursing home (Mattimore et al., 1997). One reason for this aversion to nursing home placement is the threat that it poses to external continuity without the flexibility of allowing the older adult to manipulate the environment in order to recapture structures that are familiar and could aid in coping with the aging process. The possibilities of integrating continuity theory in the design and function of residential care are enormous.

RESIDENTIAL CARE

A Historical Overview and Current Status of Residential Care

Historically, the concept of residential care pre-dated the nursing home, which first appeared in the 1960s as a form of institutionalized long-term care for the poor (see Kane, Kane, & Ladd, 1998). However, as a form of informal board and care, residential services have their genesis in efforts of the family to prevent or delay institutionalization of a loved one. Residential care facilities that have focused exclusively on older populations are perhaps best defined as closed communities where two or more unrelated adults reside and where services such as meals, medication supervision, organized activities, transportation, and assistance with activities of daily living and instrumental activities of daily living occur (Hawes, 1994). As noted earlier in this chapter, residential care has been classified by a number of different titles throughout the United States (Mitchell & Kemp, 2000). Under the generic name "board and care," in 1991 there were approximately 34,000 to 36,000 facilities with more than 600,000 beds nationwide (Hawes, 1999). Currently, residential care facilities for the elderly house and provide services to over half a million elderly people. Most of these are very old and physically frail adults who have cognitive impairment at a sufficient level to prevent them from living independently in the community (Hawes, 1999). As a formal organizational structure, since 1971 residential care facilities have been termed intermediate care facilities, and under this term were not required to meet the stringent set of medical standards required of nursing homes. However, facilities with this designation can be licensed to provide permanent living space and general services to older residents to the end of life (see Kane et al., 1998). In this chapter, nursing homes fall within the broader definition of residential care in as much as nursing homes are closed communities where one or more unrelated individuals reside. However, what distinguishes nursing home care is a focus on the ongoing medical needs of the resident. For example, by law, nursing homes must have a registered nurse on duty at all times, and operate from within a medical model. In this regard, they are designed to serve older adults who have the most severe caregiving needs requiring medical intervention to survive.

Conceptual Models of Residential Care

The question of conceptualizing residential care is challenging, given its dynamic nature and the proliferation of service delivery models within the past several years. Residential care can be defined as a formal option of care along a continuum of possible contexts for service delivery: independent living on the one hand versus 24-hour nursing home care at the opposite extreme. A significant threshold marker is the point at which the older person no longer resides in the community or can live independently. This has historically been the central component of defining residential care with emphasis on its "residential" nature (Eckert & Lyon, 1992).

Three service models of residential care are described in this section. The first, the Eden Alternative, is a model that highlights social and environmental planning to facilitate optimal living in older adults. This model emerged as a reaction to the confined nature of care present in nursing homes. The second model articulates components necessary for good quality residential care, namely housing, services, and autonomy. The third model attempts to incorporate a range of care based on client issues and problems in contrast to the intensive nature of care.

The Eden Alternative   The Eden Alternative is a model of residential care first proposed by Dr. William Thomas (Thomas, 1996), a physician director of a nursing home in the early 1990s who reacted to a number of institutionalization problems inherent in the medical model underlying nursing home care. Although the Eden Alternative is specifically about nursing home reform, a number of concepts emerged from this model and can be applied to residential care. The most important feature is likely the notion that the "home" environment epitomizes the nature of care that is most acceptable to human beings. Thus, the incorporation of home-like facilities including mechanisms to bring children into the facility are encouraged. Further, animals, birds, and plants are planned aspects of the environment so that typically, one might find hundreds of domesticated birds and substantial numbers of dogs and cats are present in any given Eden Alternative facility. Judy Thomas, a partner in the Eden Alternative, reported in an article that appeared in the *Washington Post* that Eden Alternative facilities are designed to "end the rigid hours residents must keep for meals, baths, and bedtime; let them sleep in some mornings if they choose. Throw out the time clock and let workers schedule themselves" (Levine, 1997, p. 35). Recently, Thomas (1996) described the critical components of the Eden Alternative including the following criteria: (a) understand that loneliness and helplessness account for the majority of problems in long-term care; (b) develop a "human habitat" model; (c) provide easy access to companionship; (d) provide opportunities to give and receive care; (e) imbue daily life; (f) de-emphasize programmed activities; (g) de-emphasize prescription drugs; (h) de-emphasize top-down bureaucratic authority; (i) adapt these strategies as a regular living routine; (j) develop leadership that focuses on the need to improve resident quality of life over institutionalization concerns.

The Eden Alternative represents a promising departure from the institutionalized model of long-term care by emphasizing resident choice, availability of services, and a supportive environmental structure that emphasizes connectedness among residents, as well as other living things (Levine, 1997). Thus, its philosophy emulates a "family-based" context, and although it is atheoretical (and more political) in nature, it does capture many important concepts embodied in continuity theory and SOC. Whether it can address the needs of more impaired residents with respect to cognitive and persistent behavioral problems (e.g., incontinence) that has driven institutionalization policies in the past remains to be evaluated empirically.

The Housing and Services Model   Residential care has always involved a specific context (housing), a critical component not directly articulated in many definitions. It is also noteworthy that the nature of treatment or service provision is an integral part of residential care, inasmuch as this concept of care has evolved into providing much more than a living arrangement designed to contain impairment. A comprehensive conceptualization of residential care has been a "housing and services" model (Kane et al., 1998, page 159; Wilson, 1996). This model is defined by multiple domains of care; namely, context, service, and consumer choice. The first component of the model highlights the living context and involves the distribution of private versus shared space. As in the Eden Alternative, it is assumed that the ideal environment should emulate the home. In this respect, design is critical to avoiding an institutional context that may be more efficient in service delivery but less appealing to the residents (i.e., moving from the standard institutional kitchen to a country-kitchen concept where food is available to residents in snack cupboards). The second component involves the nature of control within space, including who enters the space, where it is located, the timing of care tasks, and the opportunity for care refusal. Here, care is construed to be more restrictive than a home environment. With respect to this component, however, the model optimizes individual choice and freedom. Manifestations of this include shopping services available to residents, minimization of patronizing speech, interactions from service providers that are less compulsory (e.g., asking the resident about services before performing them). Recent research has affirmed this component of the model for better management and communication for older adults in dependent contexts (see O'Connor & Rigby, 1996; Ryan, Shumovich, Kennaley, & Pratt, 2000). The third component of this model involves the nature and availability of services (e.g., the availability of medication). Here, the model assumes that the more available services are, especially specialized services such as physical therapy and psychological services, the better the care. This third component has embodied the development of specialized facilities designed to treat individuals with similar diagnoses such as Alzheimer's disease (Davis et al., 2000). This decision model of care can be concretely exemplified in the following case scenario:

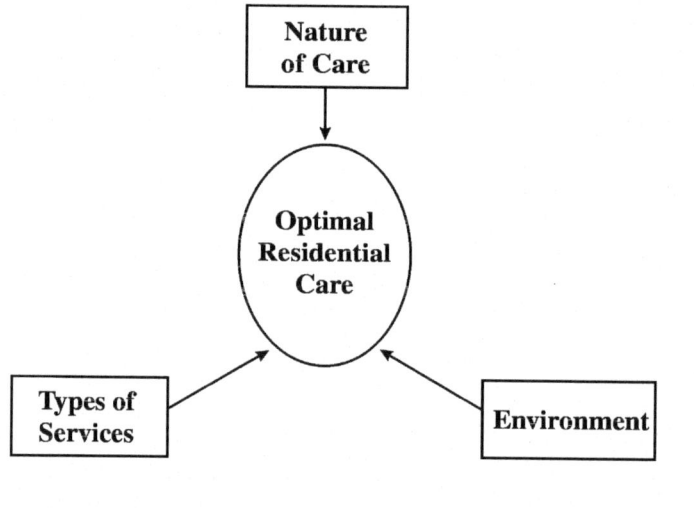

Mary's Care Needs
1) Level of Care
2) Cost of Care
3) Ability to Refuse Care

Mary's Need for Services
1) Physician
2) Nursing Care
3) Rehabilitation

Mary's Environmental Needs
1) Privacy
2) Comfort
3) Family Contacts

FIG. 1.1   Model of housing and services for Mary.

Mary is an 85-year-old widow who is currently living in her own apartment. Mary has one daughter who is married with two children who live in Mary's home. Mary recently experienced a fall, which caused her to fracture her left leg. After a visit with her physician, Mary was diagnosed with cerebral vascular dementia and the doctor suggested that she no longer drive due to her high risk of stroke-induced disorientation. Mary's daughter was concerned that Mary would no longer be able to live independently in her apartment and visited with a social worker about care options that would best meet Mary's needs at this time in Mary's life.

Using the model discussed earlier, Mary and her daughter would likely want to address the following questions. First, what kind of living space will best meet Mary's needs? For someone with mobility issues, the risk of isolation is high. Thus, a context where shared space is accessible would seem critical in a new living context. Second, what kinds of control should Mary have? It is apparent with regard to this issue that Mary is suffering from cognitive impairment; however, her ability to make decisions regarding activities of daily living and instrumental activities of daily living is intact. Thus, her need to have control within her living context should be a high priority. Options where that control does not exist, such as a nursing home environment, would not be optimal. Finally, what kinds of services should be available for Mary? This issue encompasses a number of factors including ready access to physician services should she experience another stroke-related incident.

Such questions could be used to determine whether it might be possible to re-organize Mary's current living environment to better meet her needs or whether Mary could benefit from a change in her living context. Thus, a services and delivery model deserves empirical validation in the research literature (Gramoth, Semradek, & Tornquist, 1995; Hopp, 1999). However, like the Eden Alternative, it is fundamentally atheoretical and was initially conceptualized on the basis of practical concerns. It represents an expanded alternative to allow residential care services to address a broader range of older adults with problems that vary in terms of severity.

A Model Based on Continuity Theory and SOC   Two contemporary models of adult development have been presented in this chapter; namely, continuity theory and SOC. This final section provides a conceptualization of a model that incorporates principles from these theoretical models to develop a framework to maximize the care of the older adult in a residential context. From SOC, it is apparent that residential care (as a form of long-term care) is a cultural effort to enhance active life expectancy. Thus, instead of judging long-term care as a necessary evil, it may be possible to reconceptualize it as a mechanism for extending life; that is, when absolute life expectancy is lengthened, this lengthens active life expectancy.

SOC provides information that could inform the nature and design of residential care. Clearly, residential care performs a selectivity function; that is, it removes the individual from the community where there is a maximum of decisions and choices that can easily overwhelm the individual experiencing disability. The challenge to residential care contexts is to maximize the degree of selectivity. What appears to be the case is that older adults, even in the presence of profound disability, value the opportunities for making decisions and choices, so involving the older resident (and the family) in determining how selective the environment should become would seem critical in optimizing care.

With increased disability there is a high degree of need to optimize the skills and capabilities that remain intact, while at the same time compensating for lost skills. The example below highlights this issue:

Jackie was admitted to a residential care facility because her family was no longer able to supervise her activities due to progressive Alzheimer's disease. An assessment of Jackie's cognitive functioning placed her in the moderate range of the disorder. She had a fairly high level of anxiety and agitation at times. It was noteworthy that Jackie was unable to orient herself to person, place, and time; however, she had fairly good memory for autobiographical material, particularly for playing piano tunes that she had learned as a younger adult. Jackie was admitted to the care unit and was encouraged by the staff to become involved in a number of activities. Her family indicated that she enjoyed playing the piano, so she was allowed supervised access to it. She was encouraged to play only simple tunes that she remembered and had overlearned (selection), and this became a source of entertainment to the residents as she replayed familiar old tunes (optimization). As she became progressively more demented, her piano skills worsened. In this instance she continued to sit at the piano bench listening to tape-recorded music of songs she played in the past (compensation). The residents enjoyed this music as well, and it brought satisfaction to Jackie even though she did not actually play the pieces. These strategies also helped to manage her anxiety and agitation without medication by involving her in familiar and comforting activities, thus preserving her sense of continuity.

Thus, by conceptualizing resident behaviors in terms of selection, optimization, and compensation, it may be possible to develop individualized treatment plans designed to maximize resident functioning even in the presence of declining capacity.

Principles of continuity theory have been highlighted in the two previous models of residential care and are articulated herein as they relate to this theoretical premise. For example, in the Eden Alternative model, the environment is augmented by the addition of children, animals, and plants, with the notion that this will improve functioning and satisfaction in the residents. An underlying explanation for this is that throughout life, most people interact with these things (external continuity) and thus find them significant to maintaining a stable sense of themselves (internal continuity). Introducing these objects into a care context reinstates and extends both internal and external continuity, thus enhancing satisfaction. In other words, the objects themselves are less important than what they represent in terms of establishing a sense of consistency with the outside world. It is through developing strategies and procedures based on continuity theory that optimal adjustment will occur in a residential care environment. Principles of continuity theory provide an intervention rationale which goes beyond simply adding objects, animals, or plants to the existing environment to facilitate a resident's sense of meaning in a long-term care environment.

A number of common procedures that are pervasive in residential care work argue against continuity theory. For example, it is often believed that older adults should be defined and identified by their problem behaviors or a psychiatric diagnosis ("Joe is always being manipulative and oppositional"). However, what is important in care contexts is that the resident represents a significant history that is likely influencing how he or she is adjusting to or interacting with the care environment. A person whose internal continuity involves interacting with others will likely attempt to do this even though the system may attempt to prevent it. The same is true with respect to privacy needs. Thus, it is important for the care staff to acknowledge and respect each individual's uniqueness in order to minimize discontinuities that will arise from placement in a residential care context.

In sum, both continuity theory and SOC can add dimensions and an underlying rationale for developing plans and strategies for maximizing active life expectancy within a residential care environment. It is valuable that previous models, such as the Eden Alternative, have found things that "work"; however, understanding the underlying mechanisms that make these activities work is essential for improving the efficiency and efficacy for introducing new strategies of care.

SUMMARY: THE FUTURE OF RESIDENTIAL CARE FOR THE VERY OLD

This chapter was designed to accomplish three objectives: first, to provide a brief description of the characteristics of very old adults who are at risk for loss of independence and to highlight the psychological needs of this group; second, to describe a theoretical model that can be used in the design of interventions and care options for this age group; and third, to describe residential care and to propose several new ways to conceptualize it so that it can better meet consumer needs and conform to models of adult development that highlight the underlying motivations for maximizing quality of life in residential care contexts. In this final section an attempt was made to raise a number of issues that will be important to consider in the future evolution of residential care as a service delivery option for the very old who face losses in independent functioning.

REFERENCES

American Association of Retired Persons. (1991). *Aging American: Trends and projections 1991* (DHHS Publication No. 91-28001). Washington DC: U.S. Department of Human Services.

American Association of Retired Persons. (1993). *The regulation of board and care homes: Results of a survey in 50 states.* Washington, DC: Author and Public Policy Institute.

American Association of Retired Persons. (1998). *Profile of older Americans.* Washington, DC: Author.

Atchley, R. C. (1989). A continuity theory of normal aging. *Gerontologist, 29,* 183–190.

Atchley, R. C. (2000). *Social forces and aging* (9th ed.). Belmont, CA: Wadsworth.

Baltes, P. B., & Baltes, M. M. (1990). Psychological perspectives on successful aging: The model of selective optimization with compensation. In P. B. Baltes & M. M. Baltes (Eds.). *Successful aging*: Perspectives from the behavioral sciences (pp. 1–34). New York: Cambridge University Press.

Baltes, P. D., Staudinger, U. M., & Lindenberger, U. (1999). Lifespan psychology: Theory and application to intellectual functioning. *Annual review of Psychology, 50,* 471–507.

Crimmins, E. M., Saito, Y., & Ingegneri, D. (1989). Changes in life expectancy and disability-free life expectancy in the United States. *Population and Development Review, 15,* 235–67.

Davis, K. J., Sloane, P. D., Mitchell, C. M., Preisser, J., Grant, L., Hawes, M. C., Lindeman, Q., Montgomery, R., Long, K., Phillips, L., Koch, G. (2000). Specialized dementia programs in residential care. *Gerontologist, 40,* 32–42.

Eckert, J. K., & Lyon, S. M. (1992). Board and care homes: From the margins to the mainstream in the 1990s. In M. G. Ory & A. P. Duncker (Eds), *In-home care for older people: Health and supportive services*. Newbury Park, CA: Sage.

Gramoth, L. M., Semradek, J., & Tornquist, E. M. (1995). *Enhancing autonomy in long-term care: Concepts and strategies*. New York: Spring.

Hawes, C. (1999, Summer). Managing the chronic care needs of the frail elderly in residential care settings. *Generations*, 51–55.

Hill, R. D., Thorn, B. L. & Packard, R. E. (2000). Counseling older adults: Theoretical and empirical issues in prevention and intervention. In S. D. Brown & R. W. Lent (Eds.), *Handbook of Counseling Psychology*, 3rd Ed. New York: Wiley.

Hopp, F. P. (1999). Patterns and predictors of formal and informal care among elderly persons living in board and care homes. *The Gerontologist, 39*, 167–176.

Ingebretsen, R., & Solem, P. E. (1998). Death, dying, and bereavement. In I. H. Nordhus, G. R. VandenBos, S. Berg, & P. Fromholt (Eds.), *Clinical geropsychology* (pp. 177–181. Washington, DC: American Psychological Association.

Kane, R. A., Kane, R. L., & Ladd, R. C. (1998). *The Heart of Long-Term Care*. New York: Oxford University Press.

Koplan, J. P., & Fleming, D. W. (2000). Current and future public health challenges. *Journal of the American Medical Association, 284*, 1696–1698.

Levine, S. (1997, November 21). Creating an Eden for seniors: Nursing home movement stresses quality of life. *The Washington Post*, pp. A1, A35–36.

Lubitz, J., Beebe, J. B., & Baker, C. (1995). Longevity and medicare expenditures. *New England Journal of Medicine, 332*, 99–1003.

Luborsky, B. R. (1994). The cultural adversity of physical disability: Erosion of full adult personhood. *Journal of Aging Studies, 8*, 239–254.

Manton, K. G., & Saldo, B. J. (1992). Disability and morality among the oldest old: Implications for current and future health and long term care service needs. In R. M. Suzman, D. P. Willis, & K.G. Manton (Eds.), *The oldest old*, (pp. 199–250). New York: Oxford University Press.

Mattimore, T. J., Wenger, N. S., Cesbians, N. A., Teno, J. M., Hamelon, B., Liu, H., Califf, R., Connors, A. F., Lynn, J., & Oye, K. K. (1997). Surrogate and physician understanding of patients' preferences for living permanently in a nursing home. *Journal of the American Geriatrics Society, 45*, (7), 818–824.

Mitchell, J. M., & Kemp, B. J. (2000). Quality of life in assisted living homes: A multidimensional analysis. *Journal of Gerontology: Psychological Sciences, 55*, 117–127.

Mortimer, J. A., & Graves, A. B. (1993) Education and other socioeconomic determinants of dementia and Alzheimer's Disease. *Neurology, 43*, 39–44.

O'Connor, B. P., & Rigby, H. (1996). Perceptions of baby talk, frequency of receiving baby talk, and self-esteem among community and nursing home residents. *Psychology and Aging, 11*, 147–154.

Ryan, E. B., Shumovich, M. A., Kennaley, D. E., & Pratt, M. W. (2000). Evaluations by staff, residents, and community seniors of patronizing speech in the nursing home: Impact of passive, assertive, or humorous responses. *Psychology and Aging, 15*, 272–285.

Suzman, R., Manton, K. G., & Willis, D. G. (1992). Introducing the oldest old. In R. M. Suzman, D. P. Willis, & K. G. Manton (Eds.), *The oldest old*. New York: Oxford University Press.

Taeuber, C. M., & Rosenwaike, I. (1992). A demographic portrait of America's oldest old. In R. M. Suzman, D. P. Willis, & K. G. Manton (Eds.), *The oldest old*, (pp. 17–49). New York: Oxford University Press.

Thomas, W. H. (1996). *Life worth living: How someone you love still can enjoy life in a nursing home: The Eden Alternative in action*. Boston: VanderWyk & Burnham.

Wilson, K. B. (1996). *Assisted living: Reconceptualized regulation to meet consumers' needs and preferences*. Washington, DC: American Association of Retired Persons.

Zimmerman, S. I., & Sloane, P. D. (1999, Fall). Optimum residential care for people with dementia. *Generations*, 62–58.

2

Defining Residential Care From a Developmental Perspective

Brian L. Thorn
*Silverado Senior Living, Salt Lake City,
and University of Utah*

Understanding and meeting the needs of the burgeoning population of frail elderly in our society is becoming increasingly complex. The complexity is largely attributable to the phenomenal growth in the numbers of people living into advanced age and the concomitant increase in the occurrence of disabling medical and cognitive problems. As a result, we are collectively faced with the question of how to best address these issues. The issue of caring for elderly people cuts across age and cultural boundaries because late life issues represent either a current or future reality for virtually everyone. With a sophisticated understanding and an empirically supported framework or model, we can continue to improve on our current efforts as a society to accomplish this important task. To date, the development of nursing homes and other residential facilities for the elderly have been driven primarily by pragmatic concerns. However, we believe that the pragmatic approach has been more successful at addressing some needs of the frail elderly and less successful with other needs. Specifically, psychosocial needs and subjective well-being have received less attention in geriatric residential care (GRC) settings than other needs such as medical care.

Nursing homes and assisted living facilities as we now know them have not always been around (see chap. 1); in fact, they are a relatively recent response to a growing need for more options to address late life issues. In this chapter, we discuss the genesis of geriatric residential care in the United States and present a conceptual perspective on contemporary issues. We will close the chapter with the presentation of an integrated developmental perspective for GRC that is empirically supported and responsive to the needs of the elderly on a number of different dimensions including social, medical, and psychological.

GERIATRIC RESIDENTIAL CARE IS
AN EVOLVING CONCEPT

Historically, there were few options available to individuals and families faced with the issues brought on by disabling medical conditions in late life. Just a few generations ago, relatively few people lived into their 70s and beyond. The average life expectancy in 1900 was just 47 years (Treas, 1995). The small proportion of hearty people who lived into their seventh, eight, and ninth decades of life tended to be those who were predisposed biologically and environmentally to maintain a high level of functional capacity. Still, when chronic illness or crippling accidents occurred, the vast majority of people in the early part of the 20th century were cared for by close family members, typically in the home of an adult daughter or son. Although this scenario is still often true today, fewer families are able to provide such care, and a variety of options are now available to address the needs of those older adults who are no longer able to reside on their own without the assistance of others. Predating the nursing home and contemporary multiservice retirement and assisted living communities were informal board and care arrangements in which housing, meals, and perhaps some level of assistance with activities of daily living (ADL) were provided to a generally small number of individuals in a nonfamilial setting (see chap. 1). Like family care arrangements, the board and care situations helped people with declining functional capacities remain engaged in meaningful life activities longer than if they were on their own or residing in an institutional setting such as a hospital.

Since 1900, advances in sanitation, nutrition, and medical science have increased the average life expectancy, dramatically to 75.4 years in 1990 (Treas, 1995). As the overall population figures have swelled continuously in the past century, so too has the proportion of the population grown that is made up of people in advanced age. The phenomenal increase in average life expectancy has led to some positive sociofamilial changes such as longer lasting parent–child relationships and greater likelihood of multigenerational families (Burgess, Schmeeckler, & Bengston, 1998). It has also greatly increased the number of families who must deal with the problems of aging and declining health in one or more family members.

Although many people remain healthy and vital as they age, their chances of developing a disabling physical or cognitive condition increase substantially in their 70s and even more so in their 80s. Many chronic health conditions remain incurable, but medical advances have produced treatments that make it possible to live for an extended period of time (often for many years) with an illness. The extent to which treatment allows a person to retain or regain functional capacity varies greatly according to the nature of the illness and other unique personal and environmental factors. Frequently, chronic health conditions result in reduced abilities to carry out certain daily living tasks. For some the impairment may be minor, such as an inability to perform heavy lifting or household maintenance tasks. For others, however, such as those with dementia or multiple complex health problems, there may be a drastic reduction in their ability to perform all or nearly all ADLs. Chronic illness is a risk for people at any age, but the chances of developing such an illness or a disabling condition greatly increase as individuals age. More than 80% of those who are 65 years or older have at least one chronic condition (Altcare Corporation, 1990). In the process of living with their chronic illness or condition, many people will experience acute episodes requiring hospitalization and rehabilitation as well as periods of stability or of deterioration that may require medical care and community-based or institutional long-term care (Williams & Temkin-Greener, 1996).

In many families it is no longer possible to provide in-home care for an elderly loved one, particularly when that loved one may live for many years after first developing chronic functional impairments. In the past, the time between the onset of chronic health problems in old age and death was typically much shorter than it is today with adequate medical treatment. Additionally, sociocultural developments, such as the higher prevalence of single parent families and families in which both parents work outside the home, have contributed to a situation in which it is now frequently unrealistic for a younger generation family member to provide assistance of the quantity and duration needed by many frail elderly people (Hopp, 1999). It is also true that many old people do not have living family members with whom they could reside, whereas many others would prefer not to do so and instead wish to remain in an autonomous living situation if at all possible.

Average Versus Active Life Expectancy

Active life expectancy refers not just to the expected age of death (as does *average* or *total life expectancy*), but instead looks at the interaction between aging and disability (Laditka, 1998). The greater the degree of disability and illness in a given population group, the lower their relative active life expectancy. On an individual level, a 65-year-old person would have a total life expectancy of 14–16 years but an active life expectancy of 12–13 years. Active life expectancy has been defined as "the number of years of life that can be anticipated to be healthy and essentially fully functional. The difference between the total … and active life expectancy is the years during which one or more dependency needs are likely to exist" (Williams & Temkin-Greener, 1996, p. 53). This definition suggests that once a person suffers from a disabling condition or chronic illness the active part of his or her life ends. However, this is an area that is in flux as new options apart from medical advances are helping to close the gap between active and total life expectancy.

In residential care contexts, health has been defined as "successful adaptation to stressors in the internal and external environments and an ability to fulfill social roles" (Zurakowski, 2000, p. 13), which suggests that with successful adaptation to changing circumstances, one can remain healthy in the face of physical decline. Successful residential care settings strive to facilitate adaptation of their residents to the new living situation. As an example, assisted living facilities and devices can be designed and operated so as to minimize the dependency and the subjective impact of dependency on those with mildly and moderately disabling conditions. In addition to assistance with ADLs, residential care settings should strive to help their residents maintain a sense of continuity with their earlier life (see chap. 1 for a presentation of continuity theory). Elsewhere in this chapter and volume, the same principles are applied to promote the qualities of active life engagement even in those who are severely disabled by chronic conditions, such as in nursing homes.

The interaction between aging and disability is actually a dynamic process in which there are ongoing efforts being made to both reduce the occurrence of disabling illnesses and reduce the impact of the disabilities through compensatory means. Rehabilitation therapies (physical therapy, occupational therapy, speech therapy), eye surgery for cataracts, hearing aids, ambulatory aids, emergency call buttons, prosthetic devices, medication, and mental health services are among the many examples of strategies and tools used to compensate for diminished functional ability due to declining health. For a person in late life who has spent many years as an independent adult, the experience of needing to depend on others for assistance with daily living needs can be demoralizing. In addition to compensatory or assistive strategies, residential care facilities that actively promote continuity and empowerment in the more subjective areas of life help to mitigate the negative impacts of chronic illness and disability.

In chapter 1, the lifespan developmental theory of selective optimization with compensation (SOC; Baltes, Staudinger, & Lindenberger,1999) is discussed in some detail and is identified as a theory that has been broadly supported by extensive research. SOC posits that physical and cognitive decline in late life are normal aspects of the developmental lifespan process. Likewise, to compensate for diminishing abilities with tools and strategies is a normal and typical thing for humans to do (e.g., selection, optimization, and compensation). Geriatric residential care, in all its forms, represents a societal effort to compensate for age-related decline, thereby extending active life expectancy. By providing critical assistance on a day-to-day (sometimes hour-to-hour) basis, residential care at its best enables a shift of focus away from declining or lost skills on to those skills and abilities that remain (or that can be newly developed). The following case example illustrates this point.

Berta, age 80, was diagnosed with multiple sclerosis in her 30s. She enjoyed a long marriage with a husband who was attentive, patient, and skilled at constructing assistive devices such as a ramp that helped Berta climb into their small motorhome so they could vacation together after he retired. When her husband died of a heart attack in his 60s, she found that she could not manage to perform all the tasks necessary to live on her own at home, and she could not afford to pay for 24-hour live-in assistance (even if she could have found a competent and compatible person for the job). She tried to "get by" for a time with some assistance each evening from her one son or daughter-in-law, but she found herself feeling lonely, bored, helpless, and depressed. She also worried about the "burden" she was placing on them by expecting daily help. Berta enjoyed social activities and lunch at the local senior center, but was unable to do these things without someone to help her out of the house and drive her there. She felt uncomfortable about the prospect of living with her son's family because they did not have the means or the time to provide needed assistance. Besides, she really thought she would prefer to remain responsible for her own needs as much as possible because for many years she had needed to depend on her husband for help and she hated the feeling of being helpless and dependent. An assisted living senior apartment was a good match for Berta; she was able to afford the apartment with money from the sale of her house. With the transportation and other assistance provided by the facility she was able to continue participating in activities at the senior center and could have family and friends over to her apartment for visits. She also enjoyed some of the activities sponsored by the assisted living community.

This vignette, taken from a real-life experience of an older adult, illustrates how compensatory assistance can allow a person to remain vitally engaged in life and thus extend active life expectancy. Sociological, cultural, medical, economic, and technological advances have all made such improvements in active life expectancy possible. New housing options and architectural innovations have been introduced by entrepreneurial developers and have served to increase active life expectancy for many people. Even something as simple and now commonplace as grab bars in the bathroom can greatly increase the ability of frail older people who are otherwise cognitively intact to remain actively engaged in meeting their own daily living needs and allow them to extend their active life expectancy.

Medical Advances and Public Policy Influence the Development of Residential Care

Another important factor that has influenced the development of residential care opportunities for the elderly is the nature and availability of medical services. In the first half of the 20th century, nearly all medical care was provided by general practitioners, and the array of medical treatment options was vastly limited in comparison to the present. Older people were more likely to die of their illnesses, and the available treatments were often as easily provided at home as elsewhere. With increasingly complex and high-tech medical and rehabilitative procedures being used, it has become unrealistic, impossible, or excessively inefficient in many cases to provide treatment in a person's home. This is especially true when the treatment is required on a daily or multiple-times-daily basis. Modern nursing homes and extended care rehabilitation facilities, which date back only to the 1960s, grew out of a need to address the long-term medical care needs of an increasingly large number of frail elderly (Kane, Kane, & Ladd, 1998).

Still, residential care services for the elderly would likely have remained a relative rarity for many years because many of those in need of such care were unable to pay for it. The 1960s brought an infusion of public money in the form of Medicare and Medicaid, which meant that residential medical care became available to people who otherwise would not have been able to afford it. The public and congressional debate about the need for Medicare and Medicaid increased general public awareness of, among other things, the long-term care needs of elderly people (especially poor elderly people) and the need for a societal response to a growing societal issue—namely, providing appropriate housing and care options for people in late life (Cohen, 1998).

This infusion of public money in the form of third-party reimbursements from Medicare and Medicaid into the geriatric residential care arena also heightened the need to ensure that this resource was used appropriately. Since the advent of public funding for nursing home care, federal regulation has been a potent force driving the quantity, quality, and nature of care provided to seniors in residential settings. Medicaid regulations, for example, by stipulating that medical care is the only appropriate use for Medicaid dollars, have predictably promoted the medical model in the development and organization. This has led to the subjugation of nonmedical human needs in that setting (Kane et al., 1998). Medicare funding is targeted at active treatment and rehabilitation to the exclusion of long-term care, and although the range of reimbursable nonmedical treatment options has increased somewhat over the years, the need for a broad range of facility-based treatment options for emotional concerns continues to be problematic for third-party reimbursement.

Because they have viewed their mission as primarily a medical one, nursing homes and their associated rehabilitation facilities have not ordinarily placed a high priority on the creation of a positive living environment that proactively facilitates psychosocial well-being. The medical mission and foundation in a hospital model of care has led to commonly held notions that such facilities are not part of the geriatric residential care arena (Zimmerman & Sloane, 1999). However, many residents, even those who enter the facility for the purpose of rehabilitation, spend months and possibly years residing there, and all of them have needs for dignity, privacy, and as much freedom and control as possible in their daily lives. When these basic needs are inadequately provided for, most people experience a severe disruption of continuity with their own personal history, life roles, and sense of identity. Such a disruption often leads to iatrogenic symptoms of depression, anxiety, and other mental health concerns, especially when combined with the stress of personal losses and physical decline that prompt many admission decisions. Most custodial care facilities operate on a medical model similar to nursing homes (albeit with fewer staff and fewer services) and are no more likely to provide a quality living environment.

Government intervention has sought to improve the quality of life in long-term care settings by regulating and promoting mental health and other services (Katz & Coyne, 2000; Smyer & Wilson, 1999). Federal policies have often set the standard of care by stipulating, for example, that certain allied health services (such as rehabilitation therapies and psychology services) will be paid for under Medicare and Medicaid. When more professional services are available as needed, the quality of care is generally better (Kane et al., 1998).

Regulations at the federal, state, and corporate level have done much to promote quality care and limit the occurrence of abuse in residential care settings where many people are vulnerable and unable to protect themselves from harmful individuals or situations. However, such regulations tend to be rigid, inflexible, and difficult to modify when needed, and as a result, they frequently have some unintended consequences. Most notably, regulations serve to codify policies and procedures in such a way that it becomes difficult to see how things might be better if done differently. For example, policies in some states effectively eliminate the option of residing in assisted living facilities for low income individuals by stipulating that Medicaid reimbursement for long-term care can only go to "medical" facilities (i.e., nursing homes). Such a policy results in a situation that is neither cost effective nor supportive of individual autonomy. To be fair, it is extremely difficult to write broad regulations in such a way as to provide uniquely appropriate guidance in the endlessly variable situations found in long-term care settings. Nursing homes were born as novel ideas for meeting the health care needs of a growing elderly population, but they have grown into entrenched institutions that have difficulty incorporating new ways of thinking and operating.

It is realized that the frail elderly are in need of residential care settings that focus on much more than medical care needs and, as noted above, some public policies make it difficult to adapt accordingly. Nevertheless, with the right leadership from the highest levels down, it may be possible to improve the living environment in geriatric residential care settings within the current set of state policies and regulations. The more recent creation of assisted living facilities whose mission is more focused on the provision of a quality residential environment has been a positive development in the area of geriatric residential care. As noted later, these facilities are less regulated and somewhat more variable than nursing homes even though many of them make the same mistakes as their more medically oriented counterparts by establishing a daily living environment that is characterized by rigid routines, rules, and programmed activities. The goal of the next section is to suggest a comprehensive definition of residential care that is inclusive of most facilities and homes that house and care for frail older adults who are unable to live independently.

RESIDENTIAL CARE IS A SOCIETAL RESPONSE TO A NORMATIVE LIFE SITUATION

In this book, we have chosen to use a definition of geriatric residential care that encompasses the full range of settings in which two or more nonrelated elders reside and are provided some level of daily service ranging from the simple provision of room and board to 24-hour nursing and medical care. Over the past 15–20 years, a variety of residential care options for older adults apart from nursing homes have come about in response to a significant societal need and desire to prolong the period of life in which one is able to remain essentially independent and autonomous. Most of these facilities are not federally regulated as nursing homes, but individual states generally have established some level of regulation for assisted living and similar facilities.

Traditional models of residential care have tended to be paternalistic in orientation and to unintentionally foster dependency among their residents (Collopy, 1995). In those settings where the need for assistance and medical or nursing care is the highest, the level of paternalism is also at its highest. Newer models of residential care such as retirement apartments and assisted living facilities are typically less paternalistic in orientation, but residents in those places still commonly feel that they have lost their independence and purpose in life as they are no longer able to live without daily assistance and are no longer able to participate in activities that once provided meaning to their lives. Fortunately, there are things that administrators and facility staff can do to help counter the negative psychological effects of dependency and multiple losses in the face of ongoing decline (Mitchell & Kemp, 2000). In this section, we discuss *aging in place,* the need for facilities to help residents maintain a sense of life *continuity* to facilitate well-being, and introduce the concept of *stages of decline* for elderly individuals. Chapter 3 discusses the needs of the elderly in residential care settings with greater detail and a special emphasis on psychological issues.

Stages of Decline

Extensive research on human development across the lifespan has provided support for theories that describe normal life as consisting of periods of both growth and decline (Baltes et al., 1999). Both physical and cognitive functioning begin to decline slightly in middle adulthood, but the rate of decline accelerates in the seventh, eight, and ninth decades of life (see Giambra, Arenberg, Zonderman, Kawes, & Costa, 1995). Within a normally distributed sample of people in their seventies, the average level of disability due to health or cognitive decline is in the mild to moderate range. Put another way, most people in that age range have at least one chronic illness or condition that impairs daily functioning to one degree or another. On one side of the distribution are the minority of individuals who are not significantly impaired and on the other side are those who are severely impaired in one or more areas of functioning. The mean level of impairment goes up with increasing age and the "healthy" subgroup gets smaller.

SOC theory describes how cognitive decline occurs and how we adjust to the changes with learning, choosing, and strategizing. Given that decline is a normative experience for people as they age, it is useful to think of late life as involving a process of *stages of decline.* The stages of decline are inversely comparable with the stages of growth and development during childhood and early adulthood, but there is more heterogeneity with respect to decline as some older people experience relatively little apparent decline prior to death whereas others may experience more accelerated and severe decline at earlier points in the adult lifespan.

Most people experience a period of mild or early decline characterized by one or more chronic conditions that have some impact on daily functioning but these individuals are usually able to live independently or with only occasional assistance (often provided by a spouse or other family member). As individuals get older, the physical conditions, cognitive conditions, or both, predictably worsen and individuals enter into a middle stage of decline characterized by moderate impairment and the need for regular assistance with ADL. Whether for a period of rehabilitation or for an open-ended long-term arrangement, it has been found that many people who live into advanced age will also spend some time during which they are significantly disabled with illnesses affecting either their cognitive functioning, physical functioning, or both. In a sample of people primarily in their 70s and 80s, Laditka (1998) found that 62% were either moderately or severely impaired in their ability to perform ADLs. People who are severely impaired need assistance with many or sometimes all ADLs which may also require medical care.

The onset of chronic illness and disability in late life, sometimes even in the mild stage, places people into a context of dependency that they have likely not experienced since childhood. The level of dependency, which in many cases is both physical and financial in nature, increases with advancing stages of decline. As noted in chapter 1, the point at which a person is no longer able to live independently in the community is a particularly meaningful milestone in the process of decline as the move to residential care represents a major loss of autonomy. Given what we know about stages of decline that is associated with normal and pathological (e.g., Alzheimer's disease) aging, the next section provides a conceptual framework that focuses on level of care. This framework can be used to guide programming within the variety of residential care settings described in chapter 1.

Levels of Care

The way in which people reach the milestone at which a decision is made to consider some kind of residential care takes different forms. In any case, one consideration involves matching the level of care provided with the current and future needs of the individual. The stages-of-decline concept is useful in the process of making such choices with respect to care needs. Residential care settings differ with regard to the amount of assistance and the level of care provided.

Figure 2.1 provides a graphic representation of how the stages of decline relate to levels of care and the approximate relationship of some residential care settings on these dimensions. In the early or mild stage of decline, a low level of care with few services is likely to meet the needs of most older people who generally wish to

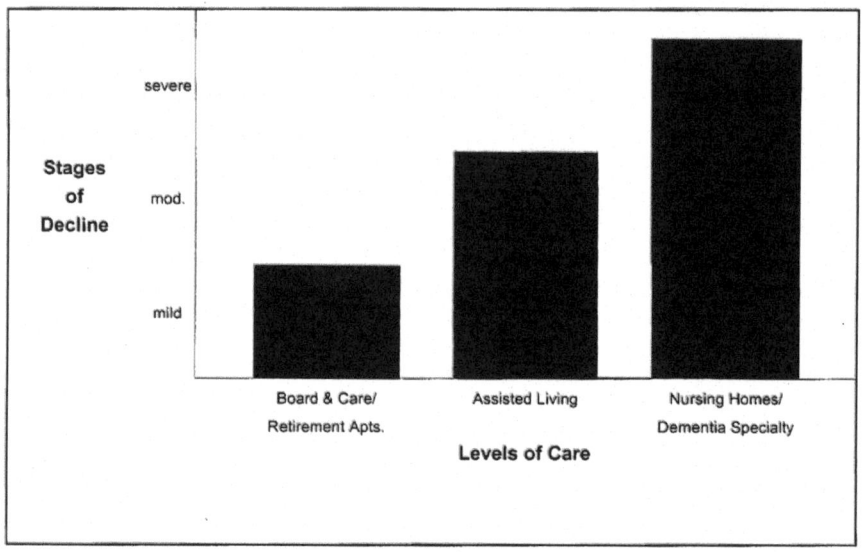

FIG. 2.1   Care needs increase as health and cognitive functioning decline.

remain as independent and self-sufficient as possible. When physical or cognitive decline advances to moderate and severe stages, direct assistance with daily living tasks and professional services (such as medical, nursing, and mental health) are needed that constitute a higher level of care. Assisted living facilities can often meet the needs of people with moderate levels of decline, whereas skilled nursing facilities are appropriate for those with severe medical needs. Some new specialized dementia facilities are providing innovative residential care services to people who suffer from cognitive decline, with or without other kinds of chronic illness and health care needs.

Research indicates that chances of manifesting clinically significant chronic illness or disease increase substantially around age 65 (Fries & Crapo, 1981). Those who remain essentially healthy beyond that time have succeeded in delaying the onset of illness, but they are still more physically vulnerable than in their younger years. Residential care versus independent living decisions frequently follow an injury or acute illness that illuminates the presence of decline and the need for assistance. In some cases, the aging individual willingly decides to move to a residential setting where his needs might be better met with the assistance of others. More commonly, the decision to move is made reluctantly with the encouragement or insistence of family or friends. The reluctance to move to a residential care facility is usually rooted in a desire to retain independence and in generally negative perceptions of nursing homes and formal GRC settings (Mattimore et al., 1997).

In their excellent book *The Heart of Long-Term Care*, Kane et al., (1998) discussed the complicated issue of combining housing (the *residential* part of GRC) with services (the *care* part of GRC). They noted that the two missions have often run at odds with each other, and particularly in nursing homes, efforts to create a home-like living environment characterized by a philosophy of consumer choice in these settings fall far short of expectations with respect to quality of life and autonomy. Daily life has been turned into a set of rigid routines where privacy is lacking and social interactions, especially those of an unstructured variety, are severely limited. The nursing home environment is much more like that of a hospital than a place where people live indefinitely and feel secure in the knowledge that quality of life and dignity will be preserved even when impairment is severe. Indeed, as we have noted, nursing homes were and are thought of as "health care settings," but in reality people do live there. Some of the routines and rules are important for the care of the residents, but others are mainly for the convenience of the management and staff or bureaucratic regulators. Most nursing home policies and regulations are well-intended, but they often run counter to the mission of providing a positive long-term living environment. The point here is not that all policies are bad, but that policies meant to address one set of problems sometimes impede the ability to address needs in other areas.

Aging in Place

Aging in place was briefly mentioned earlier in this chapter and refers to both a philosophy and a practice of providing health and personal care services to older people in the least-restrictive and most home-like setting possible, even as those people become increasingly ill and impaired (Mitchell & Kemp, 2000). Since the advent of nursing homes and public funding for long-term care, policy makers and analysts have placed a high priority on helping elderly people with declining health remain in their own home if it can be done at a reasonable and affordable cost (Kane et al., 1998). Realistically, aging in place does not necessarily mean that everyone should be able to remain living in the home they have occupied for 40 or more years and where they have raised their families. Indeed, for many people home is not directly associated with one particular house but instead refers to a chosen place of habitation where they feel safe and reasonably in control of their own lives. The important part of the aging in place concept is that as people age, they retain the need for a living environment in which they feel their identity and autonomy are preserved. Older people who retain all or nearly all of their functional capacity are able to remain in their own home or choose one of a variety of living environments. However, when physical or cognitive decline becomes prominent, a living environment that proactively helps to preserve identity and autonomy is best.

CONSIDERING A DEVELOPMENTAL PERSPECTIVE

Maintaining Life Continuity for Improved Well-Being

Researchers have found that for many elderly people the move to a GRC facility results in negative health effects (Zurakowski, 2000; Borup, Gallego, & Hefferman, 1980). Some writers have noted that the quality of medical care can be poor (Kane et al., 1998). There is also substantial evidence that the chronic illness, general physical decline, and loss of autonomy associated with residential care placement contribute to high rates of depression and anxiety which in turn can also have negative effects on overall health (Streim, 1996; Rodin, 1986). Nursing homes and other GRC facilities are social systems embedded within the larger systems of community and society, yet residents tend to feel isolated and cut off from the community at large (Zurakowski, 2000). In one large study of hospitalized elderly patients, 56% of respondents stated that they would be "very unwilling" to enter a nursing home or would "rather die" (Mattimore et al., 1997). Of course it is stressful, discouraging, and often painful to suffer the illness or chronic health problems that could trigger the placement of an older person in a long-term care facility in the first place, but the dread of spending time in such a place has more to do with the nature of life within this setting rather than with the accelerated nature of illness or age-related disability.

Tobin (1991), stated that one of the most difficult challenges for people in GRC facilities is maintaining their sense of personal identity and autonomy. Maintaining one's identity is closely associated with the maintenance of internal continuity (described in chap. 1; Atchley, 1989), a term that provides a useful conceptual framework for understanding both the problems and some of the solutions for promoting psychosocial well-being in GRC settings. In brief, continuity theory is a conceptualization of adult development and normal aging in later life. At its most basic level, the theory holds that people make choices that are consistent with their personal history and identity. Their sense of meaning and purpose in life is tied to social roles such as parent, breadwinner, homemaker, grandparent, friend, and community or church volunteer. Residential care facilities can help residents maintain a sense of continuity in their environment by providing ample opportunities and encouragement to participate in valued roles and activities or develop new ones that can be valued within the long-term care context. Generally speaking, continuity theory asserts that meaningful roles and activities cannot be chosen for the resident. Some lifetime roles such as complainer or criticizer can be difficult for staff to tolerate, but an enriched environment encourages even the most impaired resident to make choices to be themselves within a given setting even if it is, structurally, far from home (Coons & Mace, 1996).

Many authors have pointed to the need for care facility residents to have more control and a greater sense of self-efficacy in their daily lives (Johnson, Stone, Altmaier, & Berdahl, 1998; Rodin, 1986). Self-efficacy is an important part of our sense of autonomy and independence, and it is important for care facilities to promote self-efficacy in their residents precisely because autonomy and independence are cornerstones of our American society and are important facets of the identity of most individuals (a discussion of how to promote self-efficacy can be found in chap. 6 on psychosocial interventions). Promoting self-efficacy is just one way to help maintain or restore a sense of internal continuity and in doing so becomes a source of support for most people. Each individual has a unique identity and history that should be discovered, valued, and appreciated by facility staff with respect to defining a given resident as a unique individual with specific needs and strengths.

Anyone admitted to a GRC facility, regardless of their stage of decline or the level of care needed, is experiencing a significant disruption of external continuity based on this theory and they have been separated from the people, activities, places, and objects that made their lives meaningful and rewarding prior to admission. Those specific contextual settings and associations are the elements of life that reminded them of who they are and where they came from. Being separated from or losing those elements creates a disruption in external continuity that can in turn make it difficult to maintain a sense of internal continuity, thus contributing to interpersonal feelings of despair, anxiety, and depressed mood. One nursing home resident told me that since because is no longer able to work and help others (she had a long career as an elementary school teacher and deeply valued her roles as mother and grandmother), "I just don't feel like I'm me anymore." Such a cry for help eventually facilitated a situation in which this person was able to be helpful to other residents, and this intervention worked to restore her sense of internal continuity, alleviating her depression, and restoring her sense of self-worth.

Successfully promoting internal continuity means having the commitment as an organization to develop an individualized understanding of each resident, either from the resident directly or with help from the resident's family. To maximize such an approach, the flexibility to design activities and carry out daily care tasks should be tailored to fit and be consistent with each person's sense of self. The Eden Alternative is one example of a model of GRC that helps to promote well-being among residents by promoting individual autonomy and addressing the problems of loneliness, helplessness, and boredom (Tavormina, 1999). It could be argued that the success of the Eden Alternative is mainly derived from the attention paid to the psychosocial developmental needs of the residents and that other models addressing those same needs would be similarly successful in promoting subjective well-being. Another strength of the Eden Alternative is that it emphasizes the essential fact that the entire philosophy and culture of the organization from the top administrator to the frontline employees must be consistent in their approach to residents. Persistent and ongoing efforts are made to imbue the living environment with daily life (bring in the outside world), routines are eschewed, flexibility is valued, and individualized approaches to resident care are embraced. To date there is little research on the effects of the Eden Alternative on long-term care adjustment and quality of life, but anecdotal evidence suggests that some GRC organizations espousing this philosophy have been successful in reducing problematic behaviors, which has also reduced the facility's need for psychotropic medication. More research is needed so we can understand which elements are most helpful. It is likely that research will eventually confirm that the success of the Eden Alternative lies in its articulation of processes for facilitating the maintenance of a sense of continuity in its residents. In other words, a residential environment in which there is an infusion of community life and an active effort to eliminate loneliness, helplessness, and boredom is likely to also help its residents retain a sense of continuity with their earlier life.

For people in an early stage of decline living at home or in facilities providing a low level of care, relatively little assistance is usually needed to maintain a sense of continuity. These individuals are, in most cases, able to maintain contact with important others and participate in meaningful activities without assistance from others. However, with further decline and increased impairment of functioning, the need for high level-of-care facilities to provide proactive assistance with life continuity challenges increases. Bingo games and simple craft projects, common activities in many GRC facilities, will generally only appeal to those people who enjoyed participating in similar activities earlier in their lives. For others, consistent and persistent efforts to understand their unique personalities and backgrounds will give clues as to how they might best be assisted in efforts to maintain their identity and sense of continuity.

Quality of Life Versus Quality of Care

Quality of life (QOL) for older adults in residential care settings has been defined in a variety of ways and from a variety of perspectives including medical, sociological, and psychological points of view among others (Mitchell & Kemp, 2000). Despite their differences, virtually all definitions recognize the importance of the individual's subjective sense of well-being as well as her or his physical comfort, emotional well-being, and interpersonal connections (Logsdon, 2000). Defining QOL is difficult for researchers to do, yet it is even more difficult to measure quality of life, particularly in residential care settings where the level of care is high, the residents are in an advanced state of decline, and their ability to thoughtfully answer subjective questions is poor (such as in nursing homes; Brod, Stewart, Sands, & Walton, 1999). Perhaps it is because of this difficulty with QOL measurement that nursing home regulations and data-collection processes have focused more on the measurement of elements that could be more accurately described as *quality of care*.

Current guidelines for nursing homes do require that emotional and mood states be regularly assessed and recorded along with medical information, but well-trained mental health professionals are rarely involved in such assessments (Smyer & Wilson, 1999). In most states, assisted living facilities are not required to collect any QOL or mental health data. Regardless of who is doing the assessment, an evaluation of the presence or absence of a psychiatric condition along with data on medical needs do not constitute an adequate measure of QOL. These data sets leave out the subjective indicators of well-being and life satisfaction that have been found to be much more representative of QOL than objective indicators (Pearlman & Jonsen, 1985). Subjective measures of QOL also are more likely to tap into the concept of continuity and whether the individual feels connected to life in a meaningful way and that his or her identity is preserved. Recent research continues to demonstrate these points. In a multidimensional analysis of QOL in assisted living facilities, Mitchell and Kemp (2000) found that a sense of cohesiveness, low levels of conflict, and high levels of autonomy are the most important predictors of QOL on all measures.

Promoting QOL in GRC settings means placing social and psychological needs as the top priority and viewing the mission of creating a satisfactory living environment as the foundation of the organization. Clearly, the medical mission of nursing homes and some other GRC facilities is of critical importance and cannot be neglected on any level. In QOL terms, medical care would be best viewed as supplemental to the psychosocial aspects of the living environment.

Promoting Quality of Life at All Levels of Care

Everyone has developmental needs across the lifespan. Children need to develop a sense of security and belonging, and adolescents need to develop social roles, interpersonal relationships, and a sense of identity. Early and middle adulthood are focused on love, autonomy, achievement, and identity fulfillment. In late adulthood, the need for identity fulfillment and maintenance of social roles remain, but the co-occurring developmental process of decline forces changes in the way those needs are met. SOC theory demonstrates that the accumulation of lifetime learning facilitates individual's abilities to make adjustments in lifestyle and activities. Continuity theory gives us a framework for understanding what kinds of adjustments and activities will help people retain their sense of identity and self-worth, namely activities and environments that are consistent with their personal history and personality. This chapter has highlighted how components of these theories can be translated into practice.

Older adults who are healthy and living independently can and do make such adjustments for themselves; research shows that healthy people in late life tend to have lower rates of depression and higher levels of life satisfaction than younger adults (Kunzmann, Little, & Smith, 2000). Once people become chronically impaired due to physical decline and if they are placed in a residential care facility, then they are less able to maintain continuity with those parts of their identity that are represented by activities and contexts in the day-to-day world. Care facilities can promote positive adjustment by actively encouraging maximal freedom of choice and fostering, to the greatest extent possible, decision making on the part of the individual resident. Application of this principle becomes somewhat more difficult as residents become increasingly impaired, but some organizations are showing that it can be done (Coons & Mace, 1996).

As with health and rehabilitative care, it is important to match the level of psychosocial support services with the stage of decline and level of care needed to optimize adjustment and quality of life. People with mild–moderate physical decline and little or no cognitive decline will benefit from a less structured environment with high levels of freedom, flexibility, support services such as transportation, and an overall lower level of care. In such facilities, medical or nursing services and other professional health services such as rehabilitation therapies and psychology should be peripheral to the overall psychosocial-based residential model. Other authors have also suggested that residential care facilities of all sorts should be designed and built on a psychosocial model (Kane et al., 1998). For people with moderate–severe physical decline, adequate medical, nursing, and rehabilitative care are added while the social model remains primary. Even people with severe health problems who may not be able to participate in chosen activities or carry out decisions still have a need for "decisional autonomy," and residential care staff need to encourage decision making whenever possible on a daily basis (Collopy, 1995). Those who are at an advanced stage of physical decline but without significant cognitive decline are likely to benefit from a care environment that proactively facilitates meaningful interpersonal engagement and maintenance of social ties. It is not enough to passively allow residents to make decisions if they wish; choices and opportunities should be presented and encouraged regularly and repeatedly.

People who have advanced to the moderate–severe range of cognitive decline will have greater difficulty making meaningful decisions, but their need for psychosocial support is high. At the same time, many people with dementia or other form of cognitive decline have a relatively low need for medical care. It may seem unrealistic for severely demented individuals to retain much of a sense of autonomy, but they can benefit from a resident-oriented environment that proactively provides "means to their ends" (Collopy, 1995).

CONCLUSION

One of the primary issues highlighted in this chapter is how QOL for older adults can be maintained in long-term residential care environments. Nearly all of us will experience some level of physical or cognitive decline as we age and will need assistance with daily living tasks. When decline advances to the point that we are no longer able to remain living independently in our own home, then we need we need a living environment that helps us maintain continuity with our personal identity and our sense of autonomy. As we advance into moderate and severe stages of decline, we need commensurate higher levels of care and even more support to maintain our sense of self. Geriatric residential care facilities that provide a high quality of life are those that proactively seek to address psychosocial needs for continuity along with physical or health care needs.

Providing proactive psychosocial support aimed at helping residents to maintain a sense of life continuity is not necessarily costly or time-consuming. The essential ingredient is a resident-centered philosophy and model of care that is aimed at actively enhancing resident autonomy and the ongoing fulfillment of their unique developmental needs. All staff must be genuinely interested in each resident and share a commitment to make them comfortable and help them enjoy life even though they are impaired.

REFERENCES

Altcare Corporation (1990). *Chronic care ... Independence through innovation.* Bloomington, MN: Author.

Atchley, R. C. (1989). A continuity theory of normal aging. *Gerontologist, 29,* 183–190.

Baltes, P. D., Staudinger, U. M., & Lindenberger, U. (1999). Lifespan psychology: Theory and application to intellectual functioning. *Annual review of Psychology, 50,* 471–507.

Borup, J. H., Gallego, D. T., & Hefferman, P. G. (1980). Relocation: Its effect on health, functioning, and mortality. *Gerontologist, 20,* 468–479.

Brod, M., Stewart, A. L., Sands, L., & Walton, P. (1999). Conceptualization and measurement of quality of life in dementia: The Dementia Quality of Life Instrument (DQoL). *The Gerontologist, 39,* 25–35.

Burgess, E. O., Schmeeckle, M., & Bengtson, V. L. (1998). Aging individuals and societal contexts. In I. H. Nordhus, G. R. Vandenbos, S. Berg, & P. Fromholt (Eds.), *Clinical Geropsychology* (pp. 15–32). Washington, DC: American Psychological Association.

Cohen, M. A. (1998). Emerging trends in the finance and delivery of long-term care: Public and private opportunities and challenges. *The Gerontologist, 38,* 80–89.

Collopy, B. J. (1995). Power, paternalism, and the ambiguities of autonomy. In L. M. Gamroth, J. Semradek, & E. M. Tornquist (Eds.), *Enhancing autonomy in long-term care* (pp. 3–14). New York: Springer.

Coons, D. H., & Mace, N. L. (1996). *Quality of life in long-term care.* Binghamton, NY: Haworth.

Fries, J. F., & Crapo, L. M. (1981). *Vitality and aging.* San Francisco: Freeman.

Giambra, L. M., Arenberg, D., Zonderman, A. B., Kawas, C., & Costa, P. T. (1995). Adult life span changes in immediate visual memory and verbal intelligence. *Psychology and Aging, 10,* 123–139.

Hopp, F. P. (1999). Patterns and predictors of formal and informal care among elderly persons living in board and care homes. *The Gerontologist, 39,* 167–176.

Johnson, B. D., Stone, G. L., Altamaier, E. M., & Berdahl, L. D. (1998). The relationship of demographic factors, locus of control and self-efficacy to successful nursing home adjustment. *The Gerontologist, 38,* 209–216.

Kane, R. A., Kane, R. L., & Ladd, R. C. (1998). *The heart of long-term care.* New York: Oxford University Press.

Katz, I. R. & Coyne, J. C. (2000). The public health model for mental health care for the elderly. *JAMA, 283,* 2844–2845.

Kunzmann, U., Little, T. D., & Smith, J. (2000). Is age-related stability of subjective well-being a paradox? Cross-sectional and longitudinal evidence from the Berlin Aging Study. *Psychology and Aging, 15,* 511–526.

Laditka, S. B. (1998). Modeling lifetime nursing home use under assumptions of better health. *Journal of Gerontology: Social Sciences, 53B,* S177–S187.

Logsdon, R. G. (2000). Enhancing quality of life in long term care. In V. Molinari (Ed.), *Professional psychology in long term care,* (pp. 133–160). New York: Hatherleigh Press.

Mattimore, T. J., Wenger, N. S., Cesbiens, N. A., Teno, J. M., Hamel, M. B., Liu, H., Califf, R., Connors, A. F., Lynn, J., & Oye, R. K. (1997). Surrogate and physician understanding of patients' preferences for living permanently in a nursing home. *Journal of the American Geriatrics Society, 45,* 818–824.

Mitchell, J. M., & Kemp, B. J. (2000). Quality of life in assisted living homes: A multidimensional analysis. *Journal of Gerontology: Psychological Sciences, 55B,* P117–P127.

Pearlman, R., & Jonsen, G. (1985). The use of quality of life considerations in medical decision making. *Journal of the American Geriatrics Society, 33,* 344–352.

Rodin, J. (1986). Aging and health: Effects of the sense of control. *Science, 233,* 1271–1276.

Smyer, M. A., & Wilson, M. (1999). Critical issues and strategies in mental health consultation in nursing homes. In M. Duffy (Ed.), *Handbook of counseling and psychotherapy with older adults* (pp. 364–377). New York: Wiley.

Streim, J. (1996). Psychiatric problems in nursing homes. In J. I. Sheikh & I.D. Yalom (Eds.), *Treating the elderly* (pp. 107–128). San Francisco: Jossey-Bass.

Tavormina, C. E. (1999). Embracing the Eden Alternative in long-term care environments. *Geriatric Nursing, 20,* 1 58–161.

Tobin, S.S. (1991). *Personhood in advanced old age: Implications for practice.* New York: Springer.

Treas, J. (1995). Older Americans in the 1990s and beyond. *Population Bulletin* (pp. 11–22), *50(2).*

Williams, T. F. & Temkin-Greener, H. (1996). Older people, dependency, and trends in supportive care. In R. H. Binstock, L. E. Cluff, & O. Von Mering (Eds.), *The future of long-term care* (pp. 51–71). Baltimore: Johns Hopkins University Press.

Zimmerman, S. I. & Sloane, P. D. (1999, Fall). Optimum residential care for people with dementia. *Generations,* 62–68.

Zurakowski, T. L. (2000). The social environment of nursing homes and the health of older residents. *Holistic Nursing Practice, 14,* 12–23.

3

Biological, Psychological, and Social Issues Facing Older Adults in Residential Care

Kathleen S. King
Salt Lake City, Utah

Mary Ann Johnson
Veterans Administration Health Care System

"Home is the place where when you go there they have to take you in."
Robert Hellenga (1994). Sixteen Pleasures, p. 266. New York: Soho.

INTRODUCTION

To understand the impact of place of residence on the older adult, one needs to appreciate that each person is constantly influenced by the environment (Lawton, 1999). Most older adults resist the idea of leaving home even when realities of physical decline and loss of abilities to cope independently become apparent to everyone. Where one lives has several functions. It is a place of history that can evoke powerful emotions associated with memories and at the same time can inspire thoughts and expectations of the future. One's identity is expressed over time in the choice of furniture and decor; "one's personal history is re-created in microcosm through possessions" (Lawton, 1999, p. 358). In addition, people tend to structure their place of living in such a way as to increase their competence. The ability to control one's environment leads to a sense of familiarity and may be a major factor in why older adults wish to stay in their home even when overwhelmed by the de-

39

mands of staying there (Lawton, 1999). Thus, circumstances may require a choice to be made that includes the option of congregate living.

DEFINING RESIDENTIAL ASSISTED LIVING (RAL)

Several terms have been used to signify a community-based residence for older adults who no longer maintain a house. These include board and care, assisted living, residential care, and continuing care facilities (Hawes, 1999). The term residential assisted living (RAL) is used to represent a residence that includes specific services such as meals, housekeeping, hygiene, and sociorecreational amenities. Although the past two decades have represented increasing interest in developing alternative living arrangements for older adults, understanding those who relocate to RAL is not clear-cut. Some people may elect to move as a personal choice to eliminate responsibilities for home maintenance and maintain personal preferences for creativity and learning. Others may be compelled to move because of physical or emotional changes. Regardless of the stimulus for the move, RAL is considered to be an alternative to independent living and the least restrictive level of care compared to that obtained in a nursing home (Hopp, 1999). Leon, Cheng, and Neumann (1998) noted that with increasing numbers of older adults, most states have attempted to provide a choice for older people that includes supportive services, is cost effective, and either delays or is an alternative to nursing home care. This chapter presents a discussion of those factors that may interfere with independent living, the process of choosing and being accepted for RAL, and how a person adapts to the new environment of assisted living.

The varied reasons to explore RAL represent the diversified nature of the older population. The identification of an average or typical way that seniors respond, cope, or adapt to any late-life demand is difficult and probably impossible to discern (Silverstone, 1996). The fact that the elderly constitute a wide age span is one of the variables that hampers a clear categorization of response to change of living environments. There are differences between the "old-old" and the "young-old" in terms of age and historical background as well as physical, psychological, and cognitive functioning. Late-life transitions include adjustment to retirement and child launching, widowhood, physical disability, and the struggle between autonomy and dependency (Kuypers & Bengtson, 1983). Health and disability become much more salient factors in late-life adjustment for the very old (Costa & McCrae, 1993). Thus, the stresses encountered with aging, although universal across populations, become even more dominant in the older old group. Most people do not plan for aging, or even think about getting older and being unable to provide total self-care. The concept of health promotion as a means to prevent or adapt especially to physical changes by older people was not a dominant concern until the publication of *Healthy People 2000* by the U.S. Department of Health and Human Services in 1990.

Among the judgments an older person must make is that of appropriate living arrangements (Kane, Kane & Ladd, 1998). Although many elderly are able to remain in a their present residence, this is either not possible for or desired by some. If the person has not elected to enter a life care continuum of living and to "age in place," the decision to relocate may occur precipitously. Many reasons exist for relocation. The decision to move may be sudden and stimulated by an actual decrease of or a perceived lack of social support, such as death of a spouse or distance that removes one from the remainder of the family. A birthday, perceived to be an age of personal incapacity, can initiate a change of residence as the person encounters mounting constraints on physical or emotional capacities. Death of one's spouse, relocation of family members or living a distance from other social relationships can be factors in the choice of some type of residential care. The individual's inability to maintain independent living, including the up-keep of a home, or a sense of loneliness may cause the person to consider this move. Some older adults also do not want to be a burden on family but choose instead to purchase the level of care they need. In so doing, they may desire to alter their activities to allow for involvement in activities other than home maintenance and gain opportunity for personal expression through leisure activity. At the very least, they may wish to delay deterioration of function.

Mrs. M. acknowledged some of the conflicting feelings and perceptions related to making a decision for residential living. As the owner of two homes in different locations in the state, she recognized that at age 85 she could no longer care for or supervise the upkeep of both homes. She vacillated between priorities of personal health care and her desire for independence in traveling and "being my own boss". When she experienced increasing fatigue related to property management coupled with health problems that required emergency room and hospital interventions, she wondered how frequently she would experience the symptoms that took her to the emergency room and why no one had been able to identify and treat the cause. She also wondered whether she could continue to live in anxiety about the next attack. Although she has often spoke of her desire to move to a specific residential facility, indicating that doing so would provide her with on-sight monitoring, she has not been able to take the steps needed to achieve this desire.

Mrs. M. expresses many of the typical conflicting feelings experienced by older people who wish to remain independent but in order to do so may require more instrumental assistance with living arrangements. At the very least, some people wish to be relieved of some responsibilities associated with home ownership. One of the issues that Mrs. M. has tried to answer is the question "When will I know it is time?" Unfortunately, there are no standard answers to this question, and most older people find no professional caregivers can answer this for them. Mrs. M.'s assessment of her situation and worries about her physical problems caused her to be less certain about her ability to maintain herself independently. As she tries to maintain her independence she also fears the time when she will not be able to make decisions appropriately. Her goal is to be able to make her own decisions, and so she continues to search for the guidelines that will lead to the "right" answer. Further explanations of these factors involved in the complex process of decision making are reviewed next.

Biopsychosocial Changes of Aging Affecting Residence

The older population is characterized by variation in presentation of functional ability. One way this has been categorized is to think of the adult aging process as a series of stages. The young-old (age 65–74) vary from the other two groups of middle-old (age 75–84) and the old-old (85 and over). Most gerontologists consider that this distinction serves to differentiate a progression of changes in biological, social, and psychological functioning. However, the changes are not consistent from person to person. One's historical background, including genetics as well as lifestyle patterns, environmental influences, sociocultural issues, and one's belief system, affect how or whether these changes occur. Examples of persons over age 80 who continue to hike, bicycle, care for younger family members or maintain a work life out of the home have been publicized. The one factor that is universal is that the older individual tends to have more significant functional changes requiring modification in patterns of living. This group also requires more frequent follow-up for health care, be that health maintenance or treatment of physical or psychosocial pathologies. Because these physiological changes do not conform to any stable format, the person's status at any given time must be re-assessed. When further change or pathology appears, decisions regarding continuation at home or in RAL, lifestyle, and involvement in social activities must be made. Knowledge about the usual or "normal" physiological changes of aging continues to evolve. Some of the signs and symptoms previously thought to be normal or at least not preventable, such as loss of bone mass or atherosclerosis, are in fact pathological and related more to past physical, nutritional, and lifestyle patterns than to age alone. There are some characteristics about presentation of symptoms that are critical to understand in order to distinguish between those factors that are treatable, manageable, or correctable and those that require more intensive treatment and care.

Physiologically, the most apparent change is the loss of biological reserves—that is, the ability to respond to stimuli such as changes in ambient temperature, to mount a defense against a source of infection, or to adapt to glucose load. If a health care provider is not aware that these types of changes occur, it is possible to overreact and to treat them as though persons were presenting with pathology. Instead, instituting some health promotion measures, such as teaching about nutrition, or protective measures to compensate for these changes may be more appropriate. Unfortunately, the institution of therapies to correct a nonpathological change can result in pathology, creating more vulnerability for the elder.

In contrast to this response, a healthcare provider may inadvertently undertreat and create other problems. For example, failure to recognize conditions that can be corrected can result in lack of treatment. An assumption that urinary incontinence is "normal" for an older person or that forgetfulness is common and does not need further investigation may result in further pathology. In addition, for certain lifestyle habits such as smoking or excessive alcohol consumption, a kind of therapeutic "nihilism" exists. Some clinicians and loved ones believe it would be better to leave the elder with a few remaining pleasures rather than promote health. Lack of recognition of treatable conditions places that person at risk for withdrawal from social interaction or development of additional pathology. Failure to seek the source of the problem could mean lack of treatment or treatment of a nonexistent condition.

In addition to the previous changes, the older person may not present with the typical signs and symptoms of pathology, or the person may present with multiple symptoms that may be difficult to sort out so that the causative factor may not be discovered. For example, the person may not present with usual chest pain indicating a heart attack, but may instead have abdominal pain. Or the person may suddenly become confused due to reaction to multiple medications or presence of other systemic conditions such as gastrointestinal problems. Lethargy or sleep problems may represent cardiac problems or anxiety and depression.

A final reason why physiological issues may not be recognized and therefore be undertreated is lack of reporting by the older individual. Some older people believe that whatever they are experiencing is to be expected because of age. Consequently, they may fail to report changes in function or symptoms of pain representing treatable pathology. Worse, they may believe that nothing can be done and that no one would know how to address the problem. However, advanced age is insufficient reason to overlook any new symptom.

All these factors have the potential for decreased functioning, especially when someone is not available who knows the person and how that person reacts to various stimuli. The intent of gerontologists and geriatricians is to maintain the highest level of function possible. Any intervention must involve working with the individual and family or surrogate support system to identify risks and differentiate between normal and abnormal presentations.

Prior to admission to any RAL, knowledge of the person's physiological capacity is needed. Therefore, a complete physical examination plus evaluation of the physical status possibly indicating the need for more supervised care is required. This evaluation is focused on activities of daily living, such as ability to walk with or without a cane or walker, personal hygiene including bathing and toileting oneself, and ability to feed oneself. Concerns about the appropriateness of assisted living are raised when the person is incontinent of urine or bowels, is unable to provide self-care for these, or requires more supervision or assistance to ambulate. Cognitive disorders may exist that interfere with learning, memory, and judgment and require labor-intensive oversight to complete basic activities of daily living (Zimmerman & Slone, 1999).

The owners of an assisted living facility usually try to maintain their residents on site until the person's physical or cognitive capacities are compromised beyond the personnel or legal ability to provide those services. The facility may have a nurse employed to monitor the health status of the residents or a contract with a home health agency to provide some health care services. However, the resident may no longer qualify for continued living in that facility if the level of care required increases and there is demonstrated need for consistent, 24-hour oversight and care. Typical pathological conditions that may require a higher level of care include cardiac problems such as severe congestive heart failure, pulmonary diagnoses that require use of oxygen and are so severe the person's ability to ambulate beyond the room is compromised. Periodic reassessment is needed to determine when more pathology appears and a move from RAL is appropriate.

The Interactional Model

In order to understand why an older person requires assisted living and how that person adapts to this change, researchers need to rely on some framework that explains the person and his or her functioning. Such a framework can be found in the interactional model proposed by Lowry, Spinelli, and Lowry (1987).

The interactional model, developed initially for assessment and treatment of depression (Lowry et al., 1987), provides a framework for understanding psychosocial development and adaptation generally. Thus, the dynamics associated with a move to an RAL environment may be understood with the use of this model, defining behavior as a function of biological, psychological, and environmental factors. The interaction among these three factors can help to explain the reasons for and impact on adjustment following relocation into a more dependent environment.

The decision to move may be voluntary and perceived to be the best solution given alternatives of social isolation and concern about health status or safety. Those who may be categorized as "involuntary" may not wish to modify living arrangements even when those surroundings are problematic. The family may initiate this relocation when they recognize decreased physical function and their inability to provide the level of support needed for independent living. One consequence may be the older person's difficulty recognizing his or her limitations to function independently and subsequent difficulty with change of residence.

Adaptation Based on The Interactional Model

In addition to consideration of the normative factors leading to a change of residence, such as loss of a spouse and death or relocation of friends and relatives, at least three other elements influence the person's adaptation process. Table 3.1 represents the major factors. The first and perhaps most noticeable are the demands for adaptation due to changes in biological function. Although all people do not experience severe deficits in physical function, degrees of independence and de-

TABLE 3.1

Factors in Adaptation to Stress in Late Life

Biological	Social–Environmental	Psychological
Physical functioning	Social support	Mastery
Ability to complete ADLs & IADLs	Social interaction	Self-esteem
Level of health	Social resources (formal and informal resources)	Coping

Note. ADLs = activities of daily living; IADLs = instrumental activities of daily living. This table is adapted from two sources. From *An Interactional Model for the Assessment and Treatment of Depression*, by C. Lowry, R. Spinelli, and M. Lowry, 1987, Washington, DC: Department of Health and Human Services. Copyright 1987 by the Department of Health and Human Services. Adapted with permission. Also from "Physical, Psychological, and Social Resources as Moderators of the Relationship of Stress to Mental Health of the Very Old," by B. L. Roberts, R. Dunkel, and M. Haug, 1994, *Journal of Gerontology, 49*, p. S. Copyright 1994 by XX. Adapted with permission.

pendence do occur. One common problem appears when the person must forego driving due to visual, hearing, or musculoskeletal problems. Lack of driving privileges interferes with the person's ability to engage in common activities including shopping, banking, and social events. If pathological problems such as cardiac or neurological diagnoses also intervene, disuse of body or mind can alter the usual patterns the person has used to manage personal care, nutrition, and leisure-time activity. The risk of depression and gradual separation from society may occur simultaneously with physical changes.

The continuum of functioning and uncertainty about the future, both physically and cognitively, creates a cycle of events and concerns. The "what if" syndrome (i.e., "What if I fall or become more incapacitated?") may stimulate increased caution and fear of beginning anything new. Questions about moving, change of locale, the introduction of new people, and uncertainty regarding a fresh location can interfere with willingness to participate in usual as well as new activities, even in familiar surroundings. The energy required for adaptation to a new situation may be inadequate for meeting new challenges, beginning new projects, or learning about different patterns of functioning.

Older adults, just like younger, are at increased risk for development of depression and anxiety disorders when faced with serious medical illnesses. Estimates of incidence of depression for seniors with a medical illness range from 50%–75% (Jarvik, 1983). However, old age does present a distinct set of stresses even if they are not universal or considered "normal changes of aging" (Costa & McCrae, 1993). The unfortunate situation is that an older person often accumulates multiple medical problems requiring multiple interventions. Many elders passively accept these interventions by their health care providers such as added prescriptions or medical advice

(Silverstone, 1996). They may not voice their concerns about ability to abide by these because of complicating issues arising from their personal situation including finances and family concerns. Unfortunately, lack of communication of this critical self-perception may be perceived as acceptance by the provider without pursuing the implications for the person's existence. Thus, lack of assertiveness may jeopardize the individual and lead to further complications.

Successful adjustment in late life involves coping with the inevitable decline in vitality and health as well as coming to terms with losses. In the context of society, it can be challenging to age with dignity and an intact sense of one's personal and social worth and competence. The risk for development of feelings of demoralization and despair is significant and can lead to major depression (Stokes, 1992) or death (Lamberta & Wyman,1999).

Psychological mastery, a sense of control over one's personal and environmental life, is needed for a person to perceive his or her ability to maintain autonomy (Roberts, Dunkel, & Haug, 1994). Loss of control and self-esteem can lead to a sense of incompetence and worthlessness. The unknown environment of residential or assisted living may raise another possible source of fear of rejection or fear of inability to adapt in a new situation. Again, these changes require emotional energy to invest oneself in relationships and to cope with new stimuli.

Coping represents the resources, actions, and perceptions one mobilizes to decrease the threat and impact of stress (Costa & McCrae, 1993; Roberts et al, 1994). Coping that is emotion-based seeks to manage the emotional reaction over the process of adjustment; coping that is problem-focused seeks to manage the stress via resolution of the problem. One's willingness and ability to mobilize effective coping affects mental health and psychological well being. Age itself is not a determining factor as to how one perceives stress, implements coping, or evaluates the outcome. Rather, one's past history of behaviors and attitudes used to manage stresses seems to determine how one will react in late life (Atchley, 1989). Diversity of coping alternatives tends to be associated with satisfactory adjustment in late life. The popular myth that old people become rigid and dependent in their coping has been negated by a review of coping strategies used by seniors. This review showed that seniors tended to use a wide variety of mechanisms, and the coping strategies used in young and middle age were the ones endorsed in late life (Costa & McCrae, 1993).

Costa and McCrae (1993) also reported that certain personality factors correlated strongly with specific coping strategies that appeared to be relatively stable throughout life. For example, openness to experience is associated with individuals who are imaginative, empathic, and curious. Those who are more open to experiences may tend to use humor as a coping mechanism. Those who are low in openness are often practical, conventional, and down-to-earth and may use faith to cope with new or stressful situations. Both humor and faith are thought to be mature responses and serve the purpose of aiding persons to adapt to a given situation (Costa & McCrae, 1993). Those more at risk for adapting to stressful stimuli in late life are those who have high degrees of neuroticism or lifelong practice of negative emotional reactions. This disposition to personality affects the individual's perception of stress, coping choices and adjustment outcomes including perception of well-being and somatic complaints.

Environmental factors constitute the final portion of the triad of interaction affecting an older person's adaptation to change. These factors include those that arise from the social and physical context of living. Research suggests that social support is a factor in freedom from depression (Bisconti & Bergeman, 1999; Dimond, Lund, & Caserta, 1987). Both informal and formal resources for support influence mental health as well as ability to maintain a home. The two most common stresses facing older adults are the death or illness of significant others and recent physical changes with declining health (Roberts et al., 1994). The end result of these losses is potential diminished social and physical support, which can lead to decisions for change of living arrangements.

An examination of the demographics of older adults most likely to go into residential care points out that this population is generally older, sicker, and lacks informal sources of support and care (Baggett, 1989). The consequence is that the person is no longer able to live independently and must look to those outside the family for oversight of care. Approximately 8%–9% of older adults live in various residential alternatives to home including retirement facilities and communities, board and care homes, and assisted living (Lawton, 1999). Some of these options are for-profit, some charity and nonprofit, some are quite luxurious, some subsidized, some are purchased, some rented. A wide range of choices, amenities, and services exist depending on preferences, needs, and financial resources.

The choices for care open to older adults and their family members range from independent apartments to supervised long-term care in a nursing home. The possible sites between these two extremes constitute RAL.

The biopsychosocial changes related to accumulated losses may hinder the relocation process and interfere with or prolong adaptation to a new environment. In contrast, the strengths of the individual combined with an accepting environment can facilitate adaptation to change fostering continuity of self-identity. Some people elect to move in order to decrease perceived burden being placed on family members. If they are able to obtain needed care and closer monitoring of health problems, the move becomes at least in part a voluntary decision. In addition, the support provided by both personnel and other residents as well as family members who may be available to provide social and health care outlets offers both formal and informal outlets to assist with adaptation.

The choice of living arrangements may be hampered by the previously mentioned diversity of assisted living facilities. Knowledge about one's needs and consequently the most appropriate type of facility are necessary but not sufficient to select an appropriate residence. The selection of a new home is ideally based on location, type of services needed and offered including transportation, and the characteristics of other residents that match the person's perception of self.

Recommendations from friends and relatives may also enter into the equation. The characteristics of the new environment including rules and regulations related to meal times, visitors, and social activities are factors requiring a change in focus. How the person has adapted in the past to new situations may serve to predict how they will react and adapt to a situation reminiscent of dormitory living.

The following are presented to exemplify components of the interactional model. Typical of current demographics of the older population, women are overrepresented.

> After the death of her husband, Mrs. A, at age 82, moved from her home in Florida to be near her only child and his family in the West. The change of physical and social environments continued to astound her, but she found ways to adapt with a small number of other residents, maintaining a moderate walking habit that was gradually reduced because of cardiac disabilities. She frequently reported she would never adjust to the new environment, but realized she could no longer function alone. An "assignment" to use her writing skills to say goodbye to her late husband provided an outlet she had not previously considered to pursue her grief work. Residential living with a balcony view of the mountains, plus ready access to the hospital for needed surgery and medical problems, a clinic for periodic evaluation, and family support did not remove all the losses associated with relocation but provided a system to foster purpose in living.

This situation represents one person's ability to adapt by use of past skills (writing) and desire to maintain continuity with her family. Loss of her primary social support for over 40 years with the death of her husband stimulated the evaluation of her situation and resultant decision to move. Although she relocated to a geographic area foreign to her, she was able to achieve a sense of independence by accepting those events in the RAL complex that she identified "as me" and to avoid associations and activities that created more stress for her. Although the move was not her first choice, she also recognized that she needed more intense health care and transportation that could be best facilitated by her family and by close proximity to her providers. Her ability to exercise control over her alternatives probably contributed to satisfactory relocation adjustment.

> At the point at which Ms J.'s vision worsened to near blindness, she elected to move to residential housing, giving up her home of many years. As a nurse, she had always been independent, never married, and was involved in caring for herself as well as others. Shortly after moving to her new apartment, she broke her hip, was hospitalized, spent some time in long-term care for rehabilitation and eventually returned to her new apartment in an RAL community. Transportation service at the RAL provides her with access to church, shopping, clinic appointments, and "outings". Recovery from the fracture was slow but certain, and she regained a sense of belonging as she reestablished her social contacts in and out of the facility. A peer-counselor

group at her church provided Ms. J. with added social support throughout her relocations and health problems.

Ms J's decision was stimulated by increasing physical incapacity and her recognition as a professional person that she would be at greater risk for injury and possible abuse by remaining in her private home. Her decision was voluntarily made,
and her selection of the facility was made with preplanning, taking into account the
location, availability of the types of services she would need (meals, housekeeping, and transportation), and ease of access to her church and family. The fact that
she fell and sustained a fracture requiring hospitalization and subsequent rehabilitation did not interfere with her determination to remain as independent as possible. Her selection provided the type of support she needed, and her methods of
coping supported her through an unfortunate accident. This situation illustrates the
fact that assisted living does not eliminate dangers or untoward events. However, it
also illustrates that when such events happen there may be resources immediately
available to respond and manage needed care.

The death of her husband stimulated a daughter to urge her parents to move from
their home in the East in order for her to more closely monitor her father's health status. Mr. P. was limited by chronic cardiac and pulmonary problems and appreciated
the offer. Mrs. P. complained about the nature of the residential housing, her concerns about her own health (primarily limitations associated with arthritis), and lack
of care and attention from the staff. Although Mr. P. was more limited in his social
outlets, Mrs. P. was able to participate in activities and with urging did so. Treatment
for depression modified some of her symptoms, making her more accessible to the
amenities offered by the RAL. The daughter visited, provided transportation to
clinic appointments, monitored medications, and assured that her parent's health issues were addressed. She did not try to provide all social contacts for her mother but
made sure that needed care was provided. She noted that her mother had social outlets, but always tended to be negative; thus, her own ability to manage her feelings
was frequently compromised.

Mr. and Mrs. P. exemplify not only the distance required for relocation but the fact
that two people coming from the same background will continue to demonstrate
their past personalities and means of adaptation. Just as with Mrs. A. this couple
were without family in their previously familiar, comfortable, and pleasing environment. Their "up-rooting" required effort for them as well as for the daughter
who had lost her primary source of social support with the death of her husband.
Although some families are able to relocate to the parent's community, that is not
the usual scenario. The contrast of personalities between the couple and the need
for a new health care provider helped to address issues that perhaps had been overlooked previously because of familiarity with the couple. Encouragement and sup-

port from the daughter and the staff of the facility for Mrs. P. also provided some respite for the husband as he tried to manage his limiting physical abilities.

> Mrs. C. has fibromyalgia and has struggled with depression and anxiety most of her life. She was aware that her mother-in-law, who lived with mental retardation throughout her life, was now showing signs of dementia and lived alone. Mrs. C.'s husband was aware of his mother's problems, but many factors complicated his ability to act: geographic distance, disagreement among his siblings regarding the mother's degree of impairment, financial considerations, and his own wish to deny or at least minimize the problems. The mother-in-law abruptly began to demonstrate inability to function independently. As a result, Mr. and Mrs. C. drove to her home, packed her belongings, and moved her into their home. Her house was placed up for sale. She left behind a significant social network, including a boyfriend.

This example raises many questions about how families attempt to deal with the issues of declining functions of a loved one and increasing disabilities of relatives, especially parents. One could argue that the adult son, whose response resulted in disruption of his mother's and his own physical and social environment, could have decreased their stress in other ways. For example, he could have assessed and recognized the potentials of his mother's living circumstances. He could have involved his mother in some decision making so that she became a part of the move and not the object. His mother, albeit impaired, had little input into the decision not only to move from her home, but to another city.

Adjustment to RAL

The process of adjustment to relocation to RAL is as multifactored as the process of deciding to move. Seniors and their families are often surprised that the move is not the hoped-for answer to problems of daily living but rather creates a new set of problems and concerns. And the process of aging, even in a situation designed to provide support for activities of daily living, will bring with it the expected normative and pathological changes that will alter the person's needs for assistance over time.

Whatever the stimulus may be for relocation, a move from private residence to assisted living can create a sense of loss, particularly with respect to one's sense of autonomy or independent functioning. A study of adaptation of residents to nursing home life demonstrated some older adults require up to 4–6 months of readjustment time (Brooke, 1987). Possibly the same would be true for those moving into RAL, especially if that move was not elective.

A few factors have been associated with complications in the process of adjustment to RAL. A prominent factor is the role of personal decision making to relocate to an RAL. Forced residential relocation has been associated with complicated adjustment for some older individuals who place a high value on independent functioning (Dimond, McCance, & King, 1987). Forced relocation inherently limits one's choices and possibly one's sense of control over one's future. Lack of perceived control has been identified as a psychological vulnerability that can have a negative impact on coping and adaptation to stress (Roberts et al., 1994) and has been associated with increased visits to physicians (Chipperfield & Greenslade, 1999). Low self-esteem prior to a stress is believed to negatively affect successful adjustment. Also, for those who have impaired cognitive function, their ability to learn and remember components of a new environment is compromised. These individuals are most at risk for "relocation trauma" and often show a decline in cognitive ability soon after moving. Thus, relocation is a significant personal stress that taxes psychological and cognitive resources.

> Mrs. A. was relocated from a Midwest state to be closer to her son when it became clear that she no longer could live alone. She had long-standing psychological problems including bipolar disorder, but physically she managed well. She needed help with meals, transportation, and socialization. She moved into a retirement facility with minimal services. She quickly developed problems with being able to learn how to lock and unlock the door to her rooms, and her son was called numerous times to help her. Her inability to learn the complicated locking system became a threat to her ability to stay in the facility. Mrs. A. became frustrated and depressed and often just left her door open, resulting in a risk for her safety.

This vignette represents one of the many complications of adaptation to RAL: Although the elderly person and his or her family and friends may have good intentions, the process of relocating has many unintended consequences and requires ongoing support and guidance to make a successful adjustment.

Facility characteristics that are associated with positive quality of life after relocation include adequate staff and services. In addition, residents in facilities that have low conflict and high cohesion report high degrees of life satisfaction (Mitchell & Kemp, 2000). Ongoing informal support from family and friends in the community can help maintain those relationships and ties to the community that are so important in preserving the older resident's sense of autonomy (Luecknotte, 2000). Further, some evidence exists that seniors report higher satisfaction with smaller facilities, possibly because moderate size can promote cohesion. Some level of physical amenities and services and increased availability of personal space are also associated with satisfaction (Sikorska, 1999). This same study indicated that fewer sociorecreational activities were associated with satisfaction, possibly because cognitively intact individuals do not care for the activities that cognitively impaired individuals can participate in.

> Mrs. C. (from the earlier example) recognized that both she and her mother-in-law would do better if the mother-in-law lived independently. They looked together at several facilities and found a retirement home with assisted living that her mother-in-law liked a great deal. The son wanted to put off the move to reduce costs,

but when he understood that two relocations could complicate his mother's adjustment, he agreed to the placement. His mother managed to make friends and participate in social activities; she had some physical complications seemingly associated with the move and became very confused about her medications. Staff persisted in monitoring her and supporting her adjustment; her son and daughter-in-law took her to the church of her choice and other outings. Although still unhappy about leaving her home, she settled into her new environment and has been doing well overall in the process of adjustment.

The process of adjustment to relocation to RAL can be not only long but can require ongoing monitoring of the elder's physical, psychological, and social status. People tend to do better when there is ongoing informal support from family and friends (Hopp, 1999), and those individuals are often in the best position to know if relocated adults are managing well on the basis of their previous level of functioning. It is important to keep in mind that once the initial move to an RAL has been negotiated, individuals will still be subject to normative and pathological age-related changes that can affect functioning and require more formal services to maintain oneself in the facility.

Pre-Admission Assessment

An assisted living facility will require some indication that the person applying for this level of residence is appropriate for that facility. In order to make this judgment, an assessment of physical, psychological, and social parameters is needed. Although most facilities have their own format for obtaining this information, a professional care provider or case manager needs to determine the overall functioning of the person in order to submit a rational perspective about that individual's chances of success in the facility. Table 3.2 is an outline of suggestions for inclusion in this assessment. These parameters can also be used to guide the person and the family in considering a specific move. No assessment format, however, can assure the "right" choice will always be made or that the individual will not transfer from one living situation to another. However, a careful assessment may help diminish the trauma of a second move. For this reason, factors to be assessed should help find a match between the person and environment. A relocation that is forced tends to complicate the adjustment (Dimond, McCance, & King, 1987) and thus one's functioning, whereas the person's involvement in the decision has been shown to decrease feelings of guilt. Attitudes the person may have about long-term care and perception of RAL as a nursing home rather than an independent living facility can interfere with making informed choices. The experience of the present authors is that an opportunity for the older adult and his or her caregivers to discuss those factors with an adviser can yield a better long-term relocation than when such a decision is made under duress of time or pressure from others.

TABLE 3.2

Assessment Factors on the Person's Ability to Maintain in RAL Environment

Biological	Psychological	Social–Environmental
Health status	Psychological health	Social resources (proximity and availability)
Ability to perform ADLs	Self-esteem, mastery	
Ability to perform IADLs	Autonomy and perceived control	Confidant (continuity)
Health promotion needs	Coping Skills	Marital status
Medical problems and their management	History of psychological disorders & their treatment	Financial status & resources
Medications, number, frequency, route	History of emotional, physical abuse	Professional support and continuity
Sensory function	History of substance abuse	Leisure pursuits
Balance, strength	Values, preferences	Community involvements
Cognitive status	Decision-making processes	Health status of loved one

Note. RAL = residential assisted living; ADLs = activities of daily living; IADLs = instrumental activities of daily living.

The ultimate goal is to maintain the person in a mode of independence in a home-like environment with adequate services rather than foster a sense of dependence and inadequacy. Cognitive deficits may interfere with a reasoned choice by the individual, but attempts must be made to match the person with the environment in order to maintain a sense of continuity of self. Those involved in the choice to relocate, whether family, other informal caregivers, or professional care providers, need to be cognizant of the individual's wishes and characteristics of past function, especially when an urgent situation arises and the person may not be completely involved in the decision. An emergency hospitalization, changes in a neighborhood, loss of a caregiver through death or relocation, or sudden realization of an inability to maintain one's lifestyle because of increasing age-related physical incapacity or impaired cognitive function all have the potential for removing the person from the decision.

SUMMARY

The advent of RAL programs has provided both an opportunity and a challenge to older adults and their families who contemplate a change in living situations. Most people understand the circumstances necessitating a move to long-term care. The reasons for moving to RAL are not as clear-cut. There are no standard governmental policies that define the general characteristics of those persons who would most benefit from assisted living. One example of the difficulty an older woman had with deciding on a change of living arrangement was provided to emphasize the challenges a person faces with this decision. She represents the uncertainties that current elders encounter when attempting to remain a part of the community, retain their distinctive attributes, and sustain themselves in a safe environment. No attempt was made to provide a final answer to the appropriateness of "who", "where," or "when" in selection of an RAL. This decision is a process requiring time, thought, and discussion.

An assessment of the person's abilities as well as deficiencies can be used to guide the staff toward facilitation of strengths. Table 3.2, based on recognized changes that occur with aging, summarizes some of the critical features of a preadmission assessment. This can assist RAL staff as well as the person and family to determine the needs a person may have and the appropriateness of RAL as a living option. An ongoing assessment and observation of the individual's capacity to incorporate self into the environment, or the development of new pathologies, can thereby be based on a description of the person and not on first impressions.

The ability of the person to maintain a sense of self in a new situation has a foundation in that person's biopsychosocial and environmental characteristics as well as the nature of the aging population. No two people will react in the same fashion to the need to make a decision about living arrangements or to follow through with the decision. The Interactional Model proposed by Lowry et al. (1987) was used in this chapter to assist others in conceptualizing the nature of the decision and the person's adaptation to relocation. The model is a framework for understanding how a person may adapt in an uncertain situation while maintaining the ability to distinguish between self and nonself. The fact that one person may have difficulty with the decision and with the move does not mean all persons will have the same problem. The role of family is central for some persons but not for others. That person's past history (biological, psychological, and sociological–environmental) is central to understanding the coping methods used for adaptation. No two people automatically use the same coping resources, nor do older adults become rigid and dependent. Several examples have been used to demonstrate how multiple factors influence the process of adaptation even when the choice of an RAL appears to be the most appropriate for that person. The ability to incorporate past with present environment, to make new friends and maintain contact with others, and to adjust to changes in vitality and physical stamina have been discussed within the context of this model.

REFERENCES

Atchley, R. C. (1989). A continuity theory of normal aging. *Gerontologist, 29,* 183–190.
Baggett, S. A. (1989). *Residential care for the elderly: Critical issues in public policy.* New York: Greenwood Press.

Bisconti, T., & Bergeman, C. S. (1999). Perceived control as a mediator of the relationships among social support, psychological well-being and perceived health. *Gerontologist, 39*, 94–103.

Brooke, V. (1987). *Adjusting to living in a nursing home: Toward a nursing intervention.* Unpublished doctoral dissertation, University of Utah.

Chipperfield, J., & Greenslade, L. (1999). Perceived control as a buffer in use of health care services. *Journal of Gerontology, 543,* P146–P154.

Costa P. T., & McCrae, R. R. (1993). Psychological stress and coping in old age. In L. Goldberger & S. Brenitz (Eds.), *Handbook of stress: Theoretical and finical aspects* (pp. 403–412). New York: The Free Press.

Dimond, M., Lund, D., & Caserta, M. (1987). The role of social support in the first two years of bereavement in an elderly sample. *Gerontologist, 27*, 599–604.

Dimond, M., McCance, K., & King, K. (1987). Forced residential relocation: Its impact on the well-being of older adults. *Western Journal of Nursing Research, 9*, 445–464.

Hawes, C. (1999). A key piece of the integration puzzle: Managing the chronic care needs of the frail elderly in residential care settings *Generations, 22,* 51–55.

Hopp, F. P. (1999). Patterns and predictors of formal and informal care among elderly persons living in board and care homes. *The Gerontologist, 39*, 167–176.

Jarvik, L. F. (1983) The impact of immediate life situations on depression: Illnesses and losses. In L. Breslau & M. Haug (Eds.), *Depression and aging: Causes, care, and consequences* (pp. 114–120), New York: Springer.

Kane, R. A., Kane, R. L., & Ladd, R. (1998). *The heart of long term care.* New York: Oxford University Press.

Kuypers, J. A., & Bengtson, V (1983). Toward competence in the older family. In T. Brubaker (Ed.), *Family relationships in later life* (pp. 211–228). Beverly Hills, CA: Sage.

Lamberta, H. & Wyman, J. F. (1999). Failure to thrive. In J. K. Stone, J. F. Wyman, & S. A. Salisbury (Eds.), Clinical gerontological nursing: A guide to advanced practice (2nd ed., pp. 313–332), Philadelphia: Saunders.

Lawton, M. P. (1999). Environmental design features and the well-being of older persons. In M. Duffy (Ed.), *Handbook of counseling and psychotherapy with older adults* (pp. 350–363). New York: Wiley.

Leon, J., Cheng, C. -K., & Neumann, P. J. (1998). Alzheimer's disease care: Costs and potential savings. *Health Affairs, 17,* 206–216.

Lowry, C., Spinelli, R. & Lowry, M. (1987). An interactional model for the assessment and treatment of depression. DHHS Grant No. STC-9 1 T15 MH18889-01

Lueckenotte, A. (2000). *Gerontological nursing* (2nd ed.). St. Louis, MO: Mosby.

Mitchell, J. M., & Kemp, B. J. (2000). Quality of life in assisted living homes: A multidimensional analysis. *Journal of Gerontology, 55B,* P117–P127.

Roberts, B. L., Dunkel, R., & Haug, M. (1994), Physical, psychological, and social resources as moderators of the relationship of stress to mental health of the very old. *Journal of Gerontology, 49,* S35–S43.

Sikorska, E. (1999) Organizational determinants of resident satisfaction with assisted living. *Gerontologist, 39,* 450–456.

Silverstone, B. (1996). Older people of tomorrow: A psychosocial profile. *Gerontologist, 36,* 27–34.

Stokes, G. (1992). *On being old: The psychology of later life.* London: The Falmer Press.

U.S. Department of Health and Human Services (1990). *Healthy people 2000: Healthy older adults.* Washington, DC: Public Health Department.

Zimmerman, S. I., & Sloane, P.D. (1999, Fall). Optimum residential care for people with dementia. *Generations,* 62–68.

II

Assessment Issues in Residential Care

4

Assessment Strategies and Procedures for Residential Care Placement

Thomas Schenkenberg, Ph.D.
University of Utah

INTRODUCTION

Part II of this volume addresses assessment issues in residential placement and care. This chapter focuses on the assessment of the cognitive–neuropsychological functioning of the elderly individual who is a candidate for residential care, with an emphasis on the individual whose cognitive status might interfere with independent living. Assessment of medical and psychological functioning is addressed in the next chapter.

Although limitations in physical functioning are often the principal reasons for an individual to consider residential care, the development of significant cognitive impairment also leads to such a consideration. Even in the context of a primary physical limitation, the possibility of the subsequent development of cognitive impairment is an important concern in the elderly population. Thus, the need for assessment of the individual's cognitive status may be the primary reason for consideration of residential care or it may become necessary after the individual has been in residential care for some time.

Referral for a formal neuropsychological evaluation is important for several reasons:

1. Many developing neurologic conditions are subtle in their early phases. Neuropsychological assessment plays an important role in identifying con-

ditions (many of which are reversible) that may not be evident using other techniques.

2. The level of independence of the individual is an important concern in terms of safety and the nature of the residential setting to be recommended. Neuropsychological assessment can significantly assist in determining limitations and strengths with regard to independent functioning.

3. The individual's level of decision-making capacity is a fundamental matter in many issues confronting the candidate for residential care, both at the point of determination to proceed (or not) with residential care and later in the case of a progressive condition. Neuropsychological assessment contributes directly to determination of decision-making capacity.

4. Many conditions that affect elderly individuals are progressive in nature. Establishing baseline descriptions of functional abilities with follow-up testing for comparison purposes can contribute in fundamental ways to determination of further decline, stabilization, new findings, or the need to change the individual's residential or treatment status.

The following remarks focus on the pragmatic issues involved in neuropsychological evaluation in the context of decisions about residential care. Three categories of factors are discussed:

- General considerations in the neuropsychological evaluation of elderly individuals who are candidates for residential care;
- Objectives of the neuropsychological evaluation in the consideration of residential care; and
- Specific strategies and procedures.

GENERAL CONSIDERATIONS IN THE NEUROPSYCHOLOGICAL EVALUATION OF ELDERLY INDIVIDUALS WHO ARE CANDIDATES FOR RESIDENTIAL CARE

The elderly individual in our society is confronted with an extensive array of concerns, including possible decline in intellectual and physical functioning, physical illness, loss of independence, changes in financial status, the deaths of loved ones, changes in self-concept, and a host of additional matters. The popular media have increasingly focused on conditions that affect the elderly, such as Alzheimer's disease (e.g., Nash, 2000), resulting in increased awareness about such conditions. As life expectancy extends, increasing numbers of individuals experience clinically significant cognitive decline, and thus increasing numbers of family members and friends witness the decline of individuals they have known well. These factors have combined to produce increasing concern among the elderly about cognitive decline and its implications. Perhaps the most common comments the clinician encounters in this population are expressed concerns about not wanting to lose independence, not wanting to become a burden, and not wanting to be placed in a nursing home. It is against this backdrop that the cognitive evaluation of the candidate for residential care takes place.

It is important to point out that although a residential placement is often sought out by an individual as an attractive personal option in light of a practical analysis of one's own situation, the possibility of such a placement is often an intimidating and daunting notion for many people. Such perceptions are often not well-informed with regard to the actual nature of residential settings, but the negative perception often persists. Thus, if an individual is referred for a neuropsychological assessment, he or she is likely to be coming with a good deal of trepidation. The clinician simply must be aware of this. One of the most fundamental issues in assessing cognitive function is to be certain that one is eliciting the best possible performance from the patient. If the performance of the individual is adversely affected by anxiety or other such factors, the results of the tests (scores) are artificially lowered, and the interpretation of these lower scores may be incorrect. Further, it is well-known that the performance of elderly individuals on cognitive tasks is influenced by distraction (McDowd & Birren, 1990), and the testing setting must be designed to reduce such potential confounding influences.

In addition to test-taking anxiety, other psychological and psychiatric issues must be kept in mind when evaluating performance on cognitive tests. For example, Clarfield (1988) reviewed a series of studies involving individuals suspected of having a dementing disorder and determined that approximately 26% of the patients were found to have depression as the cause of their cognitive inefficiencies.

It is well-known that auditory and visual acuity decline with increasing age (Kline & Scialfa, 1996; Storandt & VandenBos, 1994). Indeed, the individuals selected as part of the standardization sample for the recently revised and widely-used test of memory function, the Wechsler Memory Scale III (WMS III; Wechsler, 1997b), were asked to indicate limitations with regard to auditory and visual acuity as part of the background information. In the age groups between 65 and 89, 40% of the normal participants reported difficulty hearing, and 90% reported that they required glasses for reading (Schenkenberg & Said, 2000). It is clear that unless the examiner makes certain that the patient is actually able to see and hear the instructions to the various cognitive tasks and the items themselves, the valid interpretation of the results is compromised.

More than 80% of individuals over the age of 65 have at least one chronic medical condition (Adams & Benson, 1992). The primary and secondary effects (e.g., fatigue) of such conditions can adversely influence test performance, and these must be taken into consideration in interpreting the scores that emerge from the testing process.

Many elderly individuals take a large number of medications, and often these medications are from different prescribing clinicians. These various clinicians are often not aware of the other medications being provided by the other clinicians.

Over-the-counter medications and other health products represent an additional source of possible influence on the patient's neuropsychological test performance. Although this matter has not been studied extensively, it is also clear from clinical practice that patients often "stockpile" supplies of previously prescribed medication and use medications actually prescribed for others (e.g., spouse).

Drug toxicity has been found to be responsible for the findings of possible dementia in a significant number of patients (e.g., see Larson, Reifler, Sumi, Canfield, & Chinn, 1986). Delirium (acute confusional state) from drug toxicity and delirium from other causes are major concerns in evaluating possible dementia in older adults.

The issue of medication effects on neuropsychological test results comes not only in the form of toxicity or as a result of "polypharmacy" but also in the context of appropriately prescribed medications. For example, in Parkinson's disease there are well-known fluctuations in motor function in patients who have received prolonged levodopa therapy (Djaldetti & Melamed, 1998). These fluctuations in function represent perhaps the greatest clinical challenge in the long-term management of patients with Parkinson's disease (Quinn, 1998). The relevance of these fluctuations in terms of neuropsychological test results comes in many forms. For example, these patients can experience a "wearing off" phenomenon, characterized by the loss of stable motor function (typically over the course of one to three hours after the last dose). Thus, a patient's motor function might be quite different at the beginning of a testing session than it is at the end of the session. Without an awareness of these potential medication effects, the interpretation of the results of tasks involving motor function (even indirectly) might be inaccurate, and perhaps a low score might be interpreted as a more enduring finding. This is only one example of the potential effect of even properly prescribed medication. Medication side effects must always be kept in mind in evaluating neuropsychological test results.

Neuropsychological test findings must be interpreted in a proper context. This context includes a number of factors. The history of the individual must be well-understood so that an accurate expectation of how this individual should perform on the tests is generated. In order to do this, the patient's academic, occupational, and avocational history must be understood. A variety of techniques have been developed to extrapolate to expected performance levels on the basis of demographic background data (e.g., Vanderploeg, 1994; Vanderploeg, Schinka, & Axelrod, 1996). The complexity of this process and its limitations are well-known to clinicians in this field. Nonetheless, this process of estimating how well this particular patient should be able to perform on these tasks is an important, fundamental element in the valid interpretation of the test results.

Clearly, a complete history of the patient in terms of medical–neurological conditions, current and past medications, alcohol and drug use, head injury, stroke, and other factors is critical to the interpretation of neuropsychological test results.

Because the patient's history is so vital to the understanding of the patient's current performance, and because memory difficulties can influence the accuracy of the self-reported history, it is very important to have corroborating sources for the history. These include a review of records and, with the patient's permission, independent discussion with another source, such as the spouse or adult child of the patient.

Cultural diversity and language issues must also be considered in the interpretation of neuropsychological test results (Hong, Morris, Chiu, & Benet-Martinez, 2000; Ponton & Leon-Carrion, 2000). Cohort differences with regard to test-taking attitudes and test-taking experience have not been studied extensively but bear consideration in interpreting neuropsychological test results. Other factors such as the (likely) age difference between the examiner and the candidate for residential placement can have an influence on the outcome as well.

Proper normative data for older individuals represent a major issue in the analysis of individual test performance. Until very recently such normative data for older individuals had not been collected in a rigorous manner. In recent years we have had the benefit of the recently revised WMS III (Wechsler, 1997b) and the Wechsler Adult Intelligence Scale III (WAIS III; Wechsler, 1997a) which include normative data on individuals to age 89. In addition, these tests were "co-normed" on the same, census-based standardization sample, allowing comparison of findings on one of the tests with findings on the other. It should be mentioned, however, that although the overall standardization sample as a whole reflects the general population in an overall manner (age, sex, race–ethnicity, educational level, and geographic region), interpretations of the scores of a person of a minority ethnic background cannot be fairly related to the normative data in the same manner as those of a person whose ethnic background reflects the majority of the individuals in that normative data set. Further, the individuals in the standardization sample were screened principally through self-report questionnaires concerning their medical and psychiatric history. Thus, it is quite possible that some individuals with actual impairments are included in the standardization sample.

A second large data set that addresses the issue of age-related norms is the set generated from the Mayo's Older Americans Normative Studies (MOANS). These norms extend to age 97 and provide normative data sets for tests such as the Auditory Verbal Learning Test, the Boston Naming Test, the Trail Making Test, and a number of other popular neuropsychological tests (e.g., Invik, Malec, Smith, Tangalos, & Peterson, 1996). Again, caution is recommended in light of the fact that this "normative" sample is 99.6% Caucasian and is not representative of the general population in the United States, in any event, having been recruited from the region near Rochester, Minnesota (Green, 2000).

Despite the noted limitations, the normative data available for older adults have been significantly expanded and aggregated for use by the practicing clinician (Spreen & Strauss, 1998). Further, important texts have been developed that are designed to describe the clinical neuropsychological assessment process (Filskov & Boll, 1981/1986; Heilman & Valenstein, 1993; Kolb & Wishaw, 1990; Lezak, 1995). In addition, texts have been developed that specifically guide the neuropsychological assessment of the older adult (e.g., Green, 2000). All of these resources make this process considerably more effective than it was just 15 years ago. Further, the field of behavioral neurology has experienced a renaissance in recent years, and excellent sources are available to assist in the analysis of specific syndromes and their underlying neuroanatomic foundations (e.g., Mesulam, 2000).

The neuropsychological assessment process involves multiple sources of input (history, observation, test results). The conclusions, however, are the result of a considered review of these components involving interpretation by a clinician in the context of knowledge about the nervous system and the conditions that affect it. When severe impairments are demonstrated, the recommendations regarding assisted living arrangements are rather straightforward. With moderate or mild impairments, predictions with regard to the patient's ability to live independently are more complex and require carefully considered judgements and follow-up. Follow-up evaluation is particularly important in situations involving the early stage of what may be a progressive dementia. An additional word of caution is in order. It has been noted that there is a tendency in neuropsychological evaluations for some clinicians to develop a confirmatory bias (Hazlewood et al., 1997). This is a tendency to focus on those scores that appear to imply impairment, perhaps even when other scores are quite adequate. It is clearly important to be aware of this phenomenon and to consider this matter in the interpretation of test data. It is wise to repeat tests that appear to be producing results that are at odds with other findings.

OBJECTIVES OF THE NEUROPSYCHOLOGICAL EVALUATION IN THE CONSIDERATION OF RESIDENTIAL CARE

The principal object of this type of evaluation is, of course, to fully describe the actual level of the person's current neuropsychological function (in a broad array of spheres). This assessment allows the clinician to describe the individual's strengths and weaknesses in functional terms. These, in turn, may lead to certain diagnostic considerations involving neurologic conditions. The neuropsychological assessment is most helpful to the patient in the context of a neurological evaluation by a neurologist, geriatrician, internist, or other similarly qualified physician.

Disruption of neuropsychological function is common in a wide variety of neurologic conditions. Conditions such as progressive dementing disorders, stroke (and multi-infarct dementia), head injury, and Parkinson's disease have rather characteristic presentations (by history, observation, and neuropsychological testing as well as in terms of neurological exam findings and imaging studies such as MRI and CT scans). Neuropsychological assessment can assist in the diagnostic evaluation of the candidate for residential care by assisting in identifying the nature of the underlying cause of the dysfunction and thus contributing to the course of treatment. It should be emphasized that there are many treatable and even reversible causes of dementia, such as various metabolic disorders, infections, vitamin B12 deficiency, and operable lesions such as subdural hematomas and meningiomas.

If a clinically significant decline in cognitive function is noted, the first order of business is to assertively search for the cause, with a focused effort on treatable causes (e.g., Schenkenberg & Miller, 2000). Finding such a treatable cause and attacking the problem at its source might obviate the need for further consideration of a residential placement. If the deficits are not reversible, the neuropsychological exam can contribute in many additional ways to the care of the patient and the decision about residential care. From a pragmatic point of view, several basic issues need to be addressed. If these are not addressed adequately, the recommendations will be uninformed at best and potentially counterproductive or even harmful at worst. Clearly, this is a team effort in which the neuropsychological input is coordinated with input from other sources. The analysis of the situation must include several factors, including the following:

1. Whether there is an additional person (e.g., spouse, sibling) who is available, willing, and able to care for the patient part-time;
2. Whether the option of hiring a part-time caregiver exists;
3. The nature of the financial situation and possible agency or insurance support;
4. The actual nature of the options in terms of residential care (e.g., is residential care a viable option, must the patient move some distance to have access to such care, are "levels" of care available at the facility, does the patient need to be able to manage his or her own medication in the facility, does the staff manage medication, must the patient be ambulatory, what happens if the patient declines, is the prospective resident allowed to manage his or her own funds, is the resident allowed to operate a motor vehicle using the residential setting as a base?); and
5. Whether the residential placement will involve both members of a couple or only one.

An analysis of the patient's cognitive function might, indeed, indicate that there are significant deficits that indicate that, for the patient's safety, some form of assisted living or a residential setting would be recommended. The more knowledgeable the clinician is about the actual nature of the possible setting involved, the more meaningful the recommendations can be.

Cognitive impairments such as disorientation, significant memory deficits, deficits in arithmetic ability, deficits in so-called executive functioning, disturbances in language function, certain types of apraxia (including constructional apraxia), and certain types of perceptual difficulties (including spatial neglect) can have a significant impact on the individual's ability to function safely and effectively in an independent living situation. An analysis of these deficits in combination with a clear understanding about the residential care options can lead to an informed set of recommendations about whether there is a good fit between the needs of the patient and the nature of the facility being considered. Thus, the results of the neuropsychological evaluation can assist the patient in deciding whether a particular residential setting is the best fit for him or her at that particular time. Further, in the more difficult albeit common circumstance in which the patient's safety requires such a setting but he or she does not want to voluntarily pursue residential care, the findings of the neuropsychological assessment can be helpful in demonstrating such a need to the patient or to other parties.

It is also important to assess activities of daily living (ADLs) such as grooming, toileting, feeding, and transferring (in and out of bed) as well as instrumental activities of daily living (IADLs) such as using a telephone, using transportation, shopping, and managing finances (Schenkenberg & Miller, 2000).

Several additional considerations may flow from the neuropsychological evaluation. Working in concert with the residential treatment staff, the neuropsychological evaluation might assist in guiding the course of interventions that might be used to assist the patient. It is clear that the assessment process, if it is to be maximally useful, should be fully coordinated with a program to address deficits and to maximize the relative strengths that have been identified. Interventions are discussed in a subsequent chapter of this text.

At the time a decision is being made about the need for residential treatment, many additional questions regarding legal issues frequently emerge. Estate planners and attorneys point out that many elderly individuals have not completed basic documents such as wills and trusts. Often, financial matters are generally disorganized (or have become disorganized in the months or years leading up to the need for residential care).

Further, in addition to these estate-planning matters, the issue of "advance directives" should be addressed at this time. Indeed, the federal Patient Self-Determination Act of 1990 requires health care facilities, including some types of long-term care facilities, to address advance directives with individuals who are admitted to the facility. Advance directives are documents that allow a person to direct his or her medical care should he or she become mentally incapacitated. These documents take several forms but include the living will, a document that specifies the nature of the care the patient would wish to receive and not receive in the event of mental incapacitation, and the special power of attorney, by which a person assigns (in advance) decision-making authority to another specified individual in the event of the person's mental incapacitation. Most states in the United States have enacted state laws addressing advance directives.

The issue of legal competence, or "decision-making capacity" as it is called in the clinical arena (Beauchamp & Childress, 1994), is a matter of major significance in the context of executing valid legal documents (such as wills, trusts, and living wills). The lack of decision-making capacity also defines the point at which a living will would need to be implemented.

The long-held tradition in the United States is that competence is assumed until evidence is presented to demonstrate a lack of decision-making capacity. Although the determination of legal competence is a matter for the courts, clinicians have a major contribution to make to this process.

A positive, universally accepted definition of "competence" is difficult to identify. From a clinical point of view, the President's Commission on Making Health Care Decisions (1982) offered certain guidelines for testing the competence of an individual to participate in decisions about medical care. These include demonstrating that the patient is in possession of a set of values and goals, has the ability to communicate and to understand information, and has the ability to reason and deliberate about his or her choices.

The informed clinician involved in the neuropsychological assessment of candidates for residential care should be aware of the issues that are at stake related to decision-making capacity (either at the time of the evaluation or in the future). The clinician can make it a point to address the criteria mentioned earlier, perhaps guiding this process in a manner that involves a data-based approach to addressing the issues. The evaluation also represents a reference point for future evaluations related to decision-making capacity. This is not a hypothetical matter. In a study involving 150 referrals to a hospital ethics committee, it was determined that 39% of these referrals involved issues related to the decision-making capacity of the patient (Schenkenberg, 1997). This determination will always be a matter of judgement, one that hopefully balances the patient's rights to free agency with a careful analysis of cognitive impairments that might interfere with the ability to understand, communicate, and deliberate about choices. It should be mentioned that it is possible for a patient to have decision-making capacity in one aspect of decision making but not in another. This might occur, for example, in a situation in which the patient is not capable of handling finances but can understand, deliberate about, and communicate decisions about a specific medical intervention.

It is important to conceptualize the neuropsychological evaluation at the initial stage of considering residential care as simply one point in a continuing process of assessing the patient's cognitive capacities. With advancing years, progression of an underlying illness, or with improvement in an underlying condition, subsequent evaluations may be needed. Whether the question concerns a clinical matter (perhaps related to the effectiveness of an intervention strategy) or an issue having to do with legal competence (in the case of implementing the provisions of an advance directive), the availability of a baseline evaluation of the patient's performance is invaluable.

SPECIFIC STRATEGIES AND PROCEDURES

It is beyond the scope of this chapter to discuss the (literally) hundreds of tests, techniques, and strategies that are used in the contemporary practice of clinical neuropsychology. The texts by Lezak (1995) and Green (2000) describe many of the principal tests used in the neuropsychological evaluation of adults and elderly patients, respectively. Further, guidelines have been established for the practice of neuropsychology (e.g., American Psychological Association, 1988; Binder & Thompson, 1995; Hazlewood et al., 1997). The following discussion focuses on some of the issues, commonly used strategies, and tests related to the neuropsychological evaluation in the specific context of the decisions about residential care.

First, it is important to emphasize that this process is only partially about the tests themselves. The neuropsychological evaluation is a complex procedure that involves a knowledge base about conditions that affect the nervous system, focused observational skills, careful selection of measures that provide the maximum "yield" in the specific circumstance and careful deliberation about the meaning of the results. Again, such an evaluation exists in a context of information provided by physicians, laboratory results, and imaging studies, and it is only when all of these elements converge that the patient is maximally served.

Prior to the session with the patient it is important to review all relevant records, especially if verification is needed because of memory impairment on the part of the patient. This will also allow the clinician to guide the interview with the patient into certain areas of concern that might not be mentioned by the patient. The patient must have as clear an understanding as possible of the nature of the planned session. Clarifying the need to bring reading glasses and hearing aids if they are used by the patient can avoid the need to reschedule should the patient arrive at the appointment without them.

It is important to establish a comfortable rapport with the patient. This can be difficult, especially if the patient comes to the session with worries that he or she is going to be institutionalized. However, positive rapport is critical to assessing the patient's maximal level of ability. It is important to discuss when and how and to whom the results will be communicated and to receive the proper permission for sending the report to other parties.

The patient's level of alertness, cooperation, affect, and mood must be noted. If the patient is not fully cooperating, for whatever reason, the test results are very difficult to interpret. The basic sensory issues of auditory and visual acuity must be assessed. The patient's use of language must be observed and evaluated, with special attention to possible word-finding difficulty, a common problem in certain neurological conditions. Form and content of thought must be evaluated, typically while taking the history. Fundamentals such as orientation (person, place, time, and purpose), and the patient's fund of information should be examined. The academic, occupational, social, and medical history must be elicited and verified, if necessary. If there is a question about the reliability of the information the patient is providing, it can be helpful to ask a particular question a second time in the interview. In evaluating the basic mental status it can be helpful to ask if the patient can name all of his or her own children or siblings. Inability to do so often points to significant deficits. Other basic identifying information should also be elicited from the patient (e.g., birth date, age, home address, phone number, Social Security number). Asking the patient to identify his or her current medication regimen is often very enlightening. Clearly, it is important to elicit from the patient what his or her concerns might be. Examples of memory errors and other types of mistakes that have occurred in the patient's day-to-day life should be elicited. Because depression is a common and potentially confounding variable in the assessment of older adults, it is important to specifically address this in the interview and perhaps using a measure such as the Geriatric Depression Scale (GDS; Yesavage et al., 1983) or the Beck Depression Inventory II (BDI II; Beck, Steer, & Brown, 1996). It is important to note, however, that self-report questionnaires such as the GDS may underestimate symptoms of depression, and depression must also be assessed in the clinical interview.

Many formalized, screening "mental status exams" are in wide use. A popular example of such exams is the Mini Mental State Exam (MMSE; Folstein, Folstein, & McHugh, 1975). These brief mental status exams represent attempts to quickly cover a wide range of cognitive abilities and to generate a score (the maximum score on the MMSE is 30) that reflects the general integrity of the patient's cognitive function. These mental status exams have never been promoted as substitutes for a thorough exam involving a true analysis of the many components involved in cognitive function. The items on these tests are typically not "weighted" in terms of scoring (e.g., on the MMSE the patient receives one point for knowing the year and one point for visually identifying an item held up before the patient). The MMSE is heavily loaded with language-related tasks. Thus, although these brief exams can be helpful, the scores must be interpreted carefully. A score of 24, for example, could be achieved with very different error patterns by two different patients, and the two scores of 24 could have very different levels of clinical importance. Age-based and education-based norms have been developed for the MMSE, and it is clear that the expectations for a "normal" score change with increasing age (Bleecker, Bolla-Wilson, Kawas, & Agnew, 1988). Caution is urged when using these tests to assess change over time. If specific test elements are not modified in successive test sessions (and some of the items such as the orientation questions cannot be modified), the patient might display an "improved" score on the basis of "practice effect" rather than on the basis of true improvement in function. A score that changes in the downward direction is certainly more convincing, and this pattern has been reported in patients with progressive dementia.

The practice of clinical neuropsychology involves considerable variability from clinician to clinician in terms of the types of tests used in an assessment. Some practitioners routinely use so-called fixed batteries which are commercially available, such as the Halstead-Reitan Neuropsycholgical Test Battery (HRNB; Reitan & Wolfson, 1993). Some fixed batteries represent a combination of tests from various sources that are aggregated and typically named after the laboratory that first developed the combination for use (e.g., the Michigan Neuropsychological Test Battery).

Still other batteries have been developed to assess certain conditions, such as the CERAD Battery (Morris et al., 1989), developed by the Consortium to Establish a Registry for Alzheimer's Disease (CERAD).

The CERAD Battery is probably the best known battery of its type and comprises seven measures: a verbal fluency test, 15 items on the Boston Naming Test (described later), the MMSE, a word list memory task, a constructional praxis test, a delayed word list recall task involving the word list previously presented, and a word list recognition task that involves identifying the words presented earlier in a list of words that includes words that had not been presented earlier. This battery is used in many Alzheimer's centers and has several advantages: (a) it is widely used, (b) the tasks are specifically selected because they are sensitive to the changes seen in Dementia of the Alzheimer's Type (DAT), (c) the time involved is relatively short, and (d) standardization was rigorous.

Commercially available "dementia rating scales" are also available. These batteries attempt to bring together a variety of tasks that are sensitive to the changes seen in progressive dementias. The Mattis Dementia Rating Scale (DRS; Mattis, 1988) is an example of such an instrument. These "screening" instruments must be used with caution because of limited normative data, overlaps in scores between normals and patients with mild forms of cognitive impairment (resulting in an imprecision in the cutoff score), and concerns about possible cultural and educational level influences on the scores. Further issues related to screening tests and cutoff scores are discussed later.

Whereas some practitioners use the rather formalized batteries above, many practitioners select an individualized set of tests that they customarily use in their own practices. For example, Green (2000, p. 34) lists a series of tests or subtests that she feels represents a broad set of measures for assessing cognitive function in older adults.

Another approach to test selection is referred to as the "flexible battery." In this approach the clinician selects the tests to be given on the basis of the specific referral questions and issues. Typically this approach includes a certain core battery of tests that are routinely given to which additional tests are added to address the idiosyncratic needs of the particular situation.

Thus, many approaches have been used in the neuropsychological assessment process. In the specific circumstance addressed in this chapter, certain guidelines might be recommended as core issues that should be addressed in an exam involving a candidate for residential placement. A discussion of these parameters follows.

Much effort has been expended in the development of "short forms" of various cognitive tests, "abbreviated" forms of more complete measures such as the Wechsler Abbreviated Scale of Intelligence (*WASI Manual*, 1999), and the use of so-called screening measures. The increasing demands on the time of busy clinicians, the costs involved with extensive batteries, and the problems associated with "justifying" to third party payers the length of time involved in thorough evaluation combine to bring pressure to bear on the clinician with regard to shortening the assessment procedures. Certainly, efficiency is a laudable objective, and there are many legitimate applications of the shortened measures. However, in the specific circumstance of decisions about residential placement, a great deal is at stake. This assessment might well lead to the identification of a treatable cause of cognitive impairment, to the identification of significant impairments reflecting progressive dementia or even life-threatening conditions such as brain tumor, or to the identification of the need for residential care. In any event, this assessment is very likely to influence the life of the patient in major ways and for the rest of the patient's life. Despite all of the pressures noted earlier this is no time for shortcuts.

There are many ways to accomplish a thorough evaluation of the patient, and such an evaluation does not always require extremely lengthy procedures. The objective is to accomplish the examination up to the level of confidence required by the needs of the patient and the circumstance. The endurance of the elderly patient is often mentioned in terms of a justification for abbreviated evaluations. However, many patients can manage a three- or four-hour assessment session. If fatigue is an issue, a subsequent appointment can be scheduled. The important thing to keep in mind is the pivotal nature of the implications of this assessment. Very few elderly individuals, once involved in residential care, return to another, more independent type of arrangement.

In addition to the background information, observational information, assessment of psychological issues and interview information noted earlier, a thorough neuropsychological assessment should include the investigation of certain cognitive domains. These include fundamental orientation, attention, memory function, language ability, visual–spatial and constructional skills, arithmetic skills, and problem solving (executive functioning). The tasks selected must have demonstrated reliability and validity and must have age-appropriate standardization data for the elderly population.

The WAIS III and the WMS III are very important tools in the evaluation of older adults in the context of decision making about residential care. The various subtests on these extensive batteries tap a number of the skills and abilities involved in the domains noted earlier. There are excellent standardization data up to age 89. The scoring approach in these newer versions of the tests is more appropriate for use with older adults than the previous systems which placed a premium on speed of completion for some of the tasks, rather than on accuracy. The time involved in completing both the WAIS III and the WMS III would likely exceed the endurance of many elderly individuals. Thus, if both are to be given, two sessions might be needed.

The Boston Naming Test (Kaplan, Goodglass, & Weintraub, 1983) is an excellent measure of word-finding ability (a common concern among patients with certain dementing disorders). Normative data are expanding through the MOANS project described earlier.

The Trail-Making Test (Reitan & Wolfson, 1993) is a widely used test that has improving norms that take into consideration the effects of age and educational level. The complexity of Part B of this test makes it particularly sensitive to cognitive impairment from a variety of causes.

One of the mental status exams such as the MMSE can be used to collect orientation data in a quantifiable manner, and this allows comparison with (likely) previous exams of this type conducted in general medical settings. The dementia rating scales such as the Mattis DRS described earlier have utility as well. Certain cautions discussed earlier apply to mental status exams and dementia rating scales.

The Clock Drawing Test has been in use for many years (Critchley, 1953) to evaluate certain cognitive domains, and it is commonly used in residential settings to evaluate the cognitive status of elderly individuals. This test involves asking the patient to draw the face of a clock, with all the numbers and both hands and with the hands indicating a specific time. A 10-point scoring system has been devised (e.g., Spreen & Strauss, 1998). Although this test is "sensitive" to many forms of cognitive and attentional deficits, it does not have specific localizing or lateralizing power in terms of locating the site of a lesion, unless evidence of, for example, left spatial neglect is present. In such a circumstance, the right hemisphere is implicated as the site of the lesion (Schenkenberg, Bradford, & Ajax, 1979). The sensitivity of this test for identifying general cognitive impairment has been demonstrated in patients with known dementia (Wolf-Klein, Silverstone, Levy, & Brod, 1989). This has led to the use of this test as a screening test for evaluating patients whose cognitive status is not known. One must always keep in mind that the use of any screening test involves many significant limitations. It would be ideal if a short, easily administered task was capable of identifying all cases with clinically significant cognitive impairment without misclassifying any patients who are without impairment. Such a measure simply does not exist. Typically, screening tasks are those which have multifaceted requirements embedded in the task. The Clock Drawing measure is such a task. The patient must be able to comprehend language in the instructions, follow a multi-step command, have basic visual acuity, organize the drawing, carry out the drawing (motorically as well as constructionally), deal with numbers, and recall how to set the hands in the proper position (both in terms of the specific demand of the test and from long-term memory in terms of how this is done). Other tasks that have been used as screening tests, such as the Digit Symbol subtest on the WAIS III and the Symbol Digit Modalities Test (Smith, 1982), have similar multifaceted requirements. Impairments in any one of a wide variety of systems can result in a poor performance on such tasks. Nonetheless, none of the tasks used for screening covers the range of functions that might be impaired in a patient with a dementing disorder. None of these tasks has been studied adequately in terms of norms for age, constitutional intelligence, education, psychiatric status, and cultural factors. There are many concerns about the cutoff score approach to determining whether a patient falls in the category of "impaired" or not. The cutoff score approach is typically used with screening tests and has been discussed thoroughly (Lezak, 1995). Cutoff scores are scores that theoretically separate "normal" participants from "abnormal" participants. Although this approach has some merit, it must be recognized that such an approach will fail to identify some patients who have true disorders (false negatives) and, at times, falsely identify some individuals as having a clinically significant impairment when they do not (false positives). The type of error (false negative or false positive) can be increased by setting the cutoff score lower or higher. There are serious risks of misclassification in using any screening test and cutting scores. Indeed, considering the variety of conditions that can result in true clinical impairment, it should not be surprising that the use of single screening tests has demonstrated high misclassification rates (Lezak, 1995). The limitations of these approaches must be understood if the clinician is to serve the patient properly.

Visual memory tasks such as the Benton Visual Retention Test (BVRT; Benton, 1974) tap not only memory but also constructional skills. There are multiple forms of the BVRT, an advantage in performing follow-up testing. Normative data addressing age-related issues are available (Spreen & Strauss, 1998).

There are many additional measures of a rather more specialized nature that would allow the clinician to pursue specific concerns raised by the patient or as a result of the tests of the basic domains mentioned above. These would include specialized tests of motor function, visual attention, constructional ability, executive functioning, and language. These measures have been described in detail elsewhere (Green, 2000; Lezak, 1995).

CONCLUSION

The cognitive assessment of a candidate for residential care is a complex and pivotal responsibility. There is no substitute for a thorough, considered approach to this responsibility. The results can contribute greatly to the health and well-being of the patient and can contribute significantly to the decision about residential care.

REFERENCES

Adams, P. F., & Benson, V. (1992). *Current estimates from the National Health Interview Survey,* 1991 (Vital and Health Statistics, Series 10, No. 184). Hyattsville, MD: National Center for Health Statistics.

American Psychological Association. (1988, August 12). Division 40. *Definition of a clinical neuropsychologist.* Statement adopted at the 96th Annual Convention of the APA, Atlanta, GA.

Beauchamp, T. L., & Childress, J. F. (1994). Principles of biomedical ethics. New York: Oxford University Press.

Beck, A. T., Steer, R. A., & Brown, G. K. (1996). *BDI-II Manual.* San Antonio, TX: The Psychological Corporation.

Benton, A. L. (1974). *Revised Visual Retention Test*. San Antonio, TX: The Psychological Corporation.

Binder, L. M., & Thompson, L. L. (1995). The ethics code and neuropsychological assessment practices. *Archives of Clinical Neuropsychology, 10*, 27–46.

Bleecker, M. L., Bolla-Wilson, K., Kawas, C., & Agnew, J. (1988). Age-specific norms for the mini-mental state exam. *Neurology, 38*, 1565–1568.

Clarfield, A. M. (1988). The reversible dementias: Do they reverse? *Annals of Internal Medicine, 109*, 476–486.

Critchley, M. (1953). *The parietal lobes*. New York: Hafner.

Djaldetti, R., & Melamed, E. (1998). Management of response fluctuations. Practical guidelines. *Neurology, 51* (Suppl. 2), S36–S40.

Filskov, S. B., & Boll, T. J. (1981/1986). *Handbook of clinical neuropsychology* (Vols. 1 & 2). New York: Wiley.

Folstein, M. F., Folstein, S. E., & McHugh, P. R. (1975). Mini-mental state. A practical method for grading the cognitive state of patients for the clinician. *Journal of Psychiatric Research, 12*, 189–198.

Green, J. (2000). *Neuropsychological evaluation of the older adult: A clinician's guidebook*. San Diego, CA: Academic Press.

Hazlewood, M. G., Adams, K. L., Mendoza, J. E., Ryan, J. J., Schenkenberg, T., Souheaver, G. T., Vanderploeg, R. D., & Wetzel, L. (1997). *Neuropsychology program/resource guide*. Milwaukee, WI: National Center for Cost Containment.

Heilman, K. M., & Valenstein, E. (Eds.). (1993). *Clinical neuropsychology*. New York: Oxford University Press.

Hong, Y-y., Morris, M. W., Chiu, C-y, & Benet-Martinez, V. (2000). Multicultural minds. *American Psychologist, 55*, 709–720.

Invik, R., Malec, J., Smith, G., Tangalos, E., & Peterson, R. (1996). Neuropsychological test norms above age 55: COWAT, BNT, MAE Token, WRAT-R, Reading, AMNART, Stroop, TMT, JLO. *The Clinical Neuropsychologist, 10*, 1–11.

Kaplan, E. F., Goodglass, H., & Weintraub, S. (1983). *The Boston Naming Test*. Philadelphia: Lea & Febiger.

Kline, D., & Scialfa, C. (1996). Visual and auditory aging. In J. E. Birren & K. Schaie (Eds.), *Handbook of the psychology of aging*, (4th ed., pp. 181–203). San Diego, CA: Academic Press.

Kolb, B., & Wishaw, Q. (1990). *Fundamentals of neuropsychology* (3rd ed). New York: Freeman.

Larson, E. B., Reifler, B. V., Sumi, S. M., Canfield, C. G., & Chinn, N. M. (1986). Diagnostic tests in the evaluation of dementia: A prospective study of 200 elderly outpatients. *Archives of Internal Medicine, 146*, 1917–1922.

Lezak, M. D. (1995). *Neuropsychological assessment* (3rd ed). New York: Oxford University Press.

Mattis, S. (1988). *Dementia Rating Scale*. Odessa, FL: Psychological Assessment Resources.

McDowd, J. M., & Birren, J. E. (1990). Aging and attentional processes. In J. E. Birren & K. W. Schaie (Eds.), *Handbook of the psychology of aging* (3rd ed.) New York: Academic Press.

Mesulam, M. –M. (2000). *Principles of behavioral and cognitive neurology*. New York: Oxford University Press.

Morris, J. C., Heyman, A., Mohs, R. C., et al. (1989). The Consortium to Establish a Registry for Alzheimer's Disease (CERAD). Part I. Clinical and neuropsychological assessment of Alzheimer's disease. *Neurology, 39*, 1159–1165.

Nash, J. M. (2000, July 17). The new science of Alzheimer's. *Time*, 55–57.

Patient Self-Determination Act. 101st U.S.C. (1990). Omnibus Reconciliation Act of 1990; Pub L No. 101–508.

Ponton, M. O., & Leon-Carrion, J. (2000). *Neuropsychology and the Hispanic patient.* Hillsdale, NJ: Lawrence Erlbaum Associates.

President's Commission on Making Health Care Decisions (1982). In T. L. Beauchamp & J. F. Childress *Principles of biomedical ethics* (pp. 67–119). New York: Oxford University Press.

Quinn, N. P. (1998). Classification of fluctuations in patients with Parkinson's disease. *Neurology, 51* (Suppl. 2), S25–S29.

Reitan, R. M., & Wolfson, D. (1993). *The Halstead-Reitan Neuropsychological Test Battery: Theory and clinical interpretation.* Tucson, AZ: Neuropsychology Press.

Schenkenberg, T. (1997). Salt Lake City VA Medical Center's first 150 ethics committee case consultations. *Healthcare Ethics Committee Forum, 9,* 147–158.

Schenkenberg, T., Bradford, D. C., & Ajax, E. T. (1979), Line bisection and unilateral visual neglect in patients with neurologic impairment. *Neurology, 30,* 509–517.

Schenkenberg, T., & Miller, P. (2000). Cognitive decline in the elderly: Impact on independent functioning. In R. D. Hill, L. Backman, & A. S. Neely (Eds.), *Cognitive rehabilitation in older adults* (pp. 207–223). New York: Oxford University Press.

Schenkenberg, T., & Said, K. (2000). *Sensory acuity in the WAIS-III and WMS-III normative standardization sample.* Unpublished manuscript.

Smith, A. (1982). *Symbol digit modalities test: Manual.* (Revised). Los Angeles: Western Psychological Services.

Spreen, O., & Strauss, E. (1998). *A compendium of neuropsychological tests* (2nd ed.). New York: Oxford University Press.

Storandt, M., & VandenBos, G. R. (1994). *Dementia and depression in older adults.* Washington, DC: American Psychological Association.

Vanderploeg, R. (1994). *Clinician's guide to neuropsychological assessment.* Hillsdale, NJ: Lawrence Erlbaum Associates.

Vanderploeg, R., Schinka, J., & Axelrod, B. (1996). Estimation of WAIS-R premorbid intelligence: Current ability and demographic data used in a best-performance fashion. *Psychological Assessment, 8,* 404–411.

WASI Manual. (1999). San Antonio, TX: The Psychological Corporation.

Wechsler, D. (1997a). *WAIS-III Administration and Scoring Manual.* San Antonio, TX: The Psychological Corporation.

Wechsler, D. (1997b). *WMS-III Administration and Scoring Manual.* San Antonio, TX: The Psychological Corporation.

Wolf-Klein, G. P., Silverstone, F. A., Levy, A. P., & Brod, M. S. (1989). Screening for Alzheimer's disease by clock drawing. *Journal of the American Geriatric Association, 37,* 730–734.

Yesavage, J., Brink, T., Rose, T., Lum, O. Huang, O., Adey, V., & Leirer, V. (1983). Development and validation of a geriatric depression screening scale: A preliminary report. *Journal of Psychiatric Research, 17,* 37–49.

5

The Relationship Between Medical and Psychological Problems in Residential Care

Tim Grange and Anthony Morrison
Infinia Corporation, Salt Lake City, Utah

INTRODUCTION

In the previous chapters of this text, a framework for residential care was described that focused on psychological and social factors that optimize the quality of care. The purpose of this chapter is to briefly describe the relationship between physical illness and psychological symptoms, as they are manifest in residential care settings. After examining some general health considerations related to older adults and residential placement, some basic medical assessment issues are described. The bulk of this chapter highlights illnesses and diseases that have psychological symptoms as part of their typical presentation and are commonly found among those in residential care settings.

Modern medicine and the aging of the baby boomers has led to an increase in the proportion of the population considered elderly (usually defined as over 65 years; U.S. Bureau of the Census, 1996). With this increase in numbers has come a growing interest in diseases and illnesses that are typically associated with aging. One benefit from the increased attention to age-related illness from the medical community has been an enhanced understanding of the adaptive processes associated with physiological deterioration that is part of "normal aging" (see Whitbourne, 1998) Although many of the youth of America may equate growing old with pain, suffering and reduced life satisfaction, research demonstrates the opposite. In the absence of significant illness, life satisfaction remains high among older adults, and psychological illness including depression is lower in those over 65 years than in a younger adult cohort (Diener & Suh, 1997; Larson, 1978).

It is known, for example, that there is a natural deterioration of sensory and motor abilities that accompanies aging, but this mild gradual eroding of physical capacity does not appear to have a significant impact on life satisfaction. Nevertheless, with increased age comes increased incidence of chronic illness, and when there is significant debilitating illness, life satisfaction predictably declines and the incidence of psychiatric issues such as depressive symptomatology increases (Jelicic & Kempen, 1999). Human aging has a generally predictable though variable course—from growth to optimal function to maintenance to dysfunction and death (Baltes, 1987, 1997). The expression of aging and disease is diverse, and when such heterogeneity is considered with respect to the host of possible diagnostic tests, the physical findings (including mental status examination and laboratory tests), and treatments, healthcare professionals face special challenges in determining the optimal treatment for the range of physical problems that can occur in any given elderly patient. Although some expressions of illness are sudden and obvious, such as a large stroke or massive myocardial infarct, many deteriorative processes alter the body and mind gradually. These insidious disease processes are less dramatic but no less destructive than the events described earlier. Although modern medicine has produced tests that can identify some disease states in the early stages, other diseases are impossible to detect because their symptoms are mild and may fall below the critical threshold of measurement for the available tests

When older adults who have been otherwise healthy become ill because of physically or mentally disabling conditions, the need for higher levels of care increases. If the family is unable to care for an older loved one in the home, the person may be placed in a nursing home or other residential care setting. The incidence of significantly disabling illness is therefore higher in these settings than it is among older adults living at home, and it is highest in nursing homes (Hopp, 1999). As already noted in previous chapters, there is a strong correlation between illness and life satisfaction, and therefore it is no surprise that life satisfaction in nursing homes is consistently lower than in any other setting (Laditka, 1998).

Among the many issues that work against life satisfaction is the financial strain associated with such placement (Cohen, 1998). A person's stay in a nursing home can be paid for by the individual, their family, with private funds, or by a third party through an insurance benefit. The most common third party funding sources are Medicare and Medicaid. For a person to qualify for Medicaid or Medicare to fund their stay in a nursing home there has to be some medically related debilitation (Prospective Assessment Payment Commission, 1995). Medicare is a federal program that provides insurance coverage to people over 65 years of age and for younger adults who are permanently disabled. Medicare, under the hospital benefit (part A) will pay for a person to reside in a skilled facility (e.g., nursing home) for up to 100 days per benefit period as long as there is the need for a skilled service (e.g., physical therapy). If a person needs to remain in a nursing home beyond the period that Medicare will cover, the person will have to pay privately or apply for Medicaid.

Medicaid is the primary funding source for those in long-term placement who do not have the personal resources to pay the cost of the facility. To qualify for Medicaid to pay for the placement, the person must have a demonstrable need for assistance due to illness or disease, and must meet the financial requirements established for each state. Given that medical illness or disease (not simply physical aging) is the most common reason why older persons are placed in or choose to live in residential facilities, it is no surprise that people in residential care have a higher frequency of medical problems than those living at home.

This chapter makes an important contribution to the text given that some of the medical conditions that contribute to older adults being placed in residential settings can cause, exacerbate, or mimic psychological disorders. For example the shortness of breath and accompanying distress that is characteristic of chronic obstructive pulmonary disease can resemble a panic attack. There are also cases where one or more medical conditions exist with an unrelated psychological disorder (i.e., comorbidity). One example of this type of comorbidity is the person who has a history of bipolar disorder and in later life develops diabetes or falls and breaks a hip necessitating residential placement. In cases of comorbidity, both or all problems must be considered simultaneously and treated aggressively to avoid potential synergistic effects that may result in the need for higher levels of care.

A situation that is closely akin to comorbidity is when a previously undiagnosed psychological disorder becomes unmasked by the onset of medical illness. The associated psychological stress that often accompanies the onset of acute physical illness can lead to the manifestation of previously well-controlled symptoms. The following brief case example illustrates this point:

An 84-year-old man who had lived on his own since the death of his wife 10 years previous slipped in his driveway and dislocated his shoulder. While in the hospital he contracted pneumonia, and after two weeks in the hospital was discharged to a skilled nursing facility for conditioning. While in the facility the staff observed that he was hypervigilent, very nervous and at times appeared to have hallucinatory experiences. One aide also observed that he had fretful sleep and seemed to have violent nightmares. A psychiatric consult was sought and it was discovered that this man was a war veteran and had had significant combat experience. He had coped for years by keeping his life very orderly and structured and by limiting the novel things he was exposed to. His accident and subsequent illness had placed him in a situation where his psychological resources were easily overwhelmed and the symptoms of his posttraumatic stress disorder (PTSO) became manifest. With acknowledgment and psychological treatment of this PTSD-related anxiety and his ultimate recovery from the pneumonia, he was able to return to his home with additional skills to control his PTSD in the future.

GENERAL PRINCIPLES OF MEDICAL EVALUATION

The vignette just given underscores the importance of obtaining a comprehensive psychosocial and medical history of the person at intake to understand the nature of the resident's behavioral disturbance and recommend a treatment plan that would have a high likelihood of improving the client's well being. The next section reviews some of the more important components of a medical evaluation. For maximal success, any attempt to understand and treat the illnesses and diseases that are manifested by older adults in residential care settings has to be driven by a comprehensive understanding of the medical and psychosocial factors that contribute to the individual's presenting symptoms. With a comprehensive understanding of the person's symptoms, the treatment team is in a good position to choose interventions that will be most beneficial to the patient. Many of the problems associated with erroneous and harmful treatment interventions are a result of the treating staff proceeding without a full understanding of the nature of an older patient's problems. The sections that follow summarize several of the more important sources of patient information that can be used to develop meaningful treatment interventions.

The History and Physical Exam (H&P)

The history and physical examination is the cornerstone of the physician's evaluation of the patient. It sets the stage for understanding what ails the patient and what kinds of treatments are indicated for a given problem. A person's medical history is unique, and assessment must be multifaceted and tailored to the individual. It should be noted that many diagnostic tests that are routine, commonly available, and very low risk make sense to administer as a routine part of every medical evaluation. Interestingly, this proves to be a difficult task in many settings because of a number of factors (e.g., the patient has had a stroke and cannot speak). Thus, it can be difficult to capture in less than several hours a truly comprehensive history and examination of any individual who has a moderately complex problem list. Furthermore, knowledge and the accuracy and completeness of the information provided by the patient may vary depending on the patient's memory, interest, environmental factors, fatigue, cognitive abilities, and motivation. For example, information may be very limited in those older patients with dementia or may be inaccurate due to confabulation, delusions, or intentional misrepresentation that are components of self-report from individuals who have cognitive impairment. To obtain an adequate history of a patient with dementia, the treating professional may need to obtain corroboration from family members who do not suffer from dementia.

Sources of Information

Because of the reasons noted earlier, in order to gather the information for an adequate history and physical evaluation the physician must rely on many sources of information that are often not accessible from the patient. These sources of information include collateral reports of those who know the patient, objective clinical and laboratory measures, and input from other treating professionals (e.g., a psychologist).

Self-Report. The patient interview is often the primary source of information and is important both in the gathering of specific information from the person's history to observation of the person providing it. The evaluator must assess how the examinee processes a request for information and whether the resident is oriented to time, place, and person. Is the resident's memory intact for short- and long-term information? Does his or her thought pattern follow a logical course, or is it tangential? Does the person produce a never-ending verbal discourse following every question, or does he or she stop after one-word answers? What are the person's existing coping skills as evidenced by a description of approaches to problems? How much insight does the person have about the nature and extent of his or her problems? Does the person own appropriate responsibility for what has happened to him or her, or is there a propensity to blame his or her misfortune on others? Is the person generally optimistic or pessimistic, and does his or her view seem to correlate with the disease prognosis.

Although development and refinement of the patient interview is often specific to the care setting, as well as the training experiences of the interviewer, there are a number of excellent resources that can be consulted by the clinician who is interested in developing a systematic interview protocol for long-term care (see Kane & Kane, 1981).

Collateral Reports From Interested Parties. Even the best personal historian will not capture all of the details of his or her medical history. For example, many older residents in residential-based care settings have memory problems that prevent them from reporting all of the significant events from their past. Some patients who are acutely ill may not even be able to report their history or even their current symptoms (e.g., a person with a delirium may be too confused to participate productively in an interview). Other individuals may be hyperaware of the details of their symptoms and history because of features of hypochondriasis, obsessive–compulsive disorder, or issues of secondary gain. Interviewing family members; therefore, can provide a rich source of information that may augment or clarify a cognitively or emotionally impaired patient's self-report.

In addition to family members who are caregivers, older adults in residential settings usually have staff from the facility where they reside who can also provide useful information. If staff are caring for the patient on an ongoing basis, such collateral reports may provide important information related to capabilities of activities of daily life (ADLs) or instrumental activities of daily life (IADLs). These additional sources of information should be sought even though this can be time consuming for the interviewer and may involve a delay in treatment decisions. When there is a gross contradiction between two or more sources, neither source of information should be taken at face value, and further investigation may therefore be needed. Previous treatment from related professionals is another good source of information. Most hospitalizations generate typed reports and test results that can be requested. It is helpful to train staff to obtain as many records as possible before a first visit. A patient's pharmacy may also have useful records of what has been dispensed. Some states, for example, can even provide records of controlled substance prescriptions on request from a treating professional, and this information can be useful in documenting a pattern of use or abuse of prescribed substances such as narcotic painkillers.

It is important to include the findings and observations from other disciplines as well in the overall conceptualization of a prospective applicant for resident care placement. Treating professionals including psychologists, social workers, physical and occupational therapists generally conduct thorough assessments of an individual to determine treatment needs related to these specialties (e.g., psychotherapy). The information obtained from other professionals can further the understanding of what the patient is experiencing and how best to treat him or her. As noted earlier in this chapter, among older adults in residential settings, comorbidity of illnesses is common and often greatly amplifies functional deficits. Attempts to understand and treat all of the illnesses and diseases that a person suffers from is essential to optimize a resident's functional adaptation to the long-term care setting and his or her sense of well being in such a setting. For example, an ophthalmologic evaluation may lead to cataract surgery, whereas an orthopedic surgeon may provide joint replacement options to those with certain arthritic limitations or related functional limitations. Cardiology, pulmonary, and renal specialists can often help evaluate such patients and provide useful guidance. Many of these specialties are covered under Medicare (part B) as outpatient treatment.

As noted earlier, psychological testing helps with identifying specific areas of adaptational strengths and weaknesses and can pinpoint depression, anxiety, and personality disorders. For example, a thorough psychological evaluation can be used to document baseline functioning for future comparison. Neuropsychological testing can identify the nature and magnitude of cognitive deficits associated with neurological events including stroke and closed head injury. Physical therapy can help to identify deficits in mobility, and findings from a comprehensive physical therapy examination can be the impetus behind appropriate interventions that all staff can assist with. Occupational therapists can similarly provide assistance of value to upper extremity functions. Speech therapists can provide analysis and treatment plans for problems involving cognition, speech, and swallowing.

The Physical Examination. The physical examination is one of the most important sources of information about the presence and course of a given disease state. This examination is usually initiated at the first physician meeting with the patient. In this exam the physician will note features of the face, head, spine, and extremities and look for asymmetries, abnormal postures, balance and movements, degenerative joints, and deconditioning. The speech pattern and the way in which questions are processed can also be observed. Special attention should be paid to cognitive functioning by asking questions that challenge the different aspects of memory, reasoning, judgment, appropriateness, concentration, abstraction, and coping skills. The Folstein Mini Mental Status Exam (MMSE; Folstein, Folstein & McHugh, 1975) is a brief mental status examination that can be administered to provide a gross assessment of cognitive functioning. It can be a useful measure because it is relatively easy to learn and has clearly defined norms for cognitive impairment (see Galasko, Corey-Bloom, & Thal, 1991; Hill & Backman, 1995); however, it is not a complete examination, and treatment decisions should never made on the basis of a single test result. The MMSE is commonly used because of its brevity and ease of administration, but it has many limitations. A more complete and precise measure of the presence and magnitude of dementia is the Dementia Rating Scale (DRS; Mattis, 1988). This instrument has a more refined metric for evaluating dysfunction across a wider range of cognitive abilities and in this respect provides more information to guide the development of meaningful treatment approaches for the patient.

In the physical examination, the examiner should note any deficits in sensory functioning including vision and hearing as deficits in these areas can lead to misperceptions about a person's abilities, dysfunctions, or both. Sensation should also be assessed, including proprioception particularly if balance is a concern. For example, peripheral neuropathy can be subtle in the early stages of Alzheimer's disease, and sensation in the toes is usually affected before the fingers. Ankle reflexes are usually diminished before the other more prominent reflexes and can be an early warning sign of neurological deterioration associated with a progressive disease state. Alternatively, increased, asymmetric or pathologic reflexes often suggest brain dysfunction. Part of the physical examination should require that the patient move his or her extremities, transfer and walk, and follow stated commands. During these tasks the physician–examiner should look for any restriction in normal, fluid movement. If restrictions in volitional movement are observed, identifying what is causing the restriction can lead to effective intervention plans. Pain should always be considered an important and potentially treatable problem. A good cardiopulmonary exam is essential and should include checks of the carotids for bruits, the abdominal aorta for size, and the foot pulses for strength. Overall, as a part of these tasks the examiner should work to understand a patient's current function and disease state in order to address potentially correctable problems and to institute preventive measures that have a high probability of lessening the likelihood of additional problems.

Common Laboratory Procedures. Because of the increasing prevalence of disease with age, it is almost always useful to have baseline laboratory studies. These are relatively safe and at times can reveal unexpected clinical problems even before such problems emerge as symptomatology detectable at the point of the physical exam (e.g., routine labs can reveal the early stages of illness in an otherwise healthy individual). There is a danger; however, in waiting for symptoms or signs to emerge before considering lab tests. For example, considerable damage may be done either subacutely (e.g., neuropathy) or catastrophically (e.g., stroke) if laboratory tests are not used to monitor a suspected condition. Furthermore, prevention of a problem such as further strokes can be facilitated by laboratory tests that are specific to certain disorders (e.g., lipid profile). Such tests can validate a suspicion of risk of disease. Laboratory tests can also be used to develop an approach to treatment that also includes prevention. Such an approach may be preferred to using laboratory tests to simply confirm the presence of a fully emerged condition where damage has been done and high costs associated with procedures or medications to ameliorate such damage is required.

With regard to specific laboratory studies, the most comprehensive understanding of a new patient often involves interpretation of supplemental blood tests conducted in conjunction with the physical examination. Because early disease-related physical changes can be asymptomatic, it is wise to have available a complete blood count (CBC), chemistry panel (comprehensive metabolic panel or chem. 20), thyroid stimulating hormone (TSH), lipid profile, stool guaiac, and a prostatic specific antigen (PSA) in men. Drug levels are needed for certain medications (e.g., lithium and Dilantin) and a routine protime is done for those on warfarin (a blood thinner used in some older adults with a history of strokes).

Other Tests. For some disease states that affect the brain, it is helpful to get radiological studies like an MRI (magnetic resonance imagery), which is a safe and often useful procedure to validate overall brain pathology. An MRI works by using powerful magnets to create an image of internal brain structures. The brain's internal structures have different densities and show up as variations in the gray color spectrum when exposed to powerful magnetic currents. An MRI is most useful for detecting space-occupying lesions in the brain such as tumors and the white matter changes associated with multiple sclerosis. An MRI examination is not as helpful in diagnosing dementia other than showing cerebral atrophy in some advanced cases. Carotid ultrasonography is a noninvasive way to evaluate the carotid arteries for plaque, and echocardiography is indicated for anyone with congestive heart failure and for certain stroke workups. Deep venous thrombosis (a blood clot that can form deep within the leg) can be difficult to diagnose without lower extremity ultrasound, which is safe and noninvasive. Most elderly are, or will be, at increased risk for fracture and should be treated for this partly preventable problem as soon as it is discovered. Finally, if desired, dual-energy x-ray absorptiometry

(DEXA), bone density of the spine, hip, or both, may be useful in following disease treatment.

In summary, the information in this section highlights the need for a comprehensive evaluation of the patient's situation and condition before making major treatment decisions. With the information available from the patient, family members, objective measures, and other treating professionals, the physician can assemble a variety of clinical information to create a solid understanding of his or her patient. The physician is then able to more accurately determine what interventions are required and what the patient's prognosis is. Although the physician can make some preliminary judgments after the history is taken and the physical examination is completed, he or she must often wait for laboratory results, professional consults, and collateral information before making nonemergency treatment decisions. Although this may take time, investing time and resources to create a comprehensive evaluation will pay off many times over through the better treatment planning and more efficient use of resources to facilitate resident well-being and life satisfaction.

CATEGORIES OF MEDICAL ILLNESS

In reviewing illnesses and diseases that can have psychological symptoms as part of their presentation, it is not the intention of this chapter to be comprehensive. Thus, this section identifies some of the more common illnesses and diseases that are seen in residential care settings that produce psychological symptomatology. Those working in the medical profession know that any given chronic physiological illness can produce depressive symptoms, anxiety, or both, as part of its presentation and that any illness or disease that affects the brain directly or indirectly can also produce alterations in personality and behavior. In the discussion of illnesses and diseases, we start with those that can be divided easily into physiological systems and then conclude with some syndromes that do not easily fit into the major physiological systems. Some of these latter symptoms are more universal than any specific illness or disease state (e.g. pain) but require inclusion because the topic would be incomplete without them.

It is useful when examining the psychological and behavioral impact of specific illnesses to subdivide their presentation of psychological sequelae into primary, secondary, and tertiary symptoms. Primary symptoms are those that are a direct result of the pathological process the person is suffering from. Secondary symptoms are those that are a result of the primary symptoms or attempts to treat the primary symptoms. Tertiary symptoms are the social, psychological, and situational consequences of the primary and secondary symptoms. Although it is not always possible to clearly identify whether a symptom is primary, secondary, or tertiary (e.g., depression may be all three), it is useful to make such a distinction when possible. In examining the psychological symptoms that are present among elderly residents in long-term care settings, identification of whether the disease symptoms are primary, secondary, or tertiary can have important treatment implications. What follows is a vignette that is descriptive of this three-tiered symptom taxonomy:

> An 80-year-old man in a nursing home was experiencing hallucinations. He had no history of hallucinations; however, his medical history included diabetes, hypertension, and Parkinson's disease. A review of his medical chart revealed that he had recently had an increase in the medication that he used to treat his Parkinson's disease, but there were no other significant findings. He was oriented to person, place, and time and did not have prominent delusions. It was determined following a review of his chart by the treating physician that the hallucinations were a result of the medication increase, and it was subsequently reduced.

In this case, the hallucinations could have been primary symptoms if the person was suffering from schizophrenia or from dementia or delirium (described earlier in this chapter). Under these circumstances the treatment of choice would likely be antipsychotic medications. If the symptoms occurred as a result of a reaction to the stress the person was experiencing from other illnesses or situational factors the hallucinations may represent a brief reactive psychosis. If this were the case the hallucinations could be considered tertiary in nature and could be treated with psychotherapy, psychosocial interventions, and antipsychotic medications.

Cardiopulmonary

Heart Disease.   Heart disease is the largest single health problem in the United States (Western Collaborative Group Study; Rosenman et al., 1975)—it is the leading cause of death and is a significant cause of older adults being placed in residential care settings. The heart is an involuntary muscle that pumps blood throughout the body . The blood carries oxygen and other nutrients that are necessary for survival and optimal functioning. If there is damage to the heart through either normal age-related deterioration or disease (see Kitzman & Edwards, 1990), the organs of the body are deprived of the substances that are necessary for life, and these organs suffer damage. If the deprivation continues for more than a few minutes the person will die. Damage to the heart may occur suddenly or it may occur gradually over a long period of time (Arking, 1991). The brain is one organ that is very vulnerable to damage from heart failure. If a person is without consistent blood flow to the brain for more than a very brief period there can be irreversible damage to brain tissue. The following case example illustrates how heart disease can affect psychological functioning:

> A 66-year-old man suffered a myocardial infarction, and it took emergency medical personnel 20 minutes to help him achieve a regular rhythm. When visited in the hospital by the psychologist a week later he could only sit up without assistance and re-

sponded appropriately to only 50% of the questions addressed to him. Over the subsequent year he went through rehabilitation and recovered some functional abilities, including the ability to drive. However, he remained concrete in his thinking and prone to impulsivity and rigidity. He also had marked memory and other cognitive deficits and suffered from depression. The anoxic brain injury resulting from the absence of normal blood flow to the brain had left him with permanent cognitive and emotional impairment.

Establishing good habits including diet and exercise have been demonstrated to help prevent heart disease; however, for some patients diet and exercise are not enough or may come too late in the disease process. For those with congestive heart failure, combination therapy with ACE-inhibitors, diuretics, aldactone, and beta-blockers will prolong life. Lipid-altering drugs, especially the statin class, have been proven to decrease the risk of heart attack in diabetics and others and should be used more in these patients. Cerebral blood flow may be compromised in the elderly. Diabetes, dyslipidemia, and hypertension can also take their toll on physiological functioning. Medications such as aspirin and Plavix are useful in some cases, so long as the aspirin dose is balanced against the risk of GI bleeding (e.g., 81 mg 3–7 days per week). Blood pressure, another factor that increases the risk of heart failure, can be managed by various medications as well as by diet and exercise.

Pulmonary Disease.   The successful delivery of oxygen to cells and through the body is dependent on the healthy functioning of the lungs, which are the core of the pulmonary system. Remarkably, the heart and lungs continue their work usually without interruption even though age-related deterioration and pulmonary disease can influence the efficiency of their continuous performance and can also have a devastating impact on overall health. In normal aging, lung function tends to decline gradually, especially for sudden, high-level output (Kenney, 1989). However, in the absence of pulmonary disease the potential for long-lasting pulmonary health is excellent, especially with some commitment to maintenance such as exercise and avoidance of maladaptive behaviors such as cigarette smoking. Attention to prevention of disease is paramount, particularly for such catastrophes as stroke, myocardial infarction, and peripheral vascular disease. Treatable conditions such as hypertension, atrial fibrillation, diabetes, dyslipidemia, hypoxia, and others must be investigated. Vaccination programs are helpful, and new pneumovax recommendations should be instituted in some high-risk older patients.

A common pulmonary illness found in older adults is chronic obstructive pulmonary disease (COPD; Cugell, 1988). COPD can have devastating consequences for a person's ability to do even the most routine of tasks. It is also common to find psychological symptoms among those with COPD. Primary symptoms can occur from the disruption of normal oxygen flow to the brain. Secondary symptoms occur as the person struggles to breathe and suffers other symptoms that can mimic a panic attack. Tertiary symptoms occur when COPD affects cognitive functioning and precipitates dementia-like symptoms (Grant et al., 1987). The inability to perform many tasks, the dependence on oxygen, and the constant struggle to breathe can lead to a reactive depression, which would be considered tertiary symptomatology.

Cerebrovascular

To the average person a stroke is the best-known form of cerebrovascular illness. In the medical community it is often referred to as a CVA (cerebrovascular accident). CVA can be divided into two major types; occlusive and hemorrhagic. In an occlusive stroke the blood vessel becomes blocked (occluded) by either a piece of plaque or a blood clot. The result of the blockage is a disruption of blood flow to the tissue beyond the occlusion causing necrosis or death of that tissue. If blood flow is restored quickly the results are reversible (e.g., Transient Ischemic Attack– TIA); however, it does not take long for permanent damage to occur. The damage that occurs results first from the absence of life-giving blood to the tissue and then from the brain swelling that follows as the tissue dies. Although the absence of blood flow to an area of the brain is devastating, the greatest damage may result from the swelling and secondary effects. For those who die from strokes it is often the swelling that is responsible for the demise of the individual. New research on reducing the impact of strokes is primarily focused on reducing the swelling that follows the initial event.

Hemorrhagic strokes occur when a blood vessel ruptures and there is bleeding in the brain. Although they are less common than occlusive strokes, hemorrhagic strokes are more often fatal. Uncontrolled hypertension can cause blood vessels to rupture and is referred to as a hypertension stroke. Aneurysms are another cause of hemorrhagic strokes. An aneurysm is a weakening in the wall of a blood vessel that results in a ballooning effect. As the weakened portion of the vessel balloons, the wall becomes thinner and can eventually rupture. Most people who experience ruptured cerebral aneurysms die within an hour, and those who do survive are often left with devastating functional deficits requiring long-term medical care for continued survival.

With any form of cerebrovascular illness there are usually dramatic changes that take place in a person's life following a CV insult. Often there is associated paralysis or other deficits. For example the person may have focal language problems or difficulties with fine motor control. Although the motor and speech impairments may be the most obvious symptoms from a stroke, there may also be emotional impairments that occur as a direct result of damage to brain tissue. The nature and magnitude of emotional impairment that can be attributed to the physiological changes associated with a stroke vary according to the location and extent of the damage. Damage to the frontal portion of the brain can result in the person having less emotional control, and therefore the patient may become emotionally labile with symptoms including crying easily and sometimes without provocation. A person may also become more aggressive and verbally abusive even without a previous history of these behaviors. Neuroscientists believe that the frontal area of the brain acts as a monitor for all of the impulses and drives that human beings possess. It is the front part of the brain (frontal lobes) that allows for decision-making. When the frontal lobes are damaged a person may be less able to inhibit the expression of feelings and emotions (see Skilbeck, 1996).

Another well-established connection between stokes and emotional impairment is the higher incidence of acute depression in people who have strokes on the left side of the brain. Although the incidence of depression is high in the early stages of stroke for the entire population of people who suffer strokes, there is a tendency toward indifference in those with right hemisphere strokes. Depression in those who have had strokes tends to become more common and more severe over time. In a 4-year follow up study (Niemi, Laaksonen, Kotila, & Waltim, 1998), depression was also found to be a larger factor in life satisfaction than ability to walk and memory abilities in recovering stroke patients.

Although strokes can be fatal or have profound residual symptoms, many people live through the stroke and resume some aspects of normalcy in their everyday routines. Nevertheless, the risk for additional strokes is usually significant after the initial event. The preventative measures noted in this chapter can be useful in avoiding further strokes. There are also medications that can reduce the risk of further strokes. As mentioned earlier, most strokes are occlusive, and these medications (e.g., warfarin) work by thinning the blood and therefore reduce the likelihood of blockage.

Neurologic

Dementia. Dementia has been defined in many different ways, creating confusion among lay and professional caregivers about what to expect when an individual receives this diagnosis. According to Lezak (1995), dementia has three major components: impairment in more than one cognitive domain, impairment that represents a deterioration of functioning, and impairment that is progressive and irreversible. She also pointed out that the symptoms of dementia must be present when the person is in a clear state of consciousness, in order to differentiate dementia from delirium (a transient state that can present with severe but reversible cognitive deficits). Others (American Psychiatric Association, 1994) use a broader definition of dementia that would include people who have had strokes or closed head injuries; however, for the purpose of this chapter Lezak's definition will be adopted.

The most common form of dementia is Alzheimer's disease. This disease is estimated to afflict 7% of the population of persons 65 years and older. Alzheimer's is marked by a steady progression of cognitive deterioration beginning with memory deficits and personality changes. The diagnosis of Alzheimer's disease is presumptive and is made when a person manifests the cognitive and personality changes that are known to be characteristic of the disease process. The diagnosis can only be confirmed with a biopsy or autopsy when senile plaques and neurofibrillary tangles that are present in the brain tissue of Alzheimer's patients are found and counted. Researchers throughout the world have exerted great effort to identify Alzheimer's disease through lab tests and other less intrusive means. Some positive results have been found with such things as the APOE gene (Bondi, Salmon, Galasko, Thomas, & Thal, 1999) that has been found to increase the risk for Alzheimer's disease in some populations; however, no solid diagnostic test has been definitively identified.

Some researchers have identified stages of Alzheimer's disease and have described cognitive and personality changes that occur during these stages. In the earliest stages of Alzheimer's disease the only noticeable symptoms a person will have are mild short-term memory loss and personality changes. As the disease progresses, cognitive and behavioral changes become more pronounced. Personality and behavior changes are often primary symptoms, but it is not uncommon to see anxiety and depression as secondary and tertiary symptoms of Alzheimer's, particularly in the early stages of the illness. Although there is no cure for the most common dementias, there have been some advances in medications that are believed to slow the progression of the illness. These drugs (Cognex , Aricept and Exelon) work by facilitating the production of the neurotransmitter acetalcholine, which has been implicated in the progression of Alzheimer's. Alzheimer's disease is considered a cortical dementia because it affects primarily the cortical or outer layer of the brain. Dementing processes that involve the deeper areas of the brain are referred to as subcortical and include such well-known illnesses as Parkinson's disease and Huntington's chorea.

Parkinson's Disease.   Parkinson's Disease results from the death of nerve cells (which deplete neurotransmitters) in an area of the brain referred to as the basal ganglia. The basal ganglia is collection of structures deep within the brain that control movement and other important functions. The early onset of Parkinson's is usually characterized by the presence of a mild tremor and loss of normal coordination and muscle strength. As the disease progresses, the motor problems become more profound and in some cases the person becomes completely rigid. The cause of Parkinson's is not fully understood, but some common theories include exposure to toxic agents and unidentified viral agents. Although there is no cure, there are a variety of treatments for the symptoms of the disease. Some medications that help increase the amount of the missing neurotransmitter have been effective at providing temporary relief from the symptoms. Surgical interventions have also been effective in providing relief from the motor symptoms, but again the effects have been temporary. Because of the nature and location of the damage caused by Parkinson's disease, depressive symptoms are common among affected individuals and are considered primary symptoms of the disease. The medications used to treat Parkinson's disease can cause secondary symptoms that closely resemble schizophrenia, including hallucinations.

Huntington's Disease.   Whereas the cause of Parkinson's disease is unclear, Huntington's disease is known to be a hereditary condition that usually has its onset after age 30. Although both Parkinson's disease and Huntington's disease involve deterioration of the basal ganglia, they affect different neurotransmitter systems. Huntington's Disease involves a deficiency in the neurotransmitter GABA along with other neurochemical defects (Reitan & Wolfson, 1988). Early symptoms include a general clumsiness with slowed fine motor movements and a tendency to drop things. As the disease progresses the irregular jerky movements are present along with grimacing facial expressions and tongue movements. Primary psychological symptoms include depression and behavioral disturbance.

Traumatic Head Injury.   The latest nomenclature from the American Psychiatric Association (1994) includes head trauma as one of the causes of dementia. A traumatic brain injury occurs when a moving object strikes the head while stationary, or when the head is moving and strikes a stationary object. The most common causes of traumatic brain injury include motor vehicle accidents, falls, and assaults. Motor vehicle accidents and falls are most often acceleration–deceleration accidents. As the head comes to a sudden stop when it encounters the stationary object, the brain moves and collides with the skull. Although the resulting damage to the brain varies according to the location and magnitude of the impact, there are some consistent areas of damage. The inside of the skull is mostly smooth, but in the areas behind the nose and above the ears there are rough bony protrusions that cause damage to the brain as it moves back and forth across the area. The result is usually a disruption of short-term memory abilities and some disinhibition.

Disinhibition occurs because of damage to the frontal lobes, and the frontal lobes, because of their size and location, are the most vulnerable and are most often affected in traumatic brain injuries. As discussed earlier, the frontal lobes play an important part in controlling impulses and behaviors, and damage to them compromises the person's ability to inhibit inappropriate urges. Traumatic brain injury can also produce other emotional and behavioral sequelae including depression and psychotic symptoms. These symptoms are often primary symptoms, but secondary and tertiary symptoms can also occur. The number of people with traumatic brain injury who are in residential care settings has increased in recent years (Rapoport & Feinstein, 2000). In some states there is not a good alternative placement for traumatically brain injured people, and therefore most of these survivors end up living in nursing homes. There are a number of problems that occur when these individuals are mixed with a traditional elderly nursing home population.

Some of these difficulties are a function of the age discrepancy, but many of the problems are directly attributable to the symptoms of traumatic brain injury, especially if the traumatic brain injury patient is experiencing seizures.

A seizure is a bout of abnormal random electrical activity in the brain caused by a large number of neurons firing at the same time. The cause of seizures is often unknown, but they are more common after trauma to the brain (e.g., stroke or closed head injury). A patient's seizure threshold can also be lowered by fever, fatigue, and some medications. Although medications are available to control seizures, many of them have deleterious side effects including cognitive impairment. Another neurologic illness that can lead to a younger person being placed in a long-term care facility is multiple sclerosis (MS).

MS.   MS is a disease that attacks the myelin (the fatty insulation) that surrounds the nerve cells and facilitates communication between cells. MS usually has a step-wise course with periods of exacerbations followed by periods of plateau and even some recovery. Although the precise causes of MS are not yet known, most researchers agree that a number of factors in combination are probably involved. These factors include environmental (possible toxins and climate) and viral sources (exposure to common viral agents may trigger MS in those who are prone). Genetic factors have also been examined, and although MS does not appear to be of primary heredity etiology, having a first-degree relative such as a parent or sibling with MS increases an individual's risk of developing the disease. It has been estimated for example, that there is a seven-fold risk above the general population for individuals with a family history.

Primary symptoms of MS include weakness, numbness, tremor, loss of vision, pain, paralysis, loss of balance, and bladder and bowel dysfunction. An example of a secondary condition is repeated urinary tract infections from bladder dysfunction. Inactivity can result in disuse weakness, poor postural alignment and trunk control, muscle imbalances, decreased bone density (increasing risk of fracture), and shallow, inefficient breathing. Bedsores can also occur due to paralysis. Depression is frequently seen among people who have been dealing with MS over a prolonged period of time. However, depression may be a primary, secondary, or tertiary symptom. Divorce and other interpersonal losses are common as MS progresses through its course and the person is less able to meet the demands of their relationships. Placement in a residential care setting usually occurs when these individuals are unable to perform ADLs.

Diabetes.   Diabetes is a term used to describe a collection of diseases that have in common the lack of or resistance to insulin—a hormone produced in the pancreas that is necessary to store eaten food for energy. The result of this metabolic failure is that the sugars go into the blood and raise the overall blood sugar level, which can adversely affect all organ systems. The most common consequences of diabetes are neuropathy, kidney disease, and blindness due to retinopathy and amputation because of circulatory problems. Most diabetes in older adults is referred to as Type II or non-insulin dependent diabetes. Type II diabetes accounts for about 85% of diabetes cases in old age (American Diabetes Association, 1997). Symptoms of diabetes include polyuria, polydipsia, and polyphagia; other symptoms are dependent on the body system affected by the disease. The psychological symptoms that accompany diabetes are usually tertiary symptoms. Depression is common among those who suffer blindness and amputation. Primary psychological symptoms are usually restricted to psychotic symptoms associated with delirium during diabetic shock. New drugs have been helpful though not curative; promising technologies are in development, and this is needed because the prevalence of diabetes is expected to rise as the population continues to age. The incidence of diabetes in its many forms is common in residential care settings.

Although there are other medical illnesses that can have psychological implications, those noted earlier account for the most common that are seen in residential settings that cater to the needs of older adults. The presence of primary, secondary, and tertiary symptoms helps explain why the incidence of psychological symptomatology is so high in residential settings. For example, a recent report from the University of Utah Health Sciences Center (Sample, 1998) stated that the rate for depressive symptoms among those recently admitted to a nursing home was 51%. The high incidence of symptoms and the many factors that can contribute the presentation of psychological symptoms among older adults in residential settings requires that the physician's treatment decisions be made carefully and with as much information as possible from a multidisciplinary team. It also requires the use of other treating professionals, especially mental health professionals (Fore, 1996).

TREATMENT OF SYMPTOMS

As noted earlier, treatment efforts are most often preceded by an attempt to gain an accurate and complete understanding of the cause of the person's symptoms. Although the focus of this section, as with the rest of this chapter, has been on the psychological and behavioral consequences of medical illness and disease, treating primary symptoms (those that are a direct result of the illness or disease) is the most effective method to ameliorate problems and facilitate individual adaptation to long-term care. The direct treatment of the disease symptoms can also be the most effective way to treat secondary and tertiary symptoms; however, direct treatment of the psychological or behavioral symptoms is also required in many cases. The focus herein is first on the treatment of the symptoms of the diseases described earlier and then concludes with a discussion of the treatment of the psychological and behavioral symptoms.

General Treatment Considerations

The treatment of psychological symptoms can take many forms, and treatment decisions will vary according to the assessment of the symptoms, their etiology, and the patient's likely response to a given intervention. In many cases listening carefully to the patient's complaints can be curative and can augment or, in some cases, replace the need for other more invasive interventions. Medical advances are providing health-care providers with more treatment options than ever before. The pace of new drugs released to the public is expected to increase. Genetic engineering has great promise for prevention and cure, and developments in this area will result in better vaccinations and medications with fewer side effects. Stronger, lighter substances available for physical prosthetic devices and remote computerized monitoring devices will become more affordable and accessible to residential care settings. Surgeries have also become less invasive, and safer medical tests provide more information about a patient's medical condition than has been the case in any previous decade. Many complications that were previously an inevitable part of certain interventions can now be prevented, postponed, or minimized. Ultimately, the goal of treatment is to help improve the quality of life, maximize independence and happiness, and minimize suffering without exhausting the individual's personal resources. The sections that follow highlight three types of behavioral manifestations either as symptoms of a disease state (secondary or tertiary) or as issues of specific concern (primary) that deserve careful attention with respect to identification and treatment by healthcare providers in long-term care. These are malnutrition, pain, and iatrogenic complaints.

Malnutrition.   Although there have been many advances in medical science the treatment of choice, when possible, will always be prevention. One of the most important preventative measure in long-term care is monitoring and addressing patient nutrition (Griep, Mets; Collys, Ponjaert-Kristoffersen, & Massart, 2000). One of the constant challenges for the staff of residential care settings that serve older adults is to make sure that residents eat and drink enough to satisfy minimal nutritional needs. When this does not happen, older patients are more susceptible to illness and disease. In all residential care settings, residents' weight, as an indirect measure of nutritional state, should be regularly checked so that interventions can be made if changes occur. Older adults often complain that they are not hungry or do not like the food that is prepared for them in a given facility. Addressing this problem may require the provision of supplements that are commonly available as nonprescription aids. However, efforts to find foods enjoyed by the patient should be made, and assistance with feeding may also be needed. There are also medications that are known to enhance appetite, and some of these include Remeron, Trazadone (antidepressants), and Oxandrin (an anabolic steroid). Amitriptyline and similar agents are usually avoided because of their strong anticholinergic effects on this age group. Treatment of depression may also ameliorate an eating problem. If the resident is overweight, a dietary consult can be obtained and, depending on cognitive ability, the resident can be educated about the dangers of obesity and assisted in developing a diet that will produce gradual weight loss while maximizing nutrition. Staff should also encourage a resident's efforts to optimize his or her food intake.

In addition to monitoring appetite and diet, encouraging a regular pattern of exercise can help an elderly resident avoid sedation and some of the negative consequences of sedation, which is often malnutrition. Habit is an important factor at any time of life and more so in older adults. Thus, helping older residents establish and maintain healthy habits, including exercising and eating right, is an important intervention that can have powerful psychological and physical benefits (Berry & Marcus, 2000).

Pain. Although pain is not in and of itself an illness or disease state, it is associated with almost all illnesses and diseases. Normally, pain is a protective mechanism the body uses to react to potentially damaging disease-related forces. The analogy of someone reaching for something hot and then quickly pulling away from the discomfort is often used to highlight how the pain reaction works; that is, pain tells people when and how to act in order to remain safe. However, there are some conditions where pain continues and secondary problems of chronic pain can develop. Chronic pain can have devastating psychological effects including depression, decreased function, and a lower quality of life (Keefe, Dunsmore, & Burnett, 1992). There are many medications and treatments available for pain, and these have varying degrees of risk and expense. Because pain is by definition subjective, there is no absolute test for pain, and the history is of primary importance. However, people report pain differently, and one may underestimate pain in those with dementia or those who are stoic by nature. Monitoring for pain is an ongoing effort associated with good health care (see Keefe et al., 1992).

The elderly are at increased risk of medication side effects, especially from GI bleeding associated with the older anti-inflammatory agents such as ibuprofen. However, several agents are generally well-tolerated from a GI standpoint, and these typically spare the COX-1 pathway while more selectively affecting the COX-2 mechanism (e.g., Vioxx, Celebrex, and Relafen). Still, these medications can cause renal and other changes and must be monitored. Acetaminophen remains a useful agent, and function can be improved by scheduling certain doses before periods of activity. Narcotics are relatively nontoxic and can be used safely in this group of older adults. However, narcotic side effects, including impaired cognition and constipation, require low starting doses and careful monitoring. The usual preparations generally last 3–5 hours, whereas sustained-release formulations provide 8–16-hour effects. A few agents have intrinsically long half-lives such as fentanyl and methadone, which provide more steady relief and less dosing. Combination therapy with anti-inflammatory agents, acetaminophen, narcotics, activity, rest, bracing and other agents is often useful and allows a customized approach to pain-related problems while minimizing side effects.

Iatrogenic Factors.   *Iatrogenic* is a term that is used to describe the illness and suffering that occurs as a result of attempts to treat illness and disease. For example, pressure sores may occur in those who cannot get out of bed while being treated for another illness and urinary tract infections are common in those with catheters. Medications are associated with many problems including their side effects, the administration of medications to the wrong patient, polypharmacy (an excessive number or amount of medication), hypopharmacy (a suboptimal number or amount) and cost. When problems occur as the result of treatment or care, they have consequences that go beyond the physical suffering they produce. Patients who have been hurt as a result of their caregiver's attempts to treat them may lose faith in the medical community and may be reluctant to seek treatment in the future. It is vital then, that treatment teams make every effort to correctly diagnose and treat patients, and that there are systems in place to help the staff of residential settings provide appropriate care for their residents. Ongoing efforts to be vigilant for these problems and to prevent and intervene early are necessary and will build trust and avoid serious complications.

SUMMARY

Aging can create numerous problems that vary widely among individuals, particularly those in residential care settings. Many of the illnesses and diseases that older adults encounter while living in residential settings have psychological or behavioral symptoms as part of their typical presentation. A physician and his or her support staff can provide appropriate care for most problems. However, a physician must often call on other treating professionals to ensure the identified patient gets the care he or she needs. By coordinating efforts, a more comprehensive and holistic treatment program can be provided. A coordinated, multidisciplinary team can provide an effective medium for serving patients with various impairments. Efforts to involve family are important and can be aided by providing them with frequent updates. Because of the variety of individual problems and the number of intervention options available, it is important to have a system for identifying and providing services efficiently. Likewise, it is important to minimize the barriers to care and to help motivate patients to participate in the course of their treatment.

REFERENCES

American Diabetes Association. (1997). *Diabetes info: Diabetes facts and figures.* Retrieved from the WorldWide Web: http://www.diabetes.org/ada/c20f.html

American Psychiatric Association. (1994). *Diagnostic and Statistical Manual of Mental Disorders*, (4th ed.). Washington DC: Author.

Arking, R. (1991). Biology of aging. Englewood Cliffs, NJ: Prentice Hall

Baltes, P. B. (1997). On the incomplete architecture of human ontogeny: Selection, optimization, and compensation as the foundation of developmental theory. *American Psychologist, 52*, 366–380.

Baltes, P. B. (1987). Theoretical propositions of life-span developmental psychology: On the dynamics between growth and decline. *Developmental Psychology, 23*, 611–626.

Berry, E. M., and Marcus, E. L. (2000). Disorders of eating in the elderly. *Journal of Adult Development. 7*, 87–99

Bondi, M. W., Salmon, D. P., Galasko, D., Thomas, R. G., & Thal, L J. (1999). Neuropsychological function and apolipoprotein E genotype in the preclinical detection of Alzheimer's disease. *Psychology and Aging, 14*, 295–303

Cohen, M. A. (1998). Emerging trends in the finance and delivery of long-term care: Public and private opportunities and challenges. *The Gerontologist, 38*, 80–89.

Cugell, D. W. (1988). COPD: A brief introduction for behavioral scientists. In A. J. McSweeny & I. Grant (Eds.), *Chronic obstructive pulmonary disease: A behavioral perspective* (pp. 1–18). New York: Marcel Dekker.

Diener, E., & Suh, M. E. (1997). Subjective well-being and age: An international analysis. In K. W. Schaie & M. P. Lawton (Eds.), *Annual review of gerontology and geriatrics* (Vol. 8, pp. 304–324). New York: Springer.

Folstein, M. F., Folstein, S. E., & McHugh, P. R. (1975). Mini-mental state. *Journal of Psychiatric Research, 12*, 189–198.

Fore, W. W. (1996). Managed care approaches to diabetes mellitus. *Hospital Practice, 31*, 115–117.

Galasko, D., Corey-Bloom, J., & Thal, L. J. (1991). Monitoring progression in Alzheimer's disease. *Journal of the American Geriatrics Society, 39*, 932–941.

Grant, I., Prigatano, G. P., Heaton, R. K., McSweeny, A. J., Wright, E. C., & Adams, K. M. (1987). Progressive neuropsychologic impairment and hypoxemia. *Archives of General Psychiatry, 44*, 999–1006.

Griep, M. I.; Mets, T. F.; Collys, K.; Ponjaert-Kristoffersen, I., & Massart, D. L. (2000). Risk of malnutrition in retirement homes elderly persons measured by the "Mini-Nutritional Assessment." *Journals of Gerontology: Biological Sciences & Medical Sciences, 55*, M57–M63.

Hill, R. D., & Backman, L. (1995). The relationship between the mini-mental state examination and cognitive functioning in normal elderly adults: A componential analysis. *Age and Aging, 24*, 440–446.

Hopp, F. P. (1999). Patterns and predictors of formal and informal care among elderly persons living in board and care homes. *Gerontologist, 39*, 167–176.

Jelicic, M., & Kempen, G. (1999). Chronic medical conditions and life satisfaction in the elderly. *Psychology and Health, 14*, 65–70.

Kane, R. A., & Kane, R. L. (1981). *Assessing the elderly: A practical guide to measurement.* Lexington, MA: Lexington.

Keefe, F. J., Dunsmore, J., & Burnett, R. (1992). Behavioral and cognitive–behavioral approaches to chronic pain: Recent advances and future directions. *Journal of Consulting and Clinical Psychology, 60*, 528–536.

Kenney, A. R. (1989). *Physiology of aging* (2nd ed). Chicago: Yearbook Medical.

Kitzman, D. W., & Edwards, W. D. (1990). Age-related changes in the anatomy of the normal human heart. *Journal of Gerontology: Medical Sciences, 45*, 33–39

Laditka, S. B. (1998). Modeling lifetime nursing home use under assumptions of better health. *Journal of Gerontology, 39*, 177–187.

Larson, R. (1978). Thirty years of research on subjective well-being of older Americans. *Journal of Gerontology, 33,* 109–125.

Lezak, M. D. (1995) *Neuropsychological Assessment* (3rd ed). New York: Oxford University Press.

Mattis, S. (1988) *Dementia Rating Scale (DRS)* Odessa, FL. Psychological Assessment Resources.

Niemi, M.L., Laaksonen, R., Kotila, M., & Waltim, O. (1988) Quality of life four years after stroke. *Stroke, 19,* 1101–1107.

Prospective Payment Assessment Commission (1995, June). *Medicare and the American health care system* [Report to Congress]. Washington, DC: U. S. Government Printing Office.

Rapoport, M. J., & Feinstein, A. (2000). Outcome following traumatic brain injury in the elderly: A critical review. *Brain Injury. 14,* 749–761

Reitan , R. M. & Wolfson, D. (1988). *Neuroanatomy and neuropathology: A clinical guide for neuropsycholgists.* Tucson, AZ: Neurpsychological Press.

Rosenman, R. H., Brand, R. J., Jenkins, D., Friedman, M., Staus, R., & Wurm, M. (1975). Coronary heart disease in the Western Collaborative Group Study: Final follow-up experience of 8½ years. *Journal of the American Medical Association, 233,* 872–877.

Sample, S. (1988.) *Health sciences report* (Vol. 22, No. 2). Salt Lake City, UT: University of Utah.

Skilbeck, C. (1996). Psychological aspects of stroke. In R. T. Woods (Ed.), *Handbook of the clinical psychology of aging* (pp. 284–301). New York: Wiley.

Bureau of the Census. (1996). *Current population reports, special studies, 65+ in the United States* (pp. 23–190). Washington DC: U. S. Government Printing Office.

Whitbourne, S. K. (1998). Physical changes in the aging individual: Clinical implications. In I. H. Nordhus, G. R. VandenBos, S. Berg, & P. Fromholt (Eds), *Clinical geropsychology.* Washington, DC: American Psychological Association.

6

Assessment for Change in Residential Care

Michael J. Lambert
Brigham Young University

Matthew J. Davis
University of Utah

Jared Morton
Dan Williams
Brigham Young University

MEASURING CHANGE IN RESIDENTIAL CARE

Addressing the needs of the frail elderly who are no longer able to live independently is a prominent theme highlighted throughout this text. Several chapters have described intervention strategies that are specific to residential care contexts including environmental planning that allows older adults to "age in place" or maintain a sense of "home" even in the presence of physical decline and disability that are associated with advanced aging.

The issue of quality of care in residential assisted living contexts is fast becoming a national priority as more adults are moving into very old age. What is apparent, however, is that there is very little research in the scientific literature that has specifically examined how one defines quality of care and, even more important, therapeutic change in residential care contexts. An issue that makes this line of research difficult is the limited number of instruments that are designed to measure ongoing functioning and change within closed residential communities for the old and very old.

Over the past decade, it has become increasingly important for geriatric health care providers within medicine, social work, and psychology to demonstrate the effectiveness of interventions designed to promote quality of life in long-term residential care settings. Residential care providers are faced with this trend as well. Providers within long-term care contexts need to show that the interventions they use improve adjustment to the vicissitudes of old age in terms that can be understood by a concerned family member as well as insurers such as Medicare. In addition to outside pressures from agencies such as the Health Care Financing Association of Health and Human Services to show that an intervention is effective, practitioners who measure change are in the best position to learn from experience and design better interventions. For example, measurement of the ability for self-care has illuminated characteristics of improvement of both residents and facilities (Walk, Flieshman, & Mandelson, 1999). For front-line staff, measuring change using formal measurement tools can increase problem awareness and concretely document the effectiveness as well as the failures of treatment efforts. Although measuring change is becoming a necessary part of practice for the individual geriatric practitioner, the demands associated with measuring change can be daunting. This is in no small part due to the difficulty of measuring change in persons living in residential care facilities who are experiencing age-related biological declines that are not amenable to improvement. How does one show the effectiveness of an intervention in impaired persons who are in a developmentally declining stage of life?

This chapter is intended to be an introduction to the topic of outcome assessment in residential care contexts as well as a resource to those who want to include outcome evaluation in long-term care. It begins by exploring the methodological considerations relevant to measuring change in impaired elderly persons. A set of measures the practitioner can use to structure the assessment of change in residential care is then recommended.

METHODOLOGICAL ISSUES IN MEASURING CHANGE

Effective residential care evaluations should document changes in functioning as a result of specific treatment efforts. Measuring change is influenced by the identified problem, the baseline functioning of the patient, the patient's potential for change, how change is defined, and the environment in which change occurs. These issues are explored in this section.

Identified Problem

Most outcome research studies have focused on change in community-dwelling older adults within limited, homogeneous diagnoses; that is, participants in these studies are often characterized with a single impairment or disorder (e.g., depression; Thompson & Gallagher-Thompson, 1997). In contrast to this approach, it is clear that clients seen in residential care settings have multiple impairments that are compounded by age-related issues of decline, such as depression due to declining cognitive functioning or anxiety associated with advanced stages of Parkinson's disease. Because the goal of most outcome research with older adults is to demonstrate the efficacy of a specific intervention (e.g., cognitive–behavioral therapy) for treating a specific issue (e.g., depression), those with multiple medical problems, psychiatric problems, or both, are often screened out. Unfortunately these multiple-problem clients make up the bulk of those in residential care settings. Although a person may enter residential care ostensibly because of functional impairment, identification of additional problems such as child–parent interpersonal conflicts, somatic concerns, anxiety, or age-related disability is common. Although many of these problems might be addressed to some extent by the simple placement of a frail older adult in a residential assisted living context, measuring change in every one of these areas is obviously a very demanding task and one that cannot be accomplished fully by an overextended staff. Given this reality, energy should be directed toward those areas that will have the largest impact on the client's ability to realize a successful adjustment to the residential care setting and are amenable to change. For these reasons, this chapter suggests measuring two major intervention target areas: functional ability and quality of life.

Point of View

Identifying the problem or impairment to be measured depends in part on whose point of view is being considered. Because every person rating an impairment is subject to seeing it through some type of filtering lens, comprehensive measurement of change must occur from multiple viewpoints, including those of the long-term care staff, the resident, and the family. Outcome measurement scales typically have five sources of information: client, trained observer, significant other(s), professional caregiver, and instrumental, a category covering information obtained from physiological indices and environmental data such as previous hospitalization records (Lambert, 1983). Ideally, all these sources of information would be represented in any measurement attempt because, as psychotherapy outcome research with community-dwelling older adults has clearly shown, the outcomes can be misunderstood and even misrepresented through failure to appreciate the effects that different perspectives can have in reflecting the degree of change or adjustment that results from any given intervention. Application of multiple measurement sources in past research studies has made it clear that multiple measures from different sources do not yield unitary results.

A multidisciplinary staffing is held for a 78-year-old man named Frank who has been living at the residential center for 3 weeks now. Frank came to the facility at the urging of family members after his wife of 30 years passed away 6 months previous and he began to have problems with self-care activities. He agreed to move to the center as he felt, "I could use some help getting around." At the meeting, staff are discussing how Frank is adapting to the living change. A nurse relays information on concerns of the family that, since entering the facility, Frank is not "coming out of his depression" as he continues to tell his daughters that he misses his wife and wants to be with her. The social worker who has been seeing Frank during his time at the facility believes that Frank has begun working through a delayed grieving process and will therefore probably show increased depression over the next couple of weeks. However, staff members note that his mood appears better as Frank has begun eating normally and initiating interactions with other residents. The physician agrees with the staff that Frank's behavior supports the conclusion that his mood has been improving but feels Franks prognosis is guarded as he has had previous episodes of depression, and testing has revealed moderate cognitive impairment.

It is our opinion that patient care would improve both for specific patients and, over time, for all patients if patient status was formally rated from several points of view. Although in long-term care facilities multiple points of view exist, measuring all points of view can be a prohibitively time-consuming task and produce conflicting outcomes—for example, the older cognitive-impaired resident who feels threatened when faced with any type of change. Careful consideration of which viewpoints will provide the most valid information can clarify what information source should be given priority. For example, after a client enters residential care, staff are more often used as raters of the need for assistance in activities of daily living because family or friends are less involved in observing these activities. Conversely, using staff to rate instrumental activities of daily living that occur in everyday life outside of a facility might provide a different perspective with respect to treatment than ratings provided by family and friends who are able to observe clients as they function at home.

Baseline Functioning

Although the aging process is one of predictable decline, with increasing impairment and baseline functioning having a negatively declining slope, there is great variation in the rate of decline of particular individuals. The individual baseline functioning level among institutionalized elderly has been found to be the best predictor of functioning 6 months after entering a structured long-term care setting (Braun, Rose, & Finch, 1991), but baseline disability in one area of functioning does not necessarily equate with disability in another area. For example, poor cognitive baseline functioning is not an accurate predictor of poor self-care ability (Backman & Hill, 1996). Therefore, it is important to measure baseline levels in each targeted area and use instruments that have a suitable metric to accurately distinguish between these disparate individual baseline levels of functioning.

As noted earlier, the structure and administration of appropriate instruments is constrained by the baseline functioning of residential care clients. Most residential care clients have some degree of impaired comprehension, shortened attention span, or impaired memory (Brod, Stewart, Sands, & Walton, 1999). Therefore, one important guideline to consider in long-term care is that outcome measures should be short and straightforward. Shorter measures reduce respondent burden. Instrument forms that are straightforward for staff to use, in terms of easy administration and simple summation scoring protocols, will increase the consistency of regular measurements taken at predetermined intervals and the subsequent overall accuracy of baseline and change scores. Some outcome measures originally designed for self-report may require interviewer administration because of the level of cognitive impairment present in a given older resident (Coast, Peters, Richards, & Gunnell, 1998). This raises the issue of "different perspectives" that may diverge with performance expectations and the ability of a resident to change.

Potential for Change

Although the residential care population is characterized by declining abilities, improvement in functioning in selected abilities is still possible. Research has reported that among institutionalized elderly, 35% showed improvement in physical functioning in response to intervention when measured 10 months apart (Finch, Kane, & Phillip, 1994). When measuring the potential for change, an initial requirement is that the instruments used must be able to record changes from baseline functioning. Although this consideration appears elementary, ceiling effects can make measurement of changes impossible (Applegate, Blass, & Williams, 1990). For example, if a group of older residents is examined for improvement in the number of self-care tasks performed independently without staff assistance and a substantial percentage of these persons have a baseline ability to perform most self-care activities, a low number of improved residents will be reported. Furthermore, the global ratings produced by many instruments may ignore specific changes that are captured by the individual questions of more specific scales and thereby conceal changes in individual areas of functioning. For example, decline in instrumental activities of daily living (e.g. balancing a checkbook) may be apparent due to the lack of need for such skills in a long-term care facility, whereas self-care behaviors (e.g. transferring oneself from the bed to a chair) may improve due to better designed furniture for impaired individuals that a facility may provide (which was not feasible when the person was living at home).

Further, individual difference characteristics such as age, education, and socioeconomic status may interact to influence the ability of a given resident to change. As an example, gender differences can affect the amount of change expected, and some research has reported that men have a slightly higher probability of improvement in bathing function than women, which is attributed to a higher baseline physical ability in elderly males (Walk et al., 1999). As the older population is largely female, measurement instruments that are biased toward men will show fewer positive results.

In addition to client and measurement scale characteristics, the domain measured can affect the potential for change. For example, cognitive impairments are highly resistant to psychosocial interventions and therefore even the best interventions will show little change in functioning. In this area, merely lengthening baseline levels of functioning might define a successful outcome. However, because attempts to measure change in cognitive status will not show much of an effect, practitioners who measure change in the area run the risk of having others interpreting the results of their intervention as ineffective, rather than simply showing the irreversible, deteriorative nature of cognitive impairment with advanced aging.

Unfortunately potential for within-individual change can be difficult to assess because the residential facility itself can influence the client's potential for change (e.g., design and structured resident routines). On the positive side, facilities with high-quality care can enhance improvement. For example, higher quality facilities have been associated with six times the improvement in bladder continence than lower quality facilities (Walk et al., 1999). The impact of living in a structured care environment, however, can also lead to functional decline as client autonomy is reduced, with subsequent increases in learned helplessness (Rodin & Langer, 1977). Additionally, the reluctance of staff to allow clients to practice self-care activities for fear of injury or other mishap can mask a given individual resident's real ability and subsequently reduce the range of improvement found, as well as the perception of potential for change from those outside the facility (e.g., family and loved ones). The residential care environment also affects scores on client-rated measurements. For example, in one study nursing home residents had self-perceived health ratings equal to community samples, despite lower observer-rated levels, a finding that may be explained by the fact that the nursing home residents were compared with an even sicker population (Eustis & Patten, 1982).

Definitions of Change in Residential Care

The potential for change also depends on how change is defined. Practitioners in residential care, as well as family and loved ones, are interested in meaningful change—that is, change that is large enough to be seen or felt not only by a statistical test of significance but also by the resident or the resident's family. Measurement instruments, then, should be capable of documenting not only change over time, but whether the level of change is clinically meaningful. Traditionally, outcome research designs with older community-dwelling adults have focused on measuring statistically significant differences between groups who either received or did not receive an intervention. However, some researchers have pointed out that statistically significant difference is not the same as clinically meaningful change. Because the great majority of older adults are in a declining state of independent functioning when they enter residential care, equating change with improvement is problematic given that it is unlikely objective improvement will occur. For example, most frail older adults who are placed in residential care will remain in such a facility until death. Thus, progressive and irreversible decline in all aspects of functioning is predictable and inevitable.

A better way to conceptualize change is to equate it with adjustment or use theories that are based on age-graded decline of functioning. In earlier chapters of this volume, selective optimization with compensation theory (SOC; Baltes, 1997) was presented. This theory can be used to guide assessments of change among the old and very old. In brief, the three main tenets of SOC—selectivity, optimization, and compensation—highlight different forms of adjustment associated with adult aging. Selectivity reflects a process whereby aging individuals choose their activities with increasing discrimination so as to conserve time and energy. Optimization is enhanced functional efficacy stemming from life learning, practice, and experience. Compensation encompasses conscious efforts to mitigate functional ability losses. The end result of these adjustment processes is facilitation of a degree of control over the aging decline. Enhancing this self-control has been documented as a key to increased quality of life in institutional environments such as residential care. Langer and Rodin (1976) showed that simple measures that give residents increased individual responsibility for decisions are associated with marked improvement. In this study, staff who were unaware that a study was being conducted rated residents who had been separated into a responsibility-induced and a comparison group. Ninety-three percent of the residents in the responsibility group were rated improved versus 21% of the comparison group.

The targeted emphasis in interventions designed for older adults in residential care is often quality of life. Through managing the coping procedures mentioned earlier it is possible to maintain quality of life even in the presence of objective physical decline. The goal of interventions, then, specific to residential care, is not to "cure or solve" issues, but to help older adults maintain a sense of dignity and autonomy and to minimize suffering in the presence of age-related decline.

Developing an approach to measure change with respect to SOC has not received much attention in the residential care literature. However, as more managed health care networks and government agencies insist on tracking patient quality of care outcomes, it appears more likely that geriatric health care providers will search for a standard way of evaluating optimal adjustment within residential care facilities. Using the change procedures presented herein, professional caregivers have a process that provides a standard for assessing change from baseline functioning while at the same time measuring whether the level of change is meaningful in this context. It is important also to use measures of change to track resident outcome by provider for the purpose of increasing the quality of services in order to justify the need for care-related resources from external governmental or private sources (Clement, 1996; Lambert & Brown, 1996). This approach to geriatric outcome research can be expected to directly modify how a residential care staff addresses specific disorders and can exert a real impact on quality of life.

Ideographic Versus Nomothetic Procedures

It is relatively tempting to stereotype the very old who are in long-term care facilities as a homogeneous group with similar problems and issues all of which are related to the process of aging. Although there are some general aspects of aging that would be considered thematic across individuals (e.g., the presence of cognitive impairment increasing as a function of advanced age), as a group, older adults are quite heterogeneous with respect to the issues they face and how they cope with those issues. Intuitively, one might consider the variety of different life experience that older adults can bring to bear on issues and problems.

Given the heterogeneity found among older persons in residential care, an individualized approach to measuring change is highly desirable. The individualized method that has received the most widespread attention and use is goal attainment scaling (GAS; Kiresuk & Smith, 1994). GAS requires treatment goals to be set up prior to intervention. These goals—formulated by the caregiving staff, a combination of geriatric practitioners, the client, and possibly the family—specify a series of likely outcomes, ranging from least to most favorable. This graduated scale must be formulated with sufficient precision so that an independent observer can determine the level at which a client is functioning at any given point in time. The particular scales and behaviors examined can vary from patient to patient and may include standardized instruments. This procedure allows for the transformation of the specific goals into an overall meaningful standard score.

Stolee, Zaza, Pedlar, and Myers (1999) used qualitative methods to evaluate the consequences of using GAS in geriatric care. GAS appeared to affect both the process of care as well as the outcome. The use of GAS resulted in shorter lengths of stay and a greater impact on functional as opposed to medical goals, especially when clients were involved in the goal-setting process. These researchers and others (e.g. Rockwood, 1995) stress the importance that outcome measurement, using a GAS protocol, can have on the specific processes underlying care provision. Stolee, Stadnyk, Myers, and Rockwood (1999) have shown that there is reasonable correspondence between standardized measures of functioning such as instrumental activities of living scales and GAS measured improvement, with GAS changes having the advantage of being more sensitive to change. They also note that GAS goals tend to focus on mobility, future care arrangements, and functional impairment. These are goals and objectives relevant to most residential care clients and their families. For these reasons, they have encouraged those involved in geriatric rehabilitation to use GAS as an outcome measurement method.

It should be noted that the GAS method suffers from the same difficulties as other individualized goal-setting procedures in that goal attainment is judged on a relative, rather than an absolute, basis, so that behavior change is confounded with expectations of change (Clark & Caudrey, 1986). Although a disadvantage of GAS is its time-consuming and cumbersome nature, the method can be modified to create a standardized measure of goals. Such an approach has been successfully applied in the care of the frail elderly and shows considerable promise (Yip et al., 1998).

A STRUCTURE FOR MEASURING CHANGE

Choosing an instrument is difficult in the absence of a guiding framework. In such a situation there is the danger of "measurement overkill," that is a tendency to include an unwieldy number of measurements rather than carefully targeting the most important areas (Kane & Kane, 1981). As mentioned previously, a core battery of scales to measure outcome in residential care has not been developed. In the absence of a core battery, a set of measures is suggested using the conceptual framework described in this chapter and adapted from Lambert's work in the field of psychotherapy (see Table 6.1). Following this ta-

TABLE 6.1

Measures for Assessing Change in Residential Care

Measure	Domain(s) measured	Data source
Global Assessment of Functioning	Psychological, social and occupational functioning	Clinician
Mini-Mental Status Examination	Cognitive functioning	Clinician
Brief Psychiatric Rating Scale	Psychiatric functioning	Clinician and Resident
Geriatric Depression Rating Scale	Depression	Resident
Outcome Questionnaire	Psychological distress and well-being, interpersonal relations	Resident
Multidimensional Observation Scale for Elderly Subjects	Interpersonal relationships	Clinician
OARS	Activities of daily living	Resident and Related Informant
Functional Activities Scale	Instrumental activities of daily living	Related Informant
Goal Attainment Scaling	Individualized to resident	Clinician, Resident and Related Informant

Note.   We use the Older Americans Resources and Services (OARS) scale over the Katz et al. (1963) activities of daily living measure, as the latter has not been shown to be sensitive to small changes (Applegate, Blass, & Williams, 1990).

ble is a brief description of each of these measures, along with instructions on how a long-term care staff might incorporate them to measure change or adjustment in residential care.

Clinician Evaluation

The Global Assessment of Functioning Scale

Author.   Diagnostic and Statistical Manual of Mental Disorders, 4th Edition (*DSM–IV*).

Publisher.   American Psychiatric Association.

Purpose.   The Global Assessment of Functioning Scale (GAF) was designed to enable clinicians to report residents' overall status for psychological, social, and occupational functioning. It is useful in measuring treatment impact and predicting outcome, particularly because it tracks and reports multiple aspects of patient status using a single score.

Description.   The GAF consists of a single 0–100 scale that indicates level of psychopathology, with a value of 100 indicating optimal patient functioning and progressively lower scores denoting less functional behavior. The continuum is divided into 10-point categories, each of which is accompanied by a description of the corresponding affect, behavior, and level of cognitive, social, and occupational functioning.

Scoring.   The GAF is scored via the caregiver's assignment of an appropriate level based on client functioning. It is assumed that caregiver familiarity with the patient's situation is the deciding factor of appropriateness.

Norms.   Studies reporting GAF norms relevant to the geriatric population are not currently available in the scientific literature.

Psychometrics.   It should be noted that the studies reporting reliability and validity for the GAF were conducted using the scale from *DSM–III-R*. The results remain applicable, as there are no significant differences between the *DSM–III-R* and the *DSM–IV* versions of the GAF. Reports of the psychometric properties of the GAF are scarce, despite its widespread use. Further statistical research, especially with older adults, is imperative and overdue.

Reliability.   A diverse team of 12 professionals calculated separate GAF scores on the basis of the admission and discharge records of 16 psychiatric inpatients. Intraclass correlation coefficients for admission and discharge were .62 and .90 ($P < .001$), respectively.

Validity.   Jones, Thornicroft, Coffey, and Dunn (1995) assessed the correlation between GAF scores and increases in patient support needs and antipsychotic medication levels. They found that a negative correlation exists, thus confirming validity.

Availability.   The GAF scale and relevant information is found in the *DSM–IV.*

The Mini-Mental State Examination (MMSE)

Authors.   Marshall F. Folstein, Susan E. Folstein, and Paul R. McHugh.

Purpose.   The MMSE was designed to provide a simple, brief, and user-friendly assessment of cognitive status.

Description.   The MMSE measures 11 tasks of cognitive ability divided into two sections. The initial section covers orientation, memory, and attention. These three aspects are tested as follows: Orientation is measured with questions of time such as the current year, season, and date, and with questions of location, such as current town and care setting name. Memory is measured through the ability to repeat three words after a time lapse. Attention and calculation are subsequently measured by counting backwards from 100 by sevens. The second section assesses the ability to name objects and follow verbal and written commands by measuring the client's ability to name a watch and a pencil, repeat a simple sentence, follow a three-stage command, read and obey a simple sentence, write a sentence, and copy a design showing intersecting pentagons. The last item is the interviewer's assessment of patient consciousness on a continuum from *alert* to *coma.*

Scoring.   Scoring is accomplished by summing the scores obtained on the individual tasks, with a total of 30 points possible.

Norms.   Means of MMSE scores calculated by age resulted in the following: For persons age 65–69, $m = 27$, $SD = 1.6$; age 70–74, $m = 27$, $SD = 1.8$; age 75–79, $m = 26$, $SD = 2.1$; age 80–84, $m = 25$, $SD = 2.2$; age 85 and up, $m = 24$, $SD = 2.9$.

Reliability.   Reliability was tested in three testing situations, using both the Pearson Product Moment Correlation and Wilcoxon T tests. When one tester administered the MMSE twice to the same person 24 hours apart, the Pearson r obtained was .887 ($p < .0001$), and the Wilcoxon T showed no significant difference. When the MMSE was administered twice to the same person 24 hours apart using two testers, the Pearson r obtained was .827 ($p < .0001$), and the Wilcoxon T again showed no significant difference. When patients with clinically stable cognitive capabilities were tested twice at an average interval of 28 days between administrations, the Pearson r obtained was .98 ($p < .0001$), and no significant difference was obtained using the Wilcoxon T.

Validity. Concurrent validity was determined by correlating MMSE scores with verbal and performance scores on the Wechsler Adult Intelligence Scale administered in a single week. For MMSE versus Verbal IQ, the Pearson r was .776 ($p < .0001$). For MMSE versus Performance IQ, the Pearson r was .660 ($p < .0001$). Significant relationships between the MMSE and other scales have also been discovered. When compared with either the 26-item Blessed Information–Memory–Concentration Test or the 6-item Blessed Orientation–Memory–Concentration Test, correlations of $-.66$ to $-.93$ have been obtained. The sign is negative because the Blessed scales report items missed, whereas the MMSE reports items correct. Noteworthy correlations have also been revealed between the MMSE and several tests used in neuropsychological assessment, between the MMSE and scales reporting activities of daily living, and between the MMSE and histopathological findings.

Availability. The Mini-Mental State Examination and the "Instructions for Administration of Mini-Mental State Examination" can be found in Folstein, Folstein, and McHugh (1975).

Clinician–Patient Report of Symptoms

The Brief Psychiatric Rating Scale (BPRS)

Authors. John E. Overall and Donald R. Gorham.

Purpose. The primary purpose in the development of the Brief Scale has been the development of an efficient, rapid evaluation procedure for use in assessing treatment change in psychiatric patients while at the same time yielding a rather comprehensive description of major symptom characteristics.

Description. The original BPRS consists of the following 16 different symptom categories: somatic concern, anxiety, emotional withdrawal, conceptual disorganization, guilt feelings, tension, mannerisms and posturing, grandiosity, depressive mood, hostility, suspiciousness, hallucinatory behavior, motor retardation, uncooperativeness, unusual thought content, and blunted affect. In 1965, two additional items, excitement and disorientation, were added. A 7-point scale is used to designate the level of pathology present in each category representing the following severity states: *not present, very mild, mild, moderate, moderately severe, severe,* and *extremely severe.* It should be noted that in five categories (tension, emotional withdrawal, mannerisms and posturing, motor retardation, and uncooperativeness) ratings are to be based on clinician observation of the patient, whereas in the remaining 11 categories, ratings are to be based on the verbal report of the participant.

Norms. Studies reporting norms relevant to geriatric populations were not encountered in the literature.

Scoring. A separate score in each of the 16 symptom areas is obtained. Overall and Gorham stated that for evaluating patient change during treatment, the use of a total pathology score, which is the simple sum of ratings on the 16 scales, is recommended, their reasoning being that although psychiatric symptomatology is multidimensional, the difference between pretreatment pathology and posttreatment pathology can be represented by a single dimension spanning the multivariate space. Both the single scale score and the total pathology score may prove useful in the assessment of geriatric outcome.

Reliability. Median Pearson Product Moment Correlations for the 18 symptom subscales, calculated from interrater reliability scores obtained in five separate studies, ranged from .63 to .88. Only two of the items, emotional withdrawal and blunted affect, were below .70. An analysis of 13 studies reporting interrater reliability for the Total Pathology Score showed that 10 of these studies reported correlations of .80 or higher.

Validity. An analysis of over 150 drug treatment studies wherein the BPRS was used as an indicator of change showed that "with only rare exception, BPRS change scores have consistently reflected treatment changes that are corroborated and supported by other clinical ratings" (Hedlund & Vieweg, 1980, p. 52).

Availability. For the original 16-item scale and detailed information regarding the BPRS, see Overall and Gorham (1962). For the current 18-item version of the scale, see Overall (1988).

Client Report of Symptoms

Geriatric Depression Scale

Authors. J. I. Sheikh and J. A. Yesavage.

Purpose. Brief rating scale of depressive symptomatology in elderly individuals. Especially applicable for use with physically ill and cognitively impaired individuals.

Description.   Available in 30-, 15-, 10-, and 4-item comprised of yes–no questions.

Norms.   Authors suggest scores over 11 are indicative of depression.

Scoring.   Response items are summed to create overall score.

Reliability.   Reliability of the 30-, 15-, and 10- item version is good, ranging from .70 to .87. The 4-item reliability is .64.

Validity.   The GDS has been validated against two other self-rated scales of depression, the HRSD and SDS. Participants were classified using research diagnostic criteria for depression. Each scale was significantly ($p < .001$) correlated to the classification variable with the following magnitudes: GDS $r = .82$, HRS-D $r = .69$, SDS $r = .83$.

Availability.   See Sheikh and Yesavage (1986).

Outcome Questionnaire (OQ-45.2 and OQ-10)

Authors.   Michael J. Lambert and Gary M. Burlingame.

Purpose.   The Outcome Questionnaire was developed to measure client progress in therapy.

Description.   Client progress is measured using a brief 10- or 45-item self-report instrument that requires clients to rate their feelings on a 5-point scale for three content domains. The first subscale is Symptom Distress, which reflects depression, anxiety, stress-related illness, and substance abuse. The second subscale, Interpersonal Relations, focuses on loneliness, intimacy, and conflict in close relationships. The final subscale, Social Role Performance, assesses distress or conflict in work, school, or homemaking roles. Each of the three subscales yields a separate score. The total score indicates a level of overall functioning.

Norms.   The mean score at intake is 67.84 ($SD = 22.09$). The mean score at termination of therapy is 60.19 ($SD = 24.24$). Fifty percent of clients are expected to show reliable change within 10 psychotherapy sessions, and 75% of clients will reach reliable change within 14 sessions.

Scoring.   Each item is scored on a 5-point Likert-type scale (range 0–4). The total score is calculated by summing individual ratings across all 45 items. This yields a total score range from 0 to180, with higher scores indicative of increased disturbance. Each subscale is calculated by summing the items unique to that domain. A cutoff score of 63 differentiates between community and clinical samples. Subscale cutoff scores are as follows: Symptom Distress = 36, Interpersonal Relations = 15, and Social Role = 12. A reliable change index (RCI) has also been derived between the community and community mental health samples. The RCI is used to determine if the change exhibited by an individual in treatment is reliable or clinically significant. In order for an individual's score to be considered clinically significant, the change score obtained must be greater than 10 for Symptom Distress, 8 for Interpersonal Relations, 7 for Social Role, and 14 for the Total Score.

Reliability.   Research has shown clinical samples have reliable changing scores, whereas nonclinical samples have scores that remain relatively constant at retest.

Validity.   Concurrent validity was estimated by calculating Pearson r coefficients on the total score and individual domain scores with other highly used outcome measures. Concurrent validity for the OQ and its individual domains were all significant ($p > .01$).

Availability.   The primary reference for the OQ is Lambert, Hatfield, Vermeersch, Hansen, Finch, Whipple & Burlingame (2000). American Professional Credentialing Services LLC, P.O. Box 477, Wharton, NJ 07885-0477; 1-888-647-2673

Measures of Interpersonal Relationships

Multidimensional Observation Scale for Elderly Subjects (MOSES)

Authors.   Edward Helmes, Kalman G. Csapo, and Judith-Ann Short.

Purpose.   The MOSES was designed to be a brief and multidimensional measure of physical needs, intellectual and cognitive functioning, and psychosocial aptitudes in the elderly to aid in placement, monitoring of patient progress, and evaluation of treatment programs. The MOSES has been shown to be sensitive to clinical change over time and, therefore, is useful for outcome measurement.

Description.   Five aspects of functioning are assessed with eight questions asked on each area. The five areas are self-care functioning, disoriented behavior, depressed/anxious mood, irritable behavior, and withdrawn behavior. Each of the eight items are scaled from 1 to 4 with higher numbers indicating more severe levels of pathology, inability to accomplish the task, or both. As regards outcome and interpersonal relationships, only the last two scales apply. The Irritable Behavior scale contains questions regarding cooperation with nursing care, the following of staff requests and instructions, irritability, reactions to frustration, verbal abuse of staff, verbal abuse of other residents, physical abuse of others, and the provocation of other residents. The Withdrawn Behavior scale measures preference for solitude, social contact initiation, response to social contacts, friendship with other residents, interest in day-to-day events, interest in outside events, the extent to which the resident keeps occupied, and the extent to which the resident helps other residents.

Norms. Studies reporting MOSES norms relevant to the geriatric population were not encountered in the literature.

Scoring. The MOSES reference contains no specific procedure for scoring. It is apparent from the primary reference that score values are simply equivalent to the number designating the alternative selected. However, even if details of scoring had been provided, it is presumed that the efficacy of such procedures would be limited in the present usage because of our recommendation that only the last two scales be used.

Reliability. Interrater reliability was assessed using intraclass correlations resulting in total values of .72 and .75 for the Irritability and Withdrawal scales, respectively. A test of internal reliability resulted in similar values of .79 and .78.

Validity. Prediction of outcome, criterion or convergent validation, and discriminant validation were all used to determine the validity of MOSES. On investigation, a lack of significant correlations with theoretically irrelevant scales indicated that a satisfactory level of discriminant validity was existent. As regards the Irritability and Withdrawal scales, convergent validity correlations were most significant in the following areas: Withdrawal scale and Robertson Mental Status, -.476 ($p < .01$); the London Psychogeriatric Rating Scale (LPRS) total score and the MOSES Irritability scale, .53 ($p < .001$); between the LPRS and the MOSES Withdrawal scale, .65 ($p < .001$); between the MOSES Irritability scale and the Emotional Lability scale of the Kingston Dementia Rating Scale, .63 ($p < .001$); between the MOSES Irritability scale and the Belligerent/Irritability scale of the Physical and Mental Impairment-of-Function Evaluation (PAMIE), .77 ($p < .001$); and between the Withdrawal/Apathetic scale of the PAMIE and the MOSES Withdrawal scale, .78 ($p < .001$).

Availability. The primary reference for the MOSES is Helmes, Csapo, and Short (1987). Further information can be obtained from Edward Helmes, Ph.D.,

Psychological Services, London Psychiatric Hospital, 850 Highbury Avenue, P.O. Box 2532, Terminal "A", London, Ontario, N6A 4HI Canada.

Measures of Activities of Daily Living

Older Americans Resources and Services (OARS)

Authors.   Linda K. George and Gerda G. Fillenbaum.

Purpose.   The OARS model has three conceptual elements: first, assessment of functioning level; second, a breakdown of needed services into their generic components and regrouping the services into patterns of actual use; and third, a matrix that assesses the impact of a patient's service packages according to functional status.

Description.   The first element is the Multidimensional Functional Assessment Questionnaire (MFAQ), which assesses the level of functioning in five domains: social resources, economic resources, physical health, mental health, and activities of daily living (ADL). These five areas represent the major areas of functioning relevant to clinical practice and service evaluation. The MFAQ consists of 99 questions, 70 of which are answered by the respondent.

The second element is the Services Assessment Questionnaire (SAQ), which elicits information about 24 broadly defined generic services (e.g. transportation, medical services, financial assistance). Information about the source of the service, the units of services received in the past 6 months, and the perceived need for some or more of the service is obtained for each generic service. The set of services generated by the SAQ represents that individual's service package. The third element, the Transition Matrix, links together the first two elements, functional status and service use. The matrix breaks down each of the five domains used in the MFAQ into two categories: impaired and unimpaired. This breakdown generates 32 unique functional status classes.

Norms.   Not applicable for this instrument.

Scoring.   For the MFAQ section, a 3-point scale is used to rate each item, while a 6-point scale, from 1 (*excellent functioning*) to 6 (*totally impaired*), is used to generate a global instrumental activities of daily living score. The SAQ section requires the list of 24 generic services from which one can assess the individual's service needs. The Matrix section is generated by rating the individual as either "adequate" or "impaired" on the five domains. This information places the individual within one of the 32 unique domains.

Reliability.   Test–retest reliability during a 5-week interval resulted in 91% of the MFAQ items being identical. Interrater reliability coefficients ranged from .67 to .87 across the five domains of functioning. Eighty percent of intrarater correlations were .80 or higher.

Validity.   Validity for the MFAQ was assessed by comparing the MFAQ interviewer ratings with the independent ratings of psychiatrists for mental health questions, physician's associates for physical health questions, and physical therapists for ADL questions. For economic resources, the external criterion was income adequacy as determined by federal budget standards. Social resources were not examined because the social workers contacted indicated that the questions in the MFAQ were identical to those they would ask. The results obtained, using Kendall's coefficient, showed correlations of .62 for economic resources, .60 for mental health, .75 for physical health, and .83 for ADL. Obviously only some of the areas that are assessed are appropriate as indices of patient outcome.

Availability.   Linda K. George, Ph.D., Box 3003, Duke University Medical Center, Durham, NC 27710.

Functional Activities Scale (FAS)

Authors.   R. I. Pfeiffer, T. T. Kurosaki, C. H. Harrah, Jr., J. M. Chance, and S. Filos.

Purpose.   This instrument was designed to identify persons who require assistance, measure response to therapy, and determine whether reported cognitive and affective changes signify functionally meaningful disease.

Description.   An informant rates the client on 10 activities: handling finances, assembling tax/insurance papers, shopping alone, playing games, using stove, preparing meals, keeping track of current events, paying attention to activities, remembering important daily routines, and traveling out of the neighborhood.

Norms.   A patient with normal functioning will score a 30, whereas a patient who is severely incapacitated will score a 0.

Scoring.   The total score is calculated by adding the points from each question. Each item is scaled from 3 (*dependent*) to 0 (*normal*). The total score ranges from 30 to 0.

Reliability.   Interrater reliability among neurologists trained in the FAQ is very high $r = .97$).

Validity.   The FAQ results were highly correlated ® = .72) to other frequently used measurements of activities of daily living.

Availability.   No specific forms or materials are necessary to use this instrument.

Individualized Assessment   Goal Attainment Scaling (GAS)

Authors.   T. J. Kiresuk and A. Smith.

Purpose.   The GAS is designed as an individualized outcome measure in geriatric rehabilitation.

Description.   Using the GAS technique, an interdisciplinary team assesses and identifies individual goals for a patient. The interdisciplinary team decides on the goals, taking into account the concerns of the client and family members. The decided on individualized goals are scaled on the basis of expected outcome (0) and possible outcomes that are better (+1 or +2) or worse (-1 or -2) than expected. At the end of the time allotted for goal completion, the patient is assessed again comparing the old score with the new score. The overall goal attainment score is calculated as follows:

$$\text{Goal Attainment Scaling} = 50 + \frac{10\Sigma\,(w_i x_i)}{[.7\Sigma w_i^2 + .3(\Sigma w_i)^2]}$$

Norms.   Not applicable for this instrument.

Scoring.   Using the formula, where wi is the weight assigned to the ith goal, and xi is the numerical value (-2 to +2) of the attainment level of the ith goal. The score is an average goal attainment score adjusted for the relative weighting assigned to the goals, the number of goals, and the expected intercorrelation among the goal scales. The intercorrelation is represented in the formula by the value of .3 for p (.7 = 1 - P). The baseline levels for each of the GAS goals are included as scale descriptors on each of the individualized goal scales (usually at the -1 or -2 level). A baseline GAS score can be calculated using these numerical values in the GAS equation.

Reliability.   Analyses show that interrater reliability between the original team and an independent nurse assessment was .93.

Validity.   The GAS correlates strongly ($r = 0.50$) with other similar measures and was found to be the most sensitive to change.

Availability. The primary reference for GAS is Kiresuk, Smith, & Cardillo (1994). This instrument does not require any materials. It can be administered and scored using the given formula.

CONCLUSION

As the baby boom generation enters old age, residential care use will increase dramatically. As a result, showing the effectiveness of interventions provided in this setting will become more important than ever. Assessing outcomes of services provided in residential care reflects our society's growing recognition that even in the declining stages of life, clinically meaningful interventions can "add life to years rather than years to life" (Clark, 1995). Measuring changes not only provides practitioners with information on what interventions are helpful, but whether an intervention has been helpful to a particular individual at a specific point in time. Further, assessing improvement over time during the process of treatment allows professional caregivers in residential care facilities to increase opportunities to modify interventions and maximize positive outcome in residents. Outside parties such as insurers or family members will have more concrete proof and a better understanding of the reasons for an intervention and the effect it had on the identified patient. Most importantly, the individual patient will benefit by more effective caregiving. Research needs to focus on the development of a core outcome battery for use in residential care that can be applied across settings. Although the recommendations made in this chapter are tentative, this chapter has highlighted the importance of implementing intervention efforts using assessment scales grounded in outcome research.

REFERENCES

Applegate, W. B., Blass, J. P., & Williams, T. F. (1990). Instruments for the functional assessment of older patients. *New England Journal of Medicine, 322,* 1207–1214.

Backman, L., & Hill, R. D. (1996). Cognitive performance and everyday functioning: Patterns in normal aging and dementia. In R. T. Woods (Ed.), *Handbook of the clinical psychology of aging.* New York: Wiley.

Baltes, P. B. (1997). On the incomplete architecture of human ontogeny: Selection, optimization, and compensation as a foundation of developmental theory. *American Psychologist, 52,* 366–380.

Braun, K. L., Rose, C. L., & Finch, M. D. (1991). Patient characteristics and outcomes in institutional and community long-term care. *The Gerontologist, 31,* 648–656.

Brod, M., Stewart, A. L., Sands, L., & Walton, P. (1999). Conceptualization and measurement of quality of life in dementia: The dementia quality of life instrument (DqoL). *The Gerontologist, 39,* 25–35.

Clark, M. S., & Caudrey, D. J. (1986). Evaluation of rehabilitation services: The use of goal attainment scaling. *International Rehabilitative Medicine, 5,* 41–45.

Clark, P. G. (1995). Quality of life, values, and teamwork in geriatric care: Do we communicate what we mean? *The Gerontologist, 35,* 402–411.

Clement, P. W. (1996). Evaluation in private practice. *Clinical Psychology: Science and Practice, 3,* 146–159.

Coast, J., Peters, T. J., Richards, S. H., & Gunnell, D. J. (1998). Use of the EUROQOL among elderly acute care patients. *Quality of Life Research, 7,* 1–10.

Eustis, N. N., & Patten, S. K. (1982). The effectiveness of long-term care. In D. J. Mangen, & W. A. Petersen, (Eds.), *Research instruments in social gerontology,* Vol. 3 (pp. 217–316). Minneapolis, MN: University of Minnesota Press.

Finch, M., Kane, R. L., Phillip, I. (1994). Developing a new metric for ADLs. *Journal of the American Geriatrics Society, 43,* 877–884.

Kane, R. A., & Kane, R. L. (1981). *Assessing the elderly.* Ravensdale, WA: Idyll Arbor, Lexington Books.

Katz, S., Ford, A. B., Moskowitz, R. W., Jackson, B. A., & Jaffe, M. W. (1963). Studies of illness in the aged. The index of ADL: A standardized measure of biological and psychosocial function. *Journal of the American Medical Association, 185,* 914–919.

Kiresuk, T. J., Smith, A., Cardillo, J. E. (1994). *Goal attainment scaling: Applications, theory, and measurement.* Mahwah, NJ: Lawrence Erlbaum Associates.

Lambert, M. J. (1983). Introduction to assessment of psychotherapy outcome: Historical perspective and current issues. In M. J. Lambert, E. R. Christensen, & S. S. DeJulio (Eds.), *The assessment of psychotherapy outcome* (pp. 3–32). New York: Wiley.

Lambert, M. J., & Brown, G. S. (1996). Data-based management for tracking outcome in private practice. *Clinical Psychology: Science and Practice, 3,* 172–178.

Langer, E. J., & Rodin, J. (1976). The effects of choice and enhanced personal responsibility for the aged: A field experiment in an institutional setting. *Journal of Personality and Social Psychology, 34,* 191–198.

Rockwood, K. (1995). Integration of research methods and outcome measures: Comprehensive care for the frail elderly. *Canadian Journal of Aging, 14,* 151–164.

Rodin, J., & Langer, E. (1977). Long-term effects on a control-relevant intervention with the institutionalized aged. *Journal of Personality and Social Psychology, 35,* 897–902.

Stolee, P., Stadnyk, K., Myers, A. M., & Rockwood, K. (1999). An individualized approach to outcome measurement in geriatric rehabilitation. *Journal of Gerontology, 54,* 641–647.

Stolee, P., Zaza, C., Pedlar, A., & Myers, A. M. (1999). Clinical experience with goal attainment scaling in geriatric care. *Journal of Aging and Health, 11,* 96–124.

Thompson, L. W., & Gallagher-Thompson, D. (1997). Psychotherapeutic interventions with older adults in outpatient and extended care settings. In R. L. Rubinstein & M. P. Lawton (Eds.), *Depression in long-term and residential care: Advances in research and treatment* (pp. 169–184). New York: Springer.

Walk, D., Fleishman, R., & Mandelson, J. (1999). Functional improvement of elderly residents of institutions. *The Gerontologist, 39,* 720–728.

Yip, A. M., Gorman, M. C., Stadnyk, K., Mills, W. G. M., MacPherson, K. M., & Rockwood, K. (1998). A standardized menu for goal attainment scaling in the care of frail elders. *The Gerontologist, 38,* 735–742.

REFERENCES TO INSTRUMENTS

American Psychiatric Association. (1994). *Diagnostic and statistical manual of mental disorders* (4th ed.). Washington, DC: Author.

Folstein, M. F., Folstein, S. E., & McHugh, P. R. (1975). "Mini-mental state." A practical method for grading the cognitive state of patients for the clinician. *Journal of Psychiatry Research, 33,* 189–198.

George, L. K., & Fillenbaum, G. G. (1985). OARS methodology: A decade of experience in geriatric assessment. *Journal of the American Geriatrics Society, 33,* 607–615.

Hall, R. C. W. (1995). Global assessment of functioning. A modified scale. *Psychosomatics, 36(3),* 267–275.

Hedlund, J. L., & Vieweg, B. W. (1980). The brief psychiatric rating scale (BPRS): A comprehensive review. *Journal of Operational Psychiatry, 11,* 48–65.

Helmes, E., Csapo, K. G., & Short, J. (1987). Standardization and validation of the multi-dimensional observation scale for elderly subjects (MOSES). *Journal of Gerontology, 42(4)*, 395–405.

Jones, S. H., Thornicroft, G., Coffey, M., & Dunn, G. (1995). A brief mental health outcome scale. Reliability and validity of the Global Assessment of Functioning (GAF). *British Journal of Psychiatry, 166*, 654–659.

Katz, S., Ford, A. B., Moskowitz, R. W., Jackson, B. A., & Jaffe, M. W. (1963). Studies of illness in the aged. The index of ADL: A standardized measure of biological and psychosocial function. *Journal of the American Medical Association, 185*, 914–919.

Kennedy, C. C., Madra, P., & Reddon, J. R. (1999). Assessing treatment outcome in psychogeriatric patients: The utility of the Global Assessment of Functioning Scale. *Clinical Gerontologist, 20(3)*, 3–11.

Lambert, M. J., Hatfield, D., Vermeersch, D. A., Hansen, N. B., Finch, A. E., Whipple, J., & Burlingame, G. M. (2000). *Administration and scoring manual for the Outcome Questionnaire (OQ-45.2)*. Wharton, NJ: American Professional Credential Services.

Lambert, M. J., Okiishi, J. C., Finch, A. E., & Johnson, L. D. (1998). Outcome assessment: From conceptualization to implementation. *Professional Psychology: Research and Practice, 29*, 63–70.

Pfeiffer, R. I., Kurosaki, T. T., Harrah, C. H., Chance, J. M., & Filos, S. (1982). Measurement of functional activities in older adults in the community. *Journal of Gerontology, 37(3)*, 323–329.

Piersma, H. L., & Boes, J. L. (1997). The GAF and psychiatric outcome. A descriptive report. *Community Mental Health Journal, 33(1)*, 35–41.

Overall, J. E. (1988). The brief psychiatric rating scale (BPRS): Recent developments in ascertainment and scaling. *Psychopharmacology Bulletin, 24(1)*, 97–99.

Overall, J. E., & Gorham, D. R. (1962). The brief psychiatric rating scale. *Psychological Reports, 10*, 799–812.

Sheikh, J. I., & Yesavage, J. A. (1986). Geriatric Depression Scale (GDS): Recent evidence and development of a shorter version. In T. L. Brink (Ed.), *Clinical gerontology: A guide to assessment and intervention* (pp. 165–173). New York: Haworth Press.

Stolee, P., Stadnyk, K., Myers, A. M., & Rockwood, K. (1999). An individualized approach to outcome measurement in geriatric rehabilitation. *Journal of Gerontology, 54(12)*, 641–647.

Travis, S. S. (1988). Observer-rated functional assessments for institutionalized elders. *Nursing Research, 37(3)*, 138–143.

van Marwijk, H. W., Wallace, P., de Bock, G. H., Hermans, J., Kaptein, A. A., & Mulder, J. D. (1995). Evaluation of the feasibility, reliability and diagnostic value of shortened versions of the geriatric depression scale. *British Journal of General Practice, 45*, 195–199.

III

Interventions in
Residential Care

7

Psychosocial Interventions: General Principles for Use in Geriatric Residential Care Facilities

Patrick Dulin
Advanced Behavioral Care

INTRODUCTION

Residents of extended care facilities struggle with a variety of mental health issues. It has been estimated that as many as 50% of nursing home residents suffer from a diagnosable mood disorder and a high number of the "healthy" residents report elevated levels of boredom and unhappiness (Smyer & Wilson, 1991). This does not mean, however, that demoralization and depression are normal and expected events for elderly individuals. There is convincing evidence that elderly adults often experience an increase in happiness as they age (Mroczek & Kolarz, 1998). It is thus clear that nursing homes could more effectively address mental health issues among residents. Fortunately, there are a variety of fundamental psychosocial techniques that can help residents feel satisfied with their lives and free from debilitating mood disorders.

The goal of this chapter is to provide research-based information regarding both the issues that geriatric residents face and the interventions proven to be helpful. There are two basic assumptions that pervade this chapter: (a) Interactions and relationships between staff and residents can contribute to, or detract from, resident health and functioning; and (b) Geriatric residents frequently struggle with a sense of helplessness which can be diminished by interventions focusing on empowerment, both environmentally and internally. The first section of this chapter discusses the importance of the staff's accurate conceptualization of residents and the therapeutic utility of personalized relationships between staff and residents.

The second section focuses on empowerment strategies that have been found to increase psychological functioning and longevity among residents of extended care facilities.

CONCEPTUALIZING RESIDENTS: THE IMPORTANCE OF ACCURACY

There are a variety of frameworks used to conceptualize residents' presenting behavioral and mood symptoms. Some are more productive and and helpful than others. I first discuss a nonproductive and potentially damaging approach that is regrettably common in residential care facilities. This is an important perspective to discuss because it is very easy to adopt if helpers are not mindful of this possibility. I will to refer to this method of conceptualizing residents as the knee-jerk approach. The knee-jerk approach is one in which staff conceptualize resident's behaviors with the first idea that comes to mind, which is often negative in nature. For example, Mr. Jones, a 79 year-old male, a recently admitted resident with a broken hip and cognitive decline, is cursing loudly and swinging at staff who are trying to shower him. The knee-jerk assessment of Mr. Jones is that he is a rude and spiteful elderly man. This is indeed a harsh judgment of Mr. Jones, and is based on very little information. Before dismissing the knee-jerk approach as something that only abusive people use, keep in mind that this is a surprisingly common interpersonal process that social psychologists refer to as the fundamental attribution error (Ross, 1977).

The fundamental attribution error refers to the propensity of people to attribute another's behavior to negative internal dispositions. A classic example of the fundamental attribution error occurs when you witness a man in front of you in the checkout line yelling at the cashier. The knee-jerk assessment of that person is that they are rude and unruly. However, it could very well be that he has a wonderful disposition, but recently was fired from his job, or the cashier was trying to shortchange him, or maybe the cashier told him he was fat and unattractive. The possibilities are endless. The point is that human beings have a strong tendency to attribute negative behavior to a bad temperament instead of situational factors like justified anger about being cheated or insulted.

Research has demonstrated that negative labeling, likely secondary to the fundamental attribution error, is prevalent in nursing homes. For instance, Suzanne Meeks (1996) studied staff members' conceptualizations of depressed residents' behavior. She found that staff focused on the residents as disruptive, noncompliant, or demanding, labels that reflect a negative internal disposition. The residents attributions about the source of their own distress was more situationally based. Residents focused on dissatisfaction with their living situation or difficulty coping with physical problems and pain as causing their distress. The level of agreement between staff and residents about the nature of presenting problems was quite low in this study, about 16%. The study highlights the tendency for staff members to blame and negatively label residents for their "difficult" behavior.

Negative dispositional labeling is likely more prevalent with regard to elderly individuals. Rodin and Langer (1980) demonstrated that younger people frequently label the elderly as incompetent, out of touch with reality, helpless, senile, and sick. Research has indicated that ageist labels such as these serve to infantalize residents and lead to increased levels of psychological dysfunction among nursing home residents. Langer and Benevento (1978) demonstrated that once residents were given a label such as "helpless," they were subsequently expected to function at a lower level. They were given easier tasks to perform, catered to, and given less responsibility for their own care. The predictable result was increased helplessness and lowered self-esteem within the residents. This and other research indicates that negative, patronizing labels can create a self-fulfilling prophecy (Ryan, Hamilton, & Kwong See, 1994). Given time, residents begin to manifest characteristics of the label.

On a more optimistic note, psychological research has shown that the fundamental attribution error is essentially fixable. People can make accurate attributions, but it requires effort focused on gathering information about the individual being assessed (Gilbert, Krull, & Penman, 1988). In the nursing home context, it is important to explore situational factors that may contribute to "difficult" behavior. For instance, with Mr. Jones, the resident who was combative when being showered, an examination of triggering factors will likely lead to an understandable reaction to uncomfortable circumstances. It is possible that Mr. Jones has always taken baths instead of showering. He may feel that he is being forced into a situation that is uncomfortable, causing fear and irritation leading to subsequent aggressive behavior. It is difficult to label Mr. Jones as "mean and unruly" when the situation is fully understood.

Another method of reducing negative labeling is to develop an approach that focuses on discovering residents' strengths. Residents are usually focused primarily on disabilities and personal limitations; after all, that is the primary reason for their placement in the facility. They may have forgotten, or no longer credit themselves with retained abilities and competencies. An exploration of their strengths, particularly the abilities they have performed throughout their life and are consistent with their sense of self can aid the helper to view them as individuals who have both strengths and deficits; not as people who are globally impaired and incompetent. As is discussed later, this process is also empowering to the resident.

In sum, time spent developing personalized relationships with residents serves the purpose of accurately conceptualizing residents and avoiding the assignment of negative, dispositional labeling. Perhaps more importantly, personalized relationships also facilitate psychological healing and growth. Following is a discussion of the therapeutic utility of developing individualized, helpful relationships and techniques for facilitating this type of relationship.

THE THERAPEUTIC UTILITY OF INDIVIDUAL RELATIONSHIPS BETWEEN STAFF AND RESIDENTS: A PRIMARY FACTOR IN TREATMENT INTERVENTION

The lack of personalized relationships between staff and residents has been shown to be one of the primary impediments to quality care of geriatric residents in nursing homes (Bowers, Esmond, & Jacobson, 2000; Mattiasson & Anderson, 1997). Barbara Bowers (2000) demonstrated that a personalized relationship between residents and a nurse aide resulted in greater attention to the resident's care needs and the provision of an informal treatment for depression. The development of personal relationships between staff and residents in this study was more significant than simply facilitating a resident's comfort with a caretaker. These personalized relationship likely served to provide the resident with support and validation; two commodities that are in short supply in nursing homes. This study highlights the notion that having a relationship with an individual staff member can serve as a psychosocial intervention in itself.

Many decades of research evaluating the beneficial factors of psychotherapy have consistently shown that aspects of the relationship between therapist and client accounts for a large portion of the effectiveness of therapy (Frank, 1974; Lambert & Bergin, 1994). Although it is not the intention of this chapter to provide instruction about providing psychotherapy to geriatric residents, there are lessons to be learned from psychotherapy research that bear directly on the issue of developing helpful relationships between staff members and residents.

The aspects of a psychotherapeutic relationship that are effective in bringing about positive change are actually not difficult to grasp. These techniques, which can be taught and used by a wide variety of care providers are discussed in the next two sections. Nurses, recreation therapists, nurse aides, and social workers can use these skills to bring about therapeutic effects for residents.

BASIC LISTENING AND VALIDATION

As a psychological consultant to nursing homes, I am frequently frustrated to find that residents are told by staff members that their concerns are invalid or inappropriate. It is often the case that staff members have not adequately heard the residents concerns in the first place. An example of this type of interaction that occurs on a daily basis, goes something like this: Resident (Joan): "I am tired of all these problems, and this place is so horrible, I wish I could just die." Staff: "Oh, come on now, Joan. You don't really want to die. You have lot's to live for." The predictable resident response to this nontherapeutic comment is arguing and resentment. After all, the resident was given the message that her concerns are invalid and that she is "being silly." Nontherapeutic, contradictory comments not only fail to be helpful, they often make the problem worse.

Remember that it is basically impossible to argue residents out of bad feelings. When residents feel that staff members are not listening and don't understand their problems, they tend to feel more alone, more irritable, and resentful. These are obviously psychological states that are aversive and likely lead to more behavior problems (and more work for staff in the long run).

Listening is an underrated psychosocial intervention, especially in the nursing home, where residents often feel abandoned and isolated. The act of someone taking the time to sit down for a few minutes and hear a resident's difficulties allows the resident to work through problematic issues and develop a more healthy perspective. There are a few skills that facilitate good listening that many people seem to know about, but seldom put into practice (Ivey, 1994). The first skill is attending. Attending refers to a set of behaviors that communicate to residents that they are being listened to. Examples of attending behaviors are looking at residents, orienting your body towards theirs, nodding your head, and letting them finish ideas without interruption. Attending behaviors connote the simple yet therapeutic message that "I am here for you and I want to understand your difficulties."

A second set of listening skills, which are easily recognized as belonging to a therapist's "bag of tricks," is called reflection. Reflection refers to the act of reflecting back to residents what you heard them say with a paraphrased comment. When reflecting with a paraphrase, simply tell residents what they told you in an abbreviated format. For example—Resident: "After my husband died and I lost my house and was forced to move in here, I haven't known what to do with myself." Staff: "It sounds like you've been through a lot and now feel lost." Notice in this example that the staff member paraphrased what the resident said and added a guess about what this may have felt like. The staff member included a reflection of affect, or feeling components of the message, which is very important when therapeutically listening to a person. When reflecting back the affective components of a statement, don't be afraid to guess about what the emotion may be. The resident will seldom be offended by a wrong guess and will most likely respond by correcting you and describing what it personally felt like.

Reflecting the affective aspects of a resident's communication is a helpful intervention because it facilitates an awareness of emotions and enhances the subsequent ability to work through them (Ivey, 1994). As has been frequently written in the psychotherapeutic arena, the first step in the process of change is to develop awareness within the client about the different emotions surrounding the problem (Mahoney, 1991). For instance, in the previous example with Joan, it is quite possible that with some exploration through reflection of affect, Joan could discover that she was not only "lost," but also felt angry and sad. Helping Joan to gain awareness into her different emotions will undoubtedly help her work through her issues about being placed in a nursing home.

Validation is another basic therapeutic technique that is simple and effective. Validation refers to the process of acknowledging the validity of another's difficulties. People are often helped by simply being heard and told by someone that their feelings are valid and that they are not having unreasonable "over the top" reactions. For instance, a validating response to Joan's frustration and wish to die would be "You know, Joan, this is a hard situation to face, I can see how you feel that way." Staff are often afraid to validate residents feelings for fear that they will make residents feel worse by agreeing with them. It is very seldom that a validating comment will lead to worse feelings. Validating comments typically create an environment in which a person can explore feelings and work through difficulties (Ivey, 1994).

A foreseeable reaction to the notion of using more listening and empathic responses towards residents is "I just don't have time for that." It is obvious that most staff members are extremely busy taking care of numerous residents with a variety of intensive needs and may find it difficult to develop a personalized, helpful relationship with each resident. However, one of the most time consuming and troublesome aspects of caring for geriatric residents is the high degree of psychological distress and subsequent behavior problems that are often labeled "attention seeking," such as frequent use of the call light. The development of helpful, personalized relationships will likely result in decreased psychological distress, which in turn leads to less "attention seeking," and in the long run, less toil for the staff. Personalized relationships with a focus on listening, communication of understanding, and validation can be thought of as preventative treatments that may initially take more of staff's time, but in the long run result in less work and a better environment for both staff and residents.

EMPOWERMENT AS A THERAPEUTIC TOOL

Perhaps the most pervasive and psychologically damaging feeling that geriatric residents struggle with is helplessness: the belief that one can no longer exercise control over basic life issues. Possessing the belief that it is possible to bring about the good things and avoid the bad is a powerful contributor to a person's overall sense of well-being, a belief that has received a great deal of attention by researchers (Rodin, 1986). A label that psychologists have used for the belief that one can effect some type of desired change in their environment is self-efficacy (Bandura, 1986). Numerous empirical studies have shown that among a variety of factors measured among nursing home residents, deficits in self-efficacy are frequently the most toxic and result in the most elevated levels of depression and poor nursing home adjustment (Herzog, Johnson, Franks, Markus, & Holmberg, 1998; Holohan & Holohan, 1987; Johnson, Stone, Altmaier, & Berdahl, 1998).

Research has repeatedly demonstrated that self-efficacy has a great deal of gravity in the prediction of both physical and mental health of elderly individuals. For instance, Herzog et al. (1998) demonstrated that among a variety of demographic and social variables measured in a study of 1400 elderly adults, self-efficacy was the strongest predictor of depression and poor physical health. Johnson et al. (1998) also found that self-efficacy was the strongest predictor of adjustment to a nursing home among a variety of psychological and demographic variables including age, education, marital status, self-efficacy, and internal locus of control. In this study, those residents with heightened levels of self-efficacy reported higher levels of positive affect (vigor) and activity levels.

Not only has self-efficacy been shown to be an important contributor to psychological health variables, it has also been demonstrated to be predictive of mortality. In a landmark study of the relationship between self-efficacy and mortality, Langer and Rodin (1976) compared residents who were encouraged to make decisions about their daily activities and engage in care taking behaviors with those who were not. They found that residents who were given the opportunity to take care of a plant and make rudimentary decisions about their daily lives were not only more active and happy than those that were not given these opportunities, they were also much more likely to be alive one year later (Rodin & Langer, 1977).

These studies, taken as a whole, converge on a central finding: Elderly adults' sense of themselves as being able to have control over their environment, make choices for themselves, and provide care to something outside themselves are all strongly related to mental health, physical health, and mortality. This is obviously a variable that deserves attention when designing treatment interventions with this population.

From an intuitive point of view it is easily understood how depression and demoralization develop within nursing home residents. Consider for a moment what it would be like to be in a situation in which you could no longer get up and go for a walk, make your own food, change your own clothes, make it to the bathroom when you feel the urge, or change yourself when you soil your clothes. Being unable to control these rudimentary activities of living that you have taken for granted during all of your adult life would obviously lead to the belief that "I can't do anything anymore," a comment that is heard on a daily basis within a nursing home. Even a small amount of empathy with the situation in which geriatric residents frequently find themselves results in an understanding of the power of helplessness to bring on depressive episodes.

To some readers, the term self-efficacy may be unwieldy, overly scientific, and difficult to relate to. Perhaps a better term that captures the spirit of the belief and ability to make changes in one's life is empowerment. After all, the aim of many interventions is to imbue residents with the power to increase the amount of good and decrease the amount of bad in their lives. The next section discusses techniques that can be used to increase empowerment in two important areas of geriatric resident's existence, their everyday environment and their internal, mental world.

Techniques for Bolstering Environmental Empowerment.

In many ways, individuals admitted to a nursing home have lost their ability to be effective in their everyday environment. In fact, an inability to care for oneself in the home is frequently the factor that precipitates placement in a residential facility. The fact that they have lost functioning and need intensive care is obvious. However, their inability to care for themselves at home does not mean they have lost the ability to care for themselves in a nursing home. This is an important distinction to make, and if not attended to, can result in the resident being labeled as entirely dependent and needy. It is thus important to encourage and empower residents to perform the self-care activities that they are still in control of.

The first step in the process of empowering residents to perform self-care is to undertake an examination of the resident's strengths. Scanning through the list of activities of daily living (ADLs) will facilitate this process. It is usually the case that the resident will be able to perform at least one or two ADLs. For instance, maybe certain residents have lost the ability to transfer and use the shower independently but are still able to wash their face, brush their teeth, and toilet themselves. A simple and helpful intervention that serves to bolster empowerment is to help residents understand which activities they can perform and discuss with them the importance of their utilization. This could help reduce the helplessness-inducing belief that they can't take care of themselves anymore. The result of a focus on strengths is the development of an orientation toward what residents can do, instead of what they are unable to do.

Another area of environmental empowerment exists with recreational activities. Although it may be difficult to provide empowerment through ADLs because of physical disabilities, it is almost always the case that a resident can choose which recreational activities they would like to engage in. First of all, make sure that residents know about the recreational activities that are available to them. Provide them with a list of activities and ask them to choose the ones they would like to engage in and at what time. Again, remind residents that they have choices about recreation and are not required to attend the activities. Keep in mind that empowerment results from individual choice making. It follows that residents will benefit most by choosing activities for themselves.

Empowerment can also be achieved through the act of caring for something or someone else. Caring for something outside the self creates the opportunity for the belief that one can make a difference in the life of another (Adler, 1937). Care-taking, or engaging in altruistic behaviors can be a particularly fruitful area to explore with geriatric residents, especially given the common geriatric resident belief of "I am no good to anyone anymore." Psychological research has demonstrated a connection between engaging in altruistic acts and positive mental health outcomes including lower mortality (Musick, Herzog, & House, 1999). A study performed by Dulin, Hill, Anderson, & Rasmussen (2000) indicated that performing altruistic activities was associated with high levels of positive affect and low levels of depression among a group of elderly individuals. It is noteworthy that within this study altruism was associated with positive mental health functioning to a greater extent than received social support. This finding underscores the notion that "doing for others" can result in better mood functioning than "receiving from others" among elderly adults.

When using care-taking behaviors as a psychosocial intervention, an examination of existing strengths is a worthwhile initial step. It will frequently be found that residents can no longer engage in the helpful activities of their past, but an exploration of retained helpful abilities can make salient the fact that they are still useful to others and able to make a difference. For instance, the resident may no longer be able to fix a broken sink, bake cookies for the grandkids, or mow the neighbor's yard, but they likely can still provide companionship, support, and advice to others. A technique that I frequently use when providing psychotherapy to depressed nursing home residents is to identify another resident to whom my client can be helpful, and then provide a minimal amount of instruction about how to be helpful. It is regrettably easy to identify someone in need of companionship or support in a nursing home. Once a helpee is identified, all that usually needs to be done is to tell the resident that the other resident could use someone to talk with and is having difficulty adjusting to the facility. It is my experience that they usually figure out how to specifically help the other resident. After using this type of intervention, their role as a helper frequently becomes the primary topic of our sessions.

It is also helpful to identify a family member who is in need of their support: a grandchild in trouble, a lonely sibling, or depressed child. There is usually someone in their family who could (and probably already does) benefit from their support and companionship. Making the fact salient that they are still needed by their family, even if they can no longer be helpful in ways they once were can have empowering effects and result in improved familial relationships.

The provision of care is not restricted to people. As mentioned earlier, the act of simply caring for a plant has been shown to result in dramatically improved mental and physical health for nursing home residents (Langer & Rodin, 1976). For those residents who have no interest in helping others, caring for a plant or animal will suffice to increase empowerment. An important lesson about how this technique can be helpful is garnered from Langer and Rodin's (1976) study. In their study, all of the residents were given plants to care for. The residents who benefitted from receiving the plant were those who were told that they, not the nurse, were responsible for its care. The residents who were told that the nurse was responsible for the plant did not benefit from the intervention. It appears that taking responsibility for something and independently providing care is the therapeutic factor within these interventions.

When encouraging care-taking behaviors among residents, it is important to take an experiential tact. In other words, residents are more likely to agree to care for a person, plant, or animal if the object in need of help is right in front of them than if it is proposed as an idea. A depressed resident will frequently say "no" to most ideas about activities, but when shown the actual object (person, plant, or animal) will have less of a proclivity to be negative. It is important to keep in mind that human beings have strong tendencies to be cooperative and helpful. Facilitating the expression of this aspect of human nature can have a variety of beneficial results (Adler, 1937), particularly among geriatric residents.

Enhancing Internal Empowerment.

Unfortunately, there are numerous individuals residing in geriatric residential facilities who are simply no longer able to perform care-taking behaviors or other externally empowering acts. For instance, individuals who are paralyzed, have amputations, or an inability to speak coherently due to aphasia may experience great difficulty engaging in both their own care and the care of others. These can be difficult people to intervene with because external activity options are vastly reduced and their level of demoralization is understandably high. There is hope, however, with severely disabled individuals. Residents such as these, although out of control of external factors, can engage in internally oriented, experiential activities that enhance a sense of control over psychological distress.

Internal empowerment refers to the ability to exert control over internal states. As with external empowerment, there is empirical evidence supporting the therapeutic utility of activities that create peace of mind and relaxation. For instance, Alexendar, Langer, Newman, Chandler, and Davies (1989) demonstrated that the use of meditation and "mindfulness" exercises (exercises that encourage the creation of new ways of thinking about situations) resulted in significant beneficial effects, both physical and psychological, compared with control groups. In this study, the meditation and mindfulness groups felt less old, reported being able to cope better with inconvenience, felt more patient, and reported higher levels of feeling in control of their lives after meditating and being more "mindful". A striking follow-up finding was the difference in mortality among the groups. Three years after the interventions were performed, 25% to 40% of the control groups had died, while 12% of the mindfulness group and 0% of the meditation group had passed away. This study presents convincing evidence that internally oriented, experiential techniques have the potential to produce impressive effects regarding both psychological and physical health.

Relaxation training is another method geriatric residents can use to exercise control over internal states. Researchers have demonstrated that relaxation training has a variety of uses with elderly populations that include reduction in anxiety (Scogin, Rickard, Keith, Wilson, & McElreath, 1992), improvement in tension headaches (Mosley, Grothues, & Meeks, 1995), and reduction in pain (Moye & Hanlon, 1996). There is also evidence that the effects of relaxation training are long-lasting. For instance, Rickard, Scogin, & Keith (1994) demonstrated that reductions in psychological symptoms and anxiety were maintained one year after the relaxation training took place.

A variety of relaxation training methods are available, but all have a few factors in common (Lantz, Buchalter, & McBee, 1997). All forms of relaxation training engage the user in a process that encourages deep breathing, the reduction of tension within the body, and a cognitive strategy (e.g., internally repeating the word "relax" during the process) for bringing about the relaxation response. Progressive muscle relaxation (Bernstein & Borkovec, 1973) is a widely used relaxation training method that enhances relaxation through the alternate tension and relaxation of specific body parts, starting with the toes and moving to the head. A study by Scogin, et al. (1992) demonstrated that progressive muscle relaxation was effective in reducing anxiety and psychological symptoms among elderly adults. This study also demonstrated that a relaxation procedure that does not require intact physical functioning was also helpful. Imaginal relaxation, which involves simply imagining that the muscle groups are tensing and relaxing, was found to be equally as effective as the actual progressive muscle relaxation procedure in reducing anxiety and other psychological symptoms. This is an important finding, as many geriatric residents are unable to alternately tense and relax muscles as a result of conditions such as stroke and arthritis.

Meditation and relaxation techniques have been shown to be teachable within a group format to geriatric residents with a wide range of cognitive functioning, including dementia. Lantz et al. (1997) described a six-session "wellness group" for use within a nursing home that uses meditation, guided imagery, and relaxation techniques. The authors of this study indicated that they were surprised at the extent to which residents with dementing illnesses benefited from the group. All members of the wellness group were perceived by staff to be less agitated, and certain individual residents became less physically aggressive and verbally disruptive. The authors also discussed an illustrative case example of an elderly gentleman who partook in their wellness group:

> Mr. I is an 84-year-old man with moderate dementia of the Alzheimer type and prominent physical aggression, which included punching, kicking, and hitting staff, most frequently during the delivery of care. He required the presence of 3 to 4 nursing assistants in order to bathe or shower, and many staff members suffered injuries as a result of his aggression. Mr. I became an immediate and regular member of the group who was able to engage in most of the tasks. During group time, he was never physically aggressive and appeared calm. Staff members who observed the group expressed surprise at his abilities, and were able to view him as someone other than an aggressor. Over time, their perceptions changed and his improved abilities to cope were reflected in a reduction in overt aggression and less resistance to care. He is now offered time to utilize breathing and meditation techniques prior to bathing, and only requires the supervision of one or two staff members. (Lantz et al., 1997, p. 554).

Groups such as this one are not difficult to implement and can be facilitated by a wide variety of care professionals. There are a variety of ways to design meditation and relaxation groups for geriatric residents, and the reader is encouraged to develop a method that fits within their particular care setting. Keep in mind, however, that research has demonstrated that for wellness groups to be maximally effective, it is important to keep the instructions simple, actively involve the residents, and set clear goals for each session (Moye & Hanlon, 1996).

Relaxation and meditation techniques, only recently implemented in extended care facilities, appear to be a very fruitful means with which to address psychological distress within geriatric residential care facilities. First of all, they provide residents with specific techniques they can use to soothe themselves and "do something" about their psychological distress. It is my experience that most residents of nursing homes will acknowledge the fact that although they can not engage in many previously enjoyed activities, they can still have an influence on their peace of mind.

Meditation and relaxation techniques are likely effective with this population because they accomplish two therapeutic outcomes. They first of all challenge the helplessness-inducing belief of "I can't do anything about my life, and I will always feel miserable." Second, they provide a specific method for reducing distress that has immediate and noticeable effects.

BARRIERS TO EFFECTIVE TREATMENT IMPLEMENTATION

As with most new ideas that enter existing organizations, there will likely be a significant amount of resistance to their implementation. Psychosocial interventions have a tendency to be placed on the "unnecessary" list within medically oriented facilities. Nursing homes typically adhere to a medical model of care, which gives primary importance to physical issues and often neglects problems that are more psychosocial in nature. It is hoped that one of the lessons learned from this chapter is that psychosocial and medical issues can not be neatly disentangled; psychosocial problems have an influence on medical–physical functioning and vice versa. Much of the research cited within this chapter supports the notion that in order to provide the most effective care for residents, psychosocial interventions must be given a high priority and must be fully supported by those in leadership roles if they are to be broadly effective.

Staff members also develop routines and habits for providing care and may be resistant to changing them in order to accommodate new interventions. They likely need to be given both encouragement and continued education about the effective use of psychosocial interventions within extended care facilities. It is my experience that most staff within extended care facilities are unaware of the interventions discussed within this chapter. Once made aware, they are frequently excited to have new tools in their "bag of tricks." Staff education regarding specific psychosocial interventions for use with a diverse array of residents can be facilitated with in-service training from psychologists or other qualified mental health personnel.

It is also plausible that staff members feel that the residents they serve are too old and incapable of making progress with psychosocial interventions. This is a common ageist belief that should be addressed and replaced with more realistic assumptions about elderly individuals. As noted elsewhere within this chapter, research has repeatedly demonstrated that elderly individuals can make remarkable progress with the appropriate use of psychosocial interventions.

A final caveat about the use of the techniques mentioned herein is that for many depressed or anxious elderly individuals, these interventions alone will not be enough. Severely depressed or anxious residents will require more intensive treatment from a qualified mental health provider. For instance, elderly individuals who have no appetite, are losing weight, severely withdrawn, and disengaged from all pleasurable activity will likely require a combination of antidepressant medication and psychotherapy to recover. Residents with severe symptoms will need to be referred to a psychologist or psychiatrist who is familiar with geriatric issues.

CONCLUSION

As noted elsewhere in this book, the current culture and interpersonal climate of nursing homes does not facilitate positive mental health functioning. In fact, there is compelling evidence that nursing homes, as they are currently operated, actually engender poor mental health functioning. Fortunately, there is much that can be done to change the overall climate through the implementation of a few simple principles and techniques.

First, staff can improve resident functioning by accurately conceptualizing the resident and avoiding rapid, pejorative judgements. Second, the use of easily learned listening and validating skills will help residents to feel understood and acknowledged, perceptions that will reduce psychological distress. Finally, residents of extended care facilities suffer from depression and demoralization largely as a result of low self-efficacy. Techniques that facilitate both external and internal empowerment will help residents feel more able and valued. Implementing such techniques will likely result in a more pleasant and enriching environment for both residents and staff.

REFERENCES

Adler, A. (1937). Mass psychology. *International Journal of Individual Psychology, Second Quarter,* 111–120.

Alexander, C. N., Langer, E. J., Newman, R. I., Chandler, H. M., & Davies, J. L. (1989). Transcendental meditation, mindfulness, and longevity: An experimental study with the elderly. *Journal of Personality and Social Psychology, 57,* 6, 950–964.

Bandura, A. (1986). *Social foundations of thought and action.* Englewood Cliffs, NJ: Prentice-Hall.

Bernstein, D. A., & Borkovec, T. D. (1973). *Progressive relaxation training: A manual for the helping professionals.* Champagne, IL: Research Press.

Bowers, B.J ., Esmond, S., & Jacobson, N. (2000). The relationship between staffing and quality in long-term care facilities: Exploring the views of nurse aides. *Journal of Nursing Care Quality, 14,* 4, 55–64.

Dulin, P., Hill, R. D., Anderson, J., & Rasmussen, D. (2001). Altruism as a predictor of life satisfaction in a sample of older adults. *Journal of Mental Health and Aging*, in press.

Frank, J. (1974). *Persuasion and healing. A comparative study of psychotherapy*. Baltimore: Johns Hopkins Press.

Gilbert, D., Krull, D. S., & Penman, B. W. (1988). Of thoughts unspoken: Social inference and the self-regulation of behavior. *Journal of Personality and Social Psychology, 55,* 685–694.

Herzog, A. R., Franks, M. M., Markus, H. R., & Holmberg, D. (1998). Activities and well-being in older age: Effects of self-concept and educational attainment. *Psychology and Aging, 13,* 2, 179–185.

Holohan, C. K., & Holohan, C. J. (1987). Life stress, hassles, and self-efficacy in aging: A replication and extension. Journal of Applied and Social Psychology, 17, 574–592.

Ivey, A. (1994). *Intentional interviewing and counseling: Facilitating client development in a multicultural society,* (3rd ed.). Pacific Grove, CA: Brooks/Cole.

Johnson, B. S., Stone, G. L., Altmaier, E. M., & Berdahl, L. D. (1998). The relationship of demographic factors, locus of control and self-efficacy to successful nursing home adjustment. *The Gerontologist, 38,* 2, 209–216.

Lambert, M. J., & Bergin, A. E. (1994). The effectiveness of psychotherapy. In A. E. Bergin & S. L. Garfield (Eds.), *Handbook of psychotherapy and behavior change* (pp. 207–243). New York: Wiley.

Langer, E. J., & Benevento, A. (1978). Self-induced dependence. *Journal of Personality and Social Psychology, 36,* 8, 886–893.

Langer, E. J. & Rodin, J. (1976). The effects of choice and enhanced personal responsibility for the aged: A field experiment in an institutional setting. *Journal of Personality and Social Psychology, 34,* 191–198.

Lantz, M. S., Buchalter, D. D., & McBee, L. (1997). The wellness group: A novel intervention for coping with disruptive behavior in elderly nursing home residents. *The Gerontologist, 37,* 4, 551–556.

Mahoney, M. J. (1991). *Human change processes*. New York: Basic Books.

Mattiasson, A. C., & Andersson, L. (1997). Quality of nursing home care assessed by competent nursing home patients. *Journal of Advanced Nursing, 26,* 1117–1124.

Meeks, S. (1996). Psychological consultation to nursing homes: Description of a six-year practice. *Psychotherapy, 33,* 1, 19–29.

Mosley, T. H., Grothues, C. A., & Meeks, W. M. (1995). Treatment of tension headache in the elderly: A controlled evaluation of relaxation training and relaxation training combined with cognitive–behavior therapy. *Journal of Clinical Geropsychology, 1,* 3, 175–188.

Moye, J., & Hanlon, S. (1996). Relaxation training for nursing home patients: Suggestions for simplifying and individualizing treatment. *Clinical Gerontologist, 16,* 3, 37–49.

Mroczek, D. K. & Kolarz, C. M. (1998). The effect of age on positive and negative affect: A developmental perspective on happiness. *Journal of Personality and Social Psychology, 75,* 1333–1339.

Musick, M. A., Herzog, A. R. & House, J. S. (1999). Volunteering and mortality among older adults: Findings from a national sample. *Journal of Gerontology: Social Sciences, 54B,* S173–S180.

Rickard, H. C., Scogin, F., & Keith, S. (1994). A one-year follow-up of relaxation training for elders with subjective anxiety. *Gerontologist, 34,* 1, 121–122.

Rodin, J. (1986). Aging and health: Effects of the sense of control. *Science, 233,* 1271–1276.

Rodin, J. & Langer, E. J. (1977). Long term effects of a control-relevant intervention with the institutionalized aged. *Journal of Personality and Social Psychology, 35,* 897–902.

Rodin, J., & Langer, E. (1980). Aging labels: The decline of control and the fall of self-esteem. *Journal of Social Issues, 36,* 12–29.

Ross, L. (1977). The intuitive psychologist and his shortcomings. In L. Berkowtiz (Ed.), *Advances in experimental social psychology,* (Vol. 10, pp. 173–220). New York: Academic Press.

Ryan, E. B., Hamilton, M. L., & Kwong See, S. K. (1994). Patronizing the old: How do younger and older adults respond to baby talk in the nursing home. *International Journal of Aging and Human Development, 39,* 21–32.

Scogin, F., Rickard, H. C., Keith, S., Wilson, J., & McElreath, L. (1992). Progressive and imaginal relaxation training for elderly persons with subjective anxiety. *Psychology and Aging, 7,* (3), 419–424.

Smyer, M. A., & Wilson, M. (1999). Critical issues and strategies in mental health consultation in nursing homes. In Duffy, M. (Ed.), *Handbook of counseling and psychotherapy with older adults* (pp. 364–377). New York: Wiley.

8

Managing Problematic Behaviors

Anthony Morrison
Infinia Corporation, Salt Lake City, Utah

INTRODUCTION

Behavior problems are a common occurrence in residential settings. For example, In U.S. nursing homes, the prevalence of behavior problems is between 64% and 83% (Allen-Burge, Stevens, & Burgio, 1999). The types of behaviors that are typically identified as problematic vary according to whom within the facility you are speaking. To the nursing staff it may be someone who constantly uses their call button, resulting in increased demands on nursing time to answer the call. To the administrator it may be a resident who hits others, which makes residents and their families more likely to look for alternative placement and may bring state investigators into the facility. To the family it may be a resident who isolates in his or her room and refuses to engage in activities, which raises concerns about depression and life satisfaction. Residents in facility settings will be identified as having problematic behavior if the behavior is inconsistent with the expectations of the reporting person or the behavior results in increased work or inconvenience for the reporting person. It is also useful to divide problematic behaviors into those that are identified as being disruptive to the facility, its residents, and staff, and those that impair the resident's quality of life (Allen-Burge et al., 1999).

TYPICAL BEHAVIOR PROBLEMS AND THEIR MOST COMMON MANIFESTATIONS

Although it is possible to write an entire book describing the types of behaviors identified as problematic with seniors in residential settings, this chapter is restricted to the most common problems and their most frequent manifestations. My intent is to help those who work or will work in these facilities to see that the problems that they encounter while performing the duties associated with their job are not unique. It is also true that an accurate description and understanding of the problem and its precipitants is the key to successful amelioration of the problematic behavior.

Frequent Use of the Call Button

The call button is an important part of a resident's world and represents the means by which a resident can call for help in an emergency or for nonemergency assistance with other activities. A person's reliance on the call button is affected by his or her capacity to do things independently and by personality variables that inform a resident's perception of their relationships with others. A person who is bedridden as a result of physical ailments has different needs than a person who can ambulate independently. In a similar way, residents who are used to having all of their needs met by others will have different expectations than residents who have been independent and self-reliant their whole life. There are regulations that require that a call button be responded to in a specified amount of time, and some facilities track the time via a computer system that can record usage and response time. However, if the staff perceive the resident as abusing or overusing the call button, then they may ignore the call or turn it off from the nursing station. Although not responding to the residents' call light violates the regulations, it has been observed in more than one facility.

For mental health professionals who consult to residential care facilities, the perceived overuse of the call button is one of the most common reasons for referral. If the staff determine that the resident is using the call button excessively, they will ask the mental health professional to help make him or her stop overusing it. Often there is little understanding on the part of the direct care staff about why the person is engaging in a behavior that is experienced as an annoyance to them. The staff may even personalize the behavior—one nurse was heard to say, "I know she was is only doing it to annoy me." The patient in question turned out to have a severe anxiety disorder which when appropriately treated resulted in a significant reduction in her use of the call button.

Although the overuse of the call button may seem like a peculiar reason to refer someone, it is often a significant issue for the staff who already feel overwhelmed. Job stress can lead to high turnover among staff if the incidence of behavior problems is high (Allen-Burge et al., 1999). For the patient, the overuse of the call button is often symptomatic of other processes that are going on in his or her life. The syndromes that can produce this behavior include anxiety, depression, adjustment reactions, dementia, delirium, and systemic illnesses that may have a fluctuating course.

Violent Behavior

Behavior that is labeled as violent can vary from a resident who uses harsh words with staff to the brutal beating of another resident or staff person. Once a resident is labeled as violent, it usually has a significant impact on how the staff as a whole respond to the person. A resident who is labeled as violent is less likely to receive the compassion of the staff and may have greater difficulty getting his or her needs met. "I'm not going in there on my own, I'm scared to," one nurse's aid said referring to a man who had been labeled as violent. Often these violent residents are identified as such because of a history of overt attacks on others. However, sometimes these labels are given inappropriately. One gentleman was referred for violent behavior because he was grabbing staff and sometimes refused to let go. It turned out that this man had had a stroke and had lost some of his motor and sensory capacity, so he could not tell how hard he was gripping things and had some difficulty with motor control. When the staff was educated about this man's deficits they were better able to work with him.

Although residents can be mislabeled as having a history of violent behavior, most facilities have had a least one situation where a resident or staff person has been beaten and injured by another resident of the facility. Some of the diseases that accompany the aging process affect a person's capacity to monitor his or her own behavior and to be able to accurately assess the degree of danger in a situation. Although many people may experience the impulse to strike out at another on occasion, most have the capacity to inhibit the impulse and to quickly review the consequences of such action. In a similar way, a person with intact cognitive functioning can accurately assess the danger that may be present in any given situation. A person whose cognitive functioning has been compromised may inaccurately perceive danger where there is none and may strike out in an attempt to protect themself. The dementias and progressive cerebrovascular diseases are the most common cause of permanent changes in brain functioning. The most common cause of transient alterations of brain functioning is delirium, which can result from many different etiologies (refer to chap. 5).

Repetitive Requests—Preservative Behavior

If you pay more than a few visits to a residential care facility you will likely encounter the resident who persistently asks the staff member sitting at the desk the same question over and over. It may sound something like this: "Is my daughter here?" "No, she said she will be here at 6:00 p.m." "Are you sure?" "Yes E … ! This is the fifth time you have asked me in the last 10 minutes." E … , looking somewhat hurt and surprised, leaves the desk, but 10 minutes later she is back asking the same question. In this particular situation the nurse involved said after E … had left that she felt awful speaking to her like that, but she felt exasperated by the constant requests for the same information.

This type of interaction is a relatively common occurrence in facility settings, and without some intervention it can have insidious consequences for the care of the residents and the morale of the staff. It is well-established that one of the biggest obstacles to providing high-quality care in the residential care industry is staff turnover. Without a consistent staff it is impossible to provide consistent, high-quality care and to create an environment that feels like home to the people who reside in a place where they are constantly having the personal needs met by someone new.

Oppositional Behavior

Behavior that is identified as oppositional typically interferes with the staff's ability to do their job the way they perceive it should be done. The morning staff who are charged with bathing residents encounter an 83-year-old lady who refuses to shower and then resists all efforts to undress her when they do finally get her into the shower room. This type of scenario creates problems for the staff and the resident. The staff have a set of tasks that they have to do to meet the regulatory requirements and the needs of the resident. When residents refuse to participate in the process and thereby prevent the staff from completing their responsibilities it creates conflict for the staff. The consequences for the resident are that she gets labeled as difficult—no one wants to be assigned to work with her, so she gets her needs met by the person with the least say, usually the newest person on the staff. She may even have her needs neglected altogether. Oppositional behavior can be manifest in many ways (e.g., the resident may refuse to participate in prescribed therapies or may refuse to eat when and where he or she is supposed to). If the staff perceive the resident as having the capacity to do what is expected and cannot see the reason for the residents' apparent unwillingness, they are more likely to view the residents' behavior as willful disobedience and engage in a power struggle with the resident.

Neglecting Self-Care

A resident who is believed to have the capacity to perform his or her own activities of daily living (ADLs) but does not do so may not be immediately identified as someone who is problematic. It is usually when the person begins to emit odors or has other outward manifestations of neglect that become disturbing to those who share their living space that the resident is referred for an evaluation. Neglect of self-care can be one of the first noticeable signs of depression in senior adults, particularly when it is accompanied by the loss of interest in things, loss of appetite, and disruption of the sleep pattern. Many of the staff who work with older adults will get help when they begin to see these symptoms become manifest. However, depression is frequently overlooked in the elderly because it often occurs without the subjective expression of sadness. It is not uncommon to see an older adult with severe depression, including all of the vegetative symptoms who does not report feeling depressed. The exact reasons for this are unclear but include generational factors—growing up in a period of time when psychological disorders were not well understood or accepted.

Yelling and Screaming

If you spend any time at all in residential care settings you will encounter residents who yell or scream. Disruptive verbal behaviors range between 10% to 30% of residents (Cohen-Mansfield & Werner, 1997a, 1997b). Often times the yelling is in the form of a request for help, but often it is a formless verbalization that communicates distress on the part of the resident. The vocalizations are disconcerting for other residents and staff and are therefore often addressed quickly. However, the manner in which they are addressed is not always optimal for the resident. For example, the nurse may get on the phone to the house physician and request an increase in a benzodiazapine. Although this may temporarily quiet the resident, if the resident is calling out because of mild confusion secondary to a delirium, it may exacerbate the cause of the residents' verbalizations.

Wandering

In many facilities there is sufficient space that a person can walk around without causing a problem for others. A resident's wandering usually does not become a problem until they start leaving the facility or start going into other resident's rooms. Although the consequences of wandering are benign for the most part, they can be devastating in other cases—for example, a confused resident who wanders onto a busy street and is hit by a car, or a resident who wanders into the room of another resident who perceives the uninvited person as a threat and attacks him or her.

Wandering is a common behavior among people with progressive dementia. The cause of wandering is not well-understood, although some researchers have opined that it results from understimulation. In facilities where there are a lot of stimulating activities, there does appear to be less wandering.

Sexual Acting Out

The role of overt sexuality in the elderly is something that is not well-understood or accepted in American society and is less understood in facility settings. There is among younger adults the general conception that senior adults do not have sexual needs and desires, and when these seniors are placed in a residential settings there is the expectation that they will check whatever sexual needs they have at the door.

It is beyond the scope of this chapter to address the facilitation of appropriate sexual needs of older adults in residential settings; therefore the focus remains on sexual expressions deemed inappropriate. The reporting of sexually inappropriate behavior occurs predominately among the male residents. Some common incidents include verbalizations of sexual need or intent, inappropriate touching of staff, repetitive masturbation, and exposing of genitalia.

As with other problematic behaviors, staff need to be careful not to make precipitous judgements about why the resident is engaging in the behavior and not to make generalizations about their character. A person who is labeled a sexual predator, like the violent resident, is at greater risk for not getting his or her health needs met. If a person is violent or sexually aggressive precautions should be taken to insure the safety of the staff, but this should not result in neglecting the resident's health needs.

Psychotic Symptoms

Psychotic symptoms are those that are characterized by a disruption of the person's connection with reality, or put another way, the individual has perceptual experiences or beliefs that are inconsistent with those recognized by the community at large as being real. For example, a person may believe he is the reincarnated Christ or that he has special powers or abilities. The most common manifestations of psychosis are delusions and hallucinations. Delusions are beliefs that are firmly held without supporting evidence or in the face of information to the contrary. Such beliefs are usually recognized as odd or peculiar by others from the person's society and are typically persecutory or grandiose in nature. Hallucinations are perceptual experiences in the absence of supporting sensory stimulation (e.g., a person who hears voices when there is no audible sound that can be discerned by those who are also within earshot). Closely akin to hallucinations are illusions, which are perceptual experiences that are a distortion of stimuli (e.g., the rustling of leaves is experienced as voices).

In the general adult population schizophrenia is the most common cause of psychotic symptoms, and auditory hallucinations are the most common type of hallucinatory experience. However, among senior adults in residential settings the most common cause of psychotic symptoms is dementia or delirium, and the most common type of hallucination is visual. The common denominator appears to be paranoia, which is the most common type of delusional content in both the younger and older adult populations.

ETIOLOGICAL FACTORS

There are various causative factors that contribute to the presence and manifestation of problematic behaviors among seniors in residential settings. A comprehensive understanding of these causative factors can lead to more effective interventions, more accurate projections of prognosis, and in some cases preventative measures. For the purpose of this chapter, etiological factors are discussed under four major categories: biological–medical, psychosocial, environmental, and situational.

Biological–Medical

General Principles and Issues.   There are a number of disease related physiological changes that can accompany the aging process and contribute to alterations in behavior patterns (e.g., an embolic stroke secondary to atherosclerosis can result in impaired reasoning and problems with inhibition). Some of the physiological changes are permanent, and others are transient. In chapter 5, medical changes that can have psychological implications are addressed in some detail. The current discussion remains cursory and limited to some of the more common causes.

Progressive Neurological Disorders.   Neurological disorders are some of the most devastating to older adults, in part because of the impact on memory and other cognitive processes that allow a person to maintain a sense of personal identity. The most common progressive neurological disorders are dementia of the Alzheimer's type and multi-infarct dementia (frequent embolic strokes usually related to atherosclerosis).

Dementia, according to the America Psychiatric Association (1994), is defined as any process that results in the significant impairment of memory and at least one other domain of cognitive functioning. Most dementias are progressive with either a steady or a fluctuating course. However, using the American Medical Association's definition, a dementia can also be a nonprogressive process—for example, a person who suffers a traumatic brain injury and experiences a significant deterioration of memory and executive functioning. As many as 50%—90% of individuals with moderate to severe dementia display clinically significant behavior problems during the course of their illness (Allen-Burge et al., 1999).

Progressive neurological disorders, like the dementias, can result in physiological changes to the brain that affect emotions and behavior. It is common to see both psychotic and depressive symptoms in a person as they progress through the stages of the most common dementia—Alzheimer's disease.

Nonprogressive Neurological Disorders.   Some neurological disorders are relatively static after their initial presentation or do not necessarily have a progressive course. Some cerebrovascular accidents would qualify as nonprogressive neurological disorders. For example, a person who survived a ruptured cerebral aneurysm could have a period of acute change followed by a period of recovery with residual deficits, but no further deterioration. Space-occupying lesions (e.g., brain tumors and abscesses) can also be nonprogressive (e.g., a meningioma that is successfully resected could result in a variety of deficit areas that after the initial period stabilize and can even show some improvement).

Although there may not be any progression of the disease process itself, there are changes in other aspects of the person's life that may alter the presentation of the symptoms. Like the effects of a progressive neurological disease, there are changes in brain structure and function as a result of nonprogressive neurological disorders that can have a profound impact on behavior. For example, anyone who has worked with the traumatic brain injury (TBI) population is aware of the personality changes and disinhibition that are characteristic of damage to the frontal lobes of the brain.

Progressive Systemic Illnesses.   Systemic illnesses can deplete the body of resources that are needed to function optimally and can exacerbate or exploit proclivities for mental illness. Perhaps the best example of this in the residential setting is multiple sclerosis (MS). Any psychologist who has consulted to residential settings has encountered the MS patient who is struggling with depression and has mild to moderate cognitive impairment that reduces his or her memory abilities and capacity to think flexibly and use abstraction. Often these MS patients are diagnosed with personality disorders because of the combined effect of their disease process and their attempts to cope with the psychological impact of an extremely debilitating illness.

The various forms of cancer can also produce changes in behavior and psychological well-being as a person struggles with severe pain, the prospect of imminent death, and the deterioration of one's body. There is also the toil of reading on the face of every person who visits the fear and apprehension of what cancer in any form can do to an individual.

Psychosocial

History of Abuse–Trauma.   The incidence of physical and emotional abuse in the United States is high, and the odds of encountering someone who has a history of abuse is equally high. Many people who have a history of abuse have found ways to manage the impact of the abuse and may even repress the memory of the abuse. However, as their emotional and physical resources become more taxed due to illness and multiple losses they become less able to defend against the residual impact of the abuse, and these symptoms may become noticeable. The symptoms are not always obvious manifestations of abuse and can be misinterpreted and misunderstood without a historical perspective.

A resident may become aggressive, excessively fearful, paranoid, or psychotic; and without an accurate understanding of why these symptoms are manifested, the resident is likely to be misunderstood and mistreated.

Pain.   Pain is associated with almost all illnesses and traumatic events. As people grow older and the incidence of illness and disease rises, the experience of pain becomes more common. In some cases the pain is quickly relieved as the illness or injury is treated. However, in many cases the treatment is protracted and the individual is treated with pain relievers. While pain relievers often help reduce the discomfort, they can also have side effects that may further complicate the person's condition. It is not uncommon to see some alteration in cognitive functioning after the administration of pain medications, and many of them are addictive.

In some cases the pain does not remit after treatment and the person develops chronic pain syndrome. Chronic pain syndrome is a classification that is used to capture those individuals who have unremitting pain that is often associated with unknown etiology. Although in many cases there is one or more known illness or trauma that could cause pain, in chronic pain cases the pain is out of the range expected, given the apparent cause. In some cases, the pain persisted despite treatment that should have relieved it, in others there is simply no explanation for the pain the individual experiences. The unremitting nature of the pain and no clear understanding of the cause, often leave the individual with little hope and considerable anguish. The rate of psychological complications, particularly depression and personality changes, is high in people with chronic pain.

Support System.   A person's support system can be problematic in as many ways as it can be helpful. As individuals get older there is a natural attenuation of their support system as significant people in their lives die or move. This erosion of the availability of significant people can have an insidious impact on a person's behavior. The most common response might be a move toward depression with increased isolation and the other vegetative symptoms. Depression is most common when there is the death of a spouse or other major figure, but it can also result from the cumulative effect of multiple losses. In some cases the loss appears not significant (e.g., a remote relative or minor acquaintance), and if it is not seen in context of multiple losses, the person may not get the care he or she needs.

Education–Vocational History.   In addition to understanding a person's medical condition and current psychosocial factors when intervening with a problematic behavior, understanding one's educational and vocational history can also be helpful. If we have some understanding of a person's intellectual ability, it will allow us to intervene in a manner that is most consistent with those abilities. Although a person's educational level is not an absolute indication of intellectual abilities, in the absence of a history of neurological compromise and without formal testing, a person's educational level and the vocational history is often the best estimate of his or her intellectual ability. For example, if we know that a person left school in the eighth grade and worked as an unskilled laborer all his life, we might avoid using interventions that rely on complex verbal reasoning.

Another way in which knowledge of a person's educational and vocational history can be useful is that it gives us some content areas to engage the patient if resistance occurs. For example, knowing that a patient enjoyed woodworking, talking about woodworking may help a patient who has difficulty engaging with a therapist in the initial stages of treatment.

Environmental   Senior adults in residential settings have generally been displaced from their own home and placed in another. Sometimes it is their own decision. For instance, an 89-year-old woman who lost her husband 20 years ago lived in the family home until it became more work than she could manage. She decided to move to a facility where her basic needs could be met and where she would be around others her own age. However, frequently the decision to move a senior adult into a residential facility is made by the family because of concerns about health and safety. Involuntary placement can also occur as a consequence of health problems (e.g., a bout of pneumonia or a broken hip requires a brief stay in a rehabilitation facility and leads to long-term placement).

The residents who are in the facilities as a result of health problems or family concerns about safety may not have much say in where and with whom they are placed in the facility. They may be placed in the room with a severely demented resident who calls out for help throughout the night or with a resident who is in persistent pain and moans constantly. Such an experience can be unnerving for a person who is used to living alone. Placement in a room with a severely impaired resident can be particularly bothersome to the newcomer with some mild cognitive decline who is afraid he or she will progress further.

It is of paramount importance that when the facility staff think about relocating a resident that they anticipate that the resident may have some difficulty with transition. There have been many instances where residents are not informed that they are being moved until the staff come in to move their belongings.

Situational   When there are significant events in a person's life, it can have a dramatic impact on the person's emotions and behaviors. Sometimes the consequent behaviors are not logically tied to the expected response. For example, a 79-year-old man was referred for sexually inappropriate behavior after the death of his sister. In this case the grieving response had led to depression and sleep and appetite changes, which in short order had compromised the cognitive functioning of this already fragile man. He had become delirious and had touched a nurse's breast while she was bathing him. Although it was true that he had been sexually inappropriate, this was not the major presenting problem with this man. He was appropriately treated for the delirium and the depression, and there was no reoccurance of "problem behavior." The natural consequences of the aging process set the stage for situationally mediated changes—a predicament that tends to be exaggerated in seniors placed in residential settings. There are physical changes, including progressive illnesses, that tax a person's resources for dealing with change. There are also multiple losses that can have the same effect. There is the loss of work, the loss of a familiar residence, the loss of independence, the loss of a familiar social network, and for many the loss of loved ones including a spouse.

The multiple changes that residents of facilities face throughout the course of their stay, along with the loss of resources to deal with these changes, make them vulnerable to changes in emotion and behavior that can become problematic. It is important for the facility staff to be aware of this vulnerability and to be prepared to intervene any time there is a significant incident in the lives of their residents. The change may be major like the death of a spouse, or it may be a relatively minor, like the marriage of a grandchild in a distant city. Although the latter may be perceived as a positive change, for the resident who can not attend, it may become the manifestation of the cumulative effect of all of the losses he or she has experienced.

INTERVENTIONS

General Principles

Regardless of the nature of the problem or its origin, if treatment is to be effective it must be driven by accurate and complete assessment. After a conceptualization is developed about what is causing the identified problem, treatment can be implemented. Treatment can take many forms depending on the perceived etiology. Treatment options include pharmacologic, psychotherapy, behavioral interventions, and environmental manipulation. Immediately following is a brief description of these intervention options followed by how they may be applied to the most common problem areas identified at the beginning of the chapter.

Pharmacologic Interventions

The use of medications to treat patients in residential settings is addressed in some detail in chapter 9. For the purposes of this chapter, I briefly discuss why the use of medications may be recommended and how these medications are thought to work. Ironically, most of the major classes of medications used in psychiatry were discovered serendipitously. That is, they were discovered while looking for or at something else. For example, inderol, a beta blocker that is used to treat explosive disorder was commonly used as a hypertensive agent, but one of the side effects was a reduction in aggression.

Most medications work by adjusting the levels of neurotransmitters in the brain. Neurotransmitters are chemical messengers that tell the nerve cells in the brain when and how often to fire/communicate. Some medications like the antidepressants Prozac and Paxil interfere with the brain's natural recycling mechanisms thereby making more of the neurotransmitter seretonin available for a longer period of time. Others like the antipsychotic Haldol block the sites that the neurotransmitter would attach to thereby preventing communication between two neurotransmitters. It is through the understanding of what these drugs do and how they work psychiatrists and mental health researchers have developed a better understanding of what causes the symptoms of mental illness.

Psychotherapy

Psychotherapy can be understood as a verbal interaction between a patient and a treating professional with the intended purpose of bringing about relief of symptoms. Although the majority of psychotherapy is individual (i.e., one patient and one therapist), psychotherapy can also be done effectively in a small group. The professional literature contains numerous references to the effectiveness of psychotherapy in ameliorating the symptoms of mental illness.

Although there are many theories on how psychotherapy should be done and as many theories about how it works, there appears to be some common principles that promote healing. It seems from comparative research that the relationship between the patient and the treating professional is the most important part of the exchange. Developing a meaningful dialogue with a concerned but objective other, allows a person to begin the investigation and working through of conflicts. The primary goal of psychotherapy, as with any therapeutic intervention, is positive change. Yalom (1995) identified 11 of what he called therapeutic factors, which he believes are the primary mechanisms by which change is effected. Some examples of these therapeutic factors include *universality*—the assurance that the patient is not unique in their struggle, and *catharsis*—the relief that comes from the expression of the problem. Professions that trained to undertake psychotherapy include psychology, psychiatry, clinical social work, and some advanced nursing degrees.

Psychosocial Interventions

The reconnecting or connecting of a resident with family and other aspects of their social support system can have a positive impact on disruptive behaviors. The impact happens because the input is from someone the resident trusts and therefore is more likely to take heed of, or it can happen because of the universal effect of substituting meaningful productive activities for monotony. The more often the resident is engaged in activities that are meaningful and stimulating to them, the less likely they are to engage in behaviors that are problematic. Social skills training can also be a useful intervention with older adults who experience challenging behaviors in residential settings. If the resident is suffering from dementia, social skills groups can be a refresher on how to appropriately interact with others and the environment.

Community involvement and volunteering can also be very therapeutic for those in residential settings. The curative value of doing something for others has been well established in all populations. Altruism, as it is often called, can take on many forms including assisting other residents within the facility. Engaging in activities that are service-oriented can also be helpful with individuals who are suffering from dementia. For example, asking an agitated resident with dementia to help with a task such as folding laundry can divert his or her attention and prove to be an effective intervention.

Most medications work by adjusting the levels of neurotransmitters in the brain. Neurotransmitters are chemical messengers that tell the nerve cells in the brain when and how often to fire or communicate. Some medications, such as the antidepressants Prozac and Paxil, interfere with the brain's natural recycling mechanisms, thereby making more of the neurotransmitter serotonin available for a longer period of time. Others, including the antipsychotic Haldol, block the sites that the neurotransmitter would attach to, thereby preventing communication between two neurotransmitters. It is through the understanding of what these drugs do and how they work that psychiatrists and mental health researchers have developed a better understanding of what causes the symptoms of mental illness.

Behavioral Interventions

When people talk of behavioral interventions in psychology, most people will usually think of a token economy, time–out techniques, or some variation of the principles that evolved out of Skinner's work. Behavior management programs, although effective when properly implemented, are often complex and time–consuming for the staff. Therefore, most of the techniques discussed herein are simpler and in most cases can be applied by one person. Although some of the interventions discussed appear to be obvious, they are often overlooked or neglected by the facility's core staff.

Listen to what the resident is saying to you. Although some may think this so obvious it need not be said, it is the single most common mistake made in working with elderly residents. Take the time to hear what the resident is saying, and the solution will be close behind. Consider, for instance, the earlier example of the elderly woman with dementia who resisted the attempts of the nurse's aids to bathe her. As the nurse's aid assigned to her listened to what was said during the first unsuccessful exchange, she learned that this lady appeared fearful of the shower. She communicated her observations to the charge nurse who passed the information on in report at shift change. The evening nurse brought the subject of the bathing up with the lady's oldest child who visited that evening. She reported that her mother had never showered and had always insisted on using a bathtub to bathe. The information was passed back through nursing report, and the next morning the resident happily bathed in the tub used for physical therapy.

Another oft-neglected principle is to treat the patient as an adult. There is a general assumption that when a person loses the capacity to live independently, or chooses to live in a residential setting, that they are no longer deserving of or require the respect that we give to other adults. Instead people treat them as objects, often not even bothering to learn their names. People call them "dear" or "sweetheart" and talk down to them as if they were children or lacked the capacity to understand what is being said. Avoid this pitfall. Learn the names of the people you work with. If you do not know the person's name, ask them, and talk to them like you would a friend or associate. If the person is suffering from dementia and cannot understand you, then simplify your language, but be careful not to adopt the patronizing tone so often heard in residential care settings.

The amount of stimulus that a person can assimilate and the amount that a person needs both change as a consequence of brain injury or disease and vary among people. Whereas with some dementia patients the challenge may be to provide them with enough stimulation, with some residents with acquired brain injury one has to be careful not to overstimulate the resident. New research has demonstrated that some of the most problematic behaviors found in patients with dementia is caused or exacerbated by lack of stimulation. Although most unimpaired adults have the capacity to extract from any situation enough stimulation to prevent boredom, dementia patients often lack this capacity. Along with this inability to actively and efficiently scan the environment for adequate stimulation is the reduced capacity to modulate their response to the lack of stimulation. For example, most individuals when in a situation that is boring, will scan other available stimuli in the environment for something more interesting; if unable to find something that is stimulating, they may resort to reverie but will probably not respond by lashing out or pacing.

For people with acquired brain injury, including traumatic brain injury and stroke, the problem with stimulation is a different one. People who are in the early stages of recovery from an insult to the brain find that they cannot easily tolerate all of the stimuli that constantly bombard their sensory organs. When this oversensitivity is coupled with the reduced capacity to tolerate frustration that accompanies most acquired brain injury, the result is a potentially volatile situation. Therefore, with individuals who are prone to overstimulation, controlling the stimulation they are exposed to can be crucial in preventing outbursts.

Maximizing consistency is another fundamental principle for those in residential settings. Consistency from those who work with senior adults living outside their own home adds to the predictability and security these residents feel. When other factors—social, medical, and environmental—are combining to erode the elderly person's feeling of security, providing them with consistency in attention and care can create a bastion that can significantly improve the person's quality of life. Part of being consistent is respecting the resident's routine. Most people over the course of their lives develop a routine for the activities of everyday life. As people get older these routines become more important to them. These routines often are not taken into account when a person is admitted to a residential care facility. The person is now expected to conform to the routine of the facility and its staff. Although there are often good reasons for the schedule of events in residential care settings, it is often possible to accommodate the previously established routines of the residents.

Although it may be difficult for a layperson to remain calm in the face of an agitated or aggressive resident, it is vital that the staff of residential care facilities do so. If the staff allow themselves to get excited and caught up in the emotion the resident's behavior, the situation can become more severe and more residents may become involved. However, if the staff model calm, controlled behavior, then they are holding a mirror up to the person of how he or she should respond.

Environmental Manipulation

The space in which a person resides can have a profound effect on a person's psychological well-being and the accompanying behavior. For many years most residential facilities looked like run-down hospitals with sterile rooms and very little that resembled the homes in which most of the residents lived in prior to their admission. More recently owners and operators of residential settings have seen the need to create residential settings that feel more like home than like a hospital. Although this type of facility may require more up-front capital, the long-term results are greater satisfaction among the residents and staff and less turnover in both groups. Less turnover and increased satisfaction usually results in higher profit margins for the facilities.

The Eden Alternative is perhaps the best known coordinated effort to improve the quality of the physical surroundings for people in residential care. The Eden Alternative has as its core concept, the goal of making the places where older adults live more vibrant and vigorous and less like the warehouses they have been in the past. One of the keys to achieving this goal is to bring plants and animals into the facilities.

In addition to the use of more home-like surroundings to improve the overall quality of life for people in residential care, there are specific environmental manipulations that can be used to extinguish or change specific problematic behaviors.

Interventions for Specific Behaviors

Frequent use of the call button.   As noted earlier, the perceived overuse of the call button is a common problem identified by staff in residential care settings. The interventions used to address this concern are driven by an understanding of the cause of the problem. The three most common causes are anxiety, memory deficits, and personality disorders. If anxiety is the cause of the overuse, effective treatment of the anxiety should result in more appropriate use of the call button. For example, a woman in her late 80s is a recent admission to a facility, and although very pleasant to interact with she persists in using her call button about every 15 minutes to request minor things such as confirming the time of a regularly scheduled activity. The staff refers her to the consulting psychologist, and she is found to have an anxiety disorder that she was able to manage through avoidance prior to her admission to the facility. The treatment is a brief course of psychotherapy, an evaluation for medication, and staff training to provide her with support and consistency. The net result is less inappropriate use of the call button.

If memory deficits are the cause of the overuse (i.e., the person forgets that the issue they are requesting assistance for has already been addressed) then a different approach is necessary. The use of environmental cues and regular unsolicited visits can often address the problem.

Residents with personality disorders can be very disruptive to any residential facility. This is particularly true of borderline and antisocial personality disorders. The borderline resident can create havoc for an untrained staff. The resident may have staff taking sides against each other and find that their efforts with the resident and other staff are undermined. Although the term borderline is frequently heard in facility settings, the diagnosis can only be made by a qualified professional, and the treatment is complex. If you suspect a resident has a personality disorder, consult a mental health professional to assess the resident and to work with the staff on how to work with them. Some key factors in the treatment are to maintain active and open communication among the staff and between the staff and the resident and to maintain consistency in the way issues are addressed with the resident.

Violent Behavior.   Violent behavior from a resident can come from the willful intent to hurt another or from the response to a perceived threat (real or imagined). Although there are people who have such a poor regard for the well-being of others that they willfully aggress against them, those individuals are in the minority. The majority of cases of aggressive or violent behavior are from those individuals who have lost the ability to accurately perceive a threat or lost the ability to inhibit the impulse to lash out at someone who offends or irritates. This loss can be temporary as in an acute psychotic episode or a delirium, or it can be the permanent result of a progressive illness such as Alzheimer's disease.

Although setting up strict and serve consequences may reduce the acting out of a willfully violent resident, such contingencies may not have the same effect, or any effect at all, on the impaired resident. For a person who lacks the capacity to inhibit their aggressive impulses, other interventions are required. Using environmental interventions to intercede during an episode of problematic behavior can be effective in some cases. An example of environmental interventions is the use of objects requiring manipulation that the resident's attention may be drawn to, thereby relieving the tension associated with the behavioral disturbance. Another potentially useful intervention is learning the antecedents associated with the violent behavior. In one facility a resident by the name of Frank had reportedly attacked three other residents over a 2-week period. Further investigation revealed that all three attacks had one thing in common—they were all in Frank's room, and the victims were all confused residents who were prone to wandering. Once a barrier in the form of a STOP sign was placed in Frank's doorway, Frank's violent episodes ceased. Finally, having a well-trained staff who is ready to intervene quickly may be the best intervention.

Repetitive Requests–Preservative Behavior.   The most common cause of repeated requests is that the resident's request has not been responded to appropriately. Once it is established that the resident's request has received an appropriate response or cannot be met (e.g., the lady with severe dementia who wants to go home), the request itself can be identified as a potential problem. Before attempting to address the request as a problem, one must first ask if the repetitiveness needs attention at all. If the repeated request is causing no significant harm, then it may make the most sense to ignore it. However, if it is causing the resident or the staff significant distress then it warrants intervention.

If the repeated requests are driven by anxiety and ignored, the resident may escalate and the behavior may become more extreme. If the requests are causing the direct care staff distress and the behavior is not addressed, there is the risk of a negative impact on the staff's perception on the resident, which could affect the care the resident gets. In an ideal world the staff that work in residential care settings would not be vulnerable to developing biases and letting those biases effect care, but the residential care world is far from ideal.

The second most common cause of repetitive requests is confusion most often caused by one of the dementias. In these situations the first intervention might be distraction. Choose an activity that is known from the resident's past to have some meaning and attempt to engage the resident in the activity. If the resident can be successfully coaxed into the activity, he or she may forget about what it was that was causing the concern.

Trying to orient a confused resident by telling that the relative they are expecting to visit has been dead for 10 years will usually not work and may even worsen the situation by increasing the resident's agitation.

Oppositional Behavior.   Residents who engage in oppositional behavior run the risk of not getting their needs met, and over time that can have devastating consequences. Dementia is probably also the most common cause of oppositional behavior. Some residents may be at a point in the progress of their disease that there is little that can be done to get them to cooperate. However, in most cases a careful evaluation and flexibility with approach can overcome oppositional behavior. A careful evaluation may reveal that a resident refusing bathing is suffering from pain that is exacerbated by the bathing experience, and lacking the capacity to articulate this simply engages in abstinent resistance not unlike a preverbal child. Providing an analgesic prior to bathing and being sensitive to the painful area or motion may reduce the resistance.

Another example might be a resident who refuses to take his medication. Once again careful evaluation reveals that he is concerned about the impact the medication will have on him based on a bad experience with a similar medication. In a case like this, reassurance from someone the resident trusts may be enough. In other cases a different medication may be necessary.

Neglecting Self-Care.   Although attention to self-care activities becomes an issue with residents with dementia, these activities are soon taken over by the staff for those residents who can no longer complete these activities on their own. However, when a resident can undertake his or her own self-care but does not this causes the staff concern. Depression is a common reason why a resident may neglect self-care. Depression is a common problem, and depressive symptoms are present in up to 50% of residents of nursing homes. In recent years there have been some important advances in the development of medications used to treat depression. Psychotherapy has also been shown to be an effective treatment for depression. However, it has historically been easier for residents to access medications than psychotherapy even though some studies have demonstrated that psychotherapy produces superior results.

Iatrogenic dependency may also be a contributing factor to the neglect of self-care among some residents. Baltes (1995) pointed out that the way residential care facilities are set up fosters dependency in some residents. A situation is created where dependency results in increased attention and time from staff, which for some residents can be more reinforcing than perceived independence.

Yelling and Screaming.   Verbally agitated behavior can be extremely disturbing to staff and other residents, and according to Dyck (1997) it can be resistant to interventions. Cohen-Mansfield & Werner (1997) reported that despite the variability in the reporting there is consensus about the impact of verbally disruptive behavior and the need to intervene effectively. When asked how they respond to a verbally disruptive resident, the most common reported intervention from nurse's aids was providing attention with verbal interaction. Other commonly used interventions were verbal reprimands, ignoring, and seclusion (Cariaga et al., 1991).

An accurate and careful appraisal of the situation will increase the likelihood that an effective intervention can be found (Cohen-Mansfield & Werner, 1997b). An experienced and consistent staff can play a key role here. If the staff know the patients, they are better able to comprehend what an impaired resident is unable to lucidly communicate. For example, while visiting a local secured dementia unit recently, a resident was observed to begin to get verbally and physically agitated. One of the nursing staff intervened and asked the patient if she was in pain. The resident affirmed that she was and was given some medication. The nurse then remarked that the resident has severe arthritis and tends to get verbally agitated when the arthritis flares up. This would not be evident to someone who did not know the resident, and the resident would not have been able to verbalize the problem.

Wandering.   Wandering is a prominent symptom of dementia. There are a number of theories about why people with dementia have the impulse to wander. One of the most popular theories is that people with dementia suffer from a lack of stimulation and wander or pace to try to relieve this impoverishment. Providing residents with adequate stimulation will likely result in a reduction in wandering.

Increased time interacting with staff has also been shown to reduce wandering (Allen-Burge et al., 1999); however, it will probably not eliminate it. Therefore, in addition to providing adequate stimulation, facilities with residents who wander need to have a safe place for them to walk.

Sexual Acting Out.   The reduction of the capacity to inhibit inappropriate impulses is a common factor in older men who are accused of sexual acting out in residential settings. However, there are other reasons for this behavior, particularly if the resident in question is still relatively intact cognitively. If the behavior results from confusion or disinhibition, some of the interventions discussed earlier will be helpful. Certainly antecedent control can quell some of the touching that results from disinhibition.

For a resident who is not obviously impaired cognitively the situation is more complex and requires thorough investigation. The resident may have antisocial tendencies and may use the sexual harassment of others as a way of dealing with boredom. However, before jumping to this possible but unlikely conclusion and branding the resident as a person to be avoided, there are other possible alternatives. For example, it may be an attempt by the resident to get the attention of the staff. Although the attention is negative, the resident may feel ineffectual in using more appropriate means of having his needs met.

One of the first interventions with a cognitively intact resident who is engaging in sexually inappropriate behavior is to talk with them about why they are doing so. Engaging a resident in a conversation about their behavior is not an easy thing to do and should be done by a mental health professional or by a staff person who has good rapport with the resident. When asked about his sexual behavior, the resident may initially deny the behavior, but as he is gently confronted with the supporting evidence, a meaningful discussion about the behavior may begin.

Psychotic Symptoms.   Overtly psychotic symptoms can be particularly concerning to the staff and the resident's family members. They can also be very alarming to the resident, but this is not always the case. It is not uncommon to hear residents comment in a matter-of-fact or unemotional way about their visual hallucinations. It is worth saying again that if the behavior is not causing the resident distress and does not affect the staff's ability to do their job, there may be no need to intervene. This is particularly true with psychotic symptoms because the only potentially effective treatment is antipsychotic drugs. Although there have been developments in the past 10 years that have produced antipsychotic drugs without the severe side-effects of the first drugs developed, there are still risks involved, particularly if the resident is already on multiple medications.

Although there are no really effective behavioral interventions for alleviating psychotic symptoms, there are things that should be avoided. Telling a resident that the voices they are hearing or the animals that they are seeing are not real will not help and may exacerbate the situation by agitating the resident further. Trying to convince a resident that no one is trying to harm them or that they should feel safe in the unfamiliar environment will probably result in the staff person being incorporated into the resident's delusional system making that person unable to be involved in the resident's care.

REFERENCES

Allen-Burge, R., Stevens, A. B., & Burgio, L. D. (1999). Effective behavioral interventions for decreasing dementia-related challenging behavior in nursing homes. *International Journal of Geriatric Psychiatry, 14,* 213–232.

American Psychiatric Association. Diagnostic and Statistical Manual of Mental Disorders, Fourth Edition, Washington, DC (1994).

American Psychological Association. (1998, December). Guidelines for the evaluation of dementia and age-related cognitive decline. *American Psychologist, 53* (12), 1298–1303.

Baltes, M. M., Dependency in Old Age: Gain and Losses. Current Directions in Psychological Science. 1995 4(1) 14–19.

Burgio, L., and Bourgeois, M. (1992). Treating severe behavioral disorders in geriatric residential settings. *Behavioral Residential Treatment,* 7(2), 145–168.

Burgio, L., Scilley, K., Hardin, J. M., Hsu, D., & Yancey, J. (1996). Environmental "white noise": An intervention for verbally agitated nursing home residents. *Journal of Gerontology,* 51B, 364–373.

Burton, L. C., German, P. S., Rovner, B. W., & Brant, L. J. (1992). Physical restraint use and cognitive decline among nursing home residents. *Journal of American Geriatric Society,* 40(8), 811–816.

Cariaga, J., Burgio, L., Flynn, W., Martin, D. A controlled study of disruptive vocalizations among geriatric residents in nursing homes. Journal of American Geriatric Society. 1991:39:501–7.

Cohen-Mansfield, J., and Werner, P. (1997). Management of verbally disruptive behaviors in nursing home residents. *Journal of Gerontology,* 52A(6), M369–M377.

Cohen-Mansfield, J., and Werner, P. (1997). Typology of disruptive vocalizations in older persons suffering from dementia. *Int. Journal of Geriatric Psychiatry, 12,* 1079–1091.

Dyck, G. (1997, March). Management of geriatric behavior problems. *Geriatric Psychiatry,* 20(1), 165–180.

Freyne, A. and Wrigley, M. (1996). Aggressive incidents towards staff by elderly patients with dementia in a long stay ward. *International Journal of Geriatric Psychiatry, 11,* 57–63.

Hussian, R.A. (1988). Modification of behaviors in dementia via stimulus manipulation. *Clinical Gerontologist,* 8(1), 37–43.

Hussian, R.A. (1980). Stimulus control in the modification of problematic behavior in elderly institutionalized patients. *International Journal of Behavioral Geriatrics,* 1(1), 33–42.

Jackson, G. A., Templeton, G. J., & Whyte, J. (1999). An overview of behavior difficulties found in long-term care settings. *International Journal of Geriatric Psychiatry, 14,* 426–430.

Loebel, J. P., Borson, S., Hyde, T., Donaldson, D., Van Tuinen, C., & Rabbitt, T. M. (1991). Relationships between requests for psychiatric consultations and psychiatric diagnosis in long term care facilities. *American Journal of Psychiatry,* 148(7), 898–903.

Mortimer, A. (1995). Reducing violence on a secure ward. *Psychiatric Bulletin*, 19, 605–608.

Patel, V. and Hope, T. (1993). Aggressive behavior in elderly people with dementia: A review. *International Journal of Geriatric Psychiatry*, 8, 457–472.

Rosenzweig, A., Prigerson, H., Miller, M., & Reynolds, C. F. III. (1997). Bereavement and late-life depression: Grief and its complications in the elderly. *Ann. Rev. Med.* 48, 421–428.

Rossby, L., Beck, C., & Heacock, P. (1992, April). Disruptive behaviors of a cognitively impaired nursing home resident. *Achieves of Psychiatric Nursing*, 6(2), 98–107.

Rovner, B. W. (1996). Behavioral disturbances of dementia in the nursing home. *International Psychogeriatrics*, 8 (suppl. 3), 435–437.

Shah, A., and De, T. (1998). The effect of an educational intervention package about aggressive behavior directed at the nursing staff of a continuing care psychogeriatric ward. *International Journal of Geriatric Psychiatry*, 13, 35–40.

Yalom, I. D., The Theory and Practice of Group Psychotherapy: (New York, Basic Books) 1995.

9

Psychopharmacology With Older Adults in Residential Care

Chris G. Davies
Holland Health Services, Inc., Mount Vernon, Washington

Brian L. Thorn
Silverado Senior Living, Salt Lake City, and University of Utah

INTRODUCTION

In the past 30 to 40 years there have been enormous advances in the efficacy of psychotropic medication, resulting in an expanded repertoire of options available for medical practitioners to use as part of the treatment for psychiatric and behavioral disturbances. Most of these medications have been developed for the general adult population, and some of them, particularly the earlier examples, can have some prominent undesirable side effects that tend to be worse in the geriatric population. Fortunately, the introduction of the SSRI antidepressants, the atypical antipsychotics, and a few other medications in the past 15 years has provided the medical community with some very effective psychopharmacological options with comparatively low side effect profiles for older adults.

These new medications are now commonly prescribed by geriatric medicine providers, and many older individuals and their caregivers are benefitting (Levy & Uncapher, 2000). However, it is our belief that psychotropic medications are frequently being used inadequately or inappropriately in geriatric residential care facilities and that the treatment of the target symptoms, behaviors, or both, can in many cases be more effectively achieved. Perhaps it is more accurate to say that the effectiveness of psychotropic medications can be greatly increased if they are viewed in a somewhat different way than they are now. The key is to think of psychopharmacology not as a sole means of treatment for "behavioral problems," but as just one among many methods for addressing the emotional, psychological, and psychiatric needs of elderly residents (and their families). In most cases, medication should play the role of a supportive partner to other nonpharmacological means of improving resident well-being and addressing behavioral issues.

Most people in our society, especially medical practitioners, are accustomed to thinking about health care from the perspective of a medical model (Ogland-Hand & Zeiss, 2000). The medical model posits that health is a matter of diagnosing and curing disease or dysfunction. Sometimes the emphasis is on disease prevention, but in any case, the disease (or condition, or problem) is the target of treatment. Most people are accustomed to seeing a doctor, having a problem diagnosed, and having a medication or other treatment prescribed to fix the problem. But a distinct problem with the medical model is that focusing narrowly on target symptoms and behaviors can cause treating professionals to overlook larger issues associated with quality of life.

A goal of this chapter is to step outside the medical model and address issues of psychopharmacology as a component of integrated mental health treatment. Instead of looking at behavioral and emotional issues as problems that need to be stopped or fixed, consider them as expressions of a person's needs, and keep in mind that even the behavior of a person with dementia has some underlying meaning. Take time and pay close attention to your residents and their immediate environment; if you can understand the psychological meaning of the symptoms and behaviors, then it will suggest ideas for how to respond interpersonally or environmentally. This concept forms a central theme of this volume and is discussed more extensively in other chapters. A therapeutic response to psychosocial or interpersonal issues, in conjunction with appropriate psychotropic medication, will help to minimize the amount of medication needed and will enhance the resident's quality of life by creating a living environment that is more responsive to personal needs. When good psychopharmacology is combined with the principles and practices discussed elsewhere in this book, the quality of the residential care staff work environment will improve along with that of the residents' care and living environment because residents will generally be less distressed.

THE BIOLOGY OF PSYCHOPHARMACOLOGY

To understand psychopharmacology, it is helpful to start with a sketch of the biological processes involved and how they are affected by the medication(s). Of course, anyone who prescribes these drugs or makes dosage changes should have a comprehensive understanding of these systems and other relevant medical knowledge and training. The brief summary in this chapter is meant only as a conceptual overview of the topic. For those who have been exposed to this material before, it will be a simple refresher.

In essence, the central nervous system (CNS; brain and spinal cord) is the control center for perception, organization, storage, retrieval, and transmission of information. Information is taken in via the five senses and transmitted to the CNS through nerve fibers called neurons. Each neuron consists of a single cell ranging from very short to long, thin strands that extend from the spine to peripheral body parts. Their primary function is to transmit information to and from the CNS. The CNS itself consists primarily of masses of neurons that transmit and process sensory information. Perception is informed by neural messages from the sense organs to the brain. Behavior is initiated and controlled by neural messages traveling from the brain through neurons to the muscles and organs of the body.

Neurons communicate with their neighbors by releasing chemicals known as neurotransmitters into a small space between them known as the synaptic cleft. The neighboring neuron has receptors that detect the particular type and quantity of neurotransmitter released into the cleft and then relay the appropriate corresponding message on down the line to the next neuron or organ. Psychotropic medications work in one of three ways: (a) by altering the amount of particular neurotransmitters, (b) by altering the function of the neurons themselves, or (c) by some combination of these two processes. The various neurotransmitters also play other roles in different regions of the body as well as the brain.

Many psychiatric conditions and psychological symptoms are correlated with characteristic changes in CNS functioning. Depression, for example, is typically accompanied by decreased levels of the neurotransmitters serotonin and norepinephrine (Levy & Uncapher, 2000). Some antidepressant medications work by increasing the amounts of these neurotransmitters available to the system. It is a complicated process to determine what CNS changes, if any, are associated with particular psychological symptoms and then develop a medication that specifically targets those symptoms without side effects. No psychotropic medication yet is so effective that it accomplishes its task, but many newer medications come closer to this goal.

Depression and other psychological symptoms and conditions are also typically associated with events and situations in a person's past, present, and perceived future psychosocial environment. Addressing a distressed individual's needs on that level with psychological intervention is equally important to addressing them medically.

AGE RELATED CHANGES IN THE BIOLOGICAL PROCESS

As noted elsewhere in this volume, physical decline in late life is a normative process. As people age, they experience changes in their CNS just as they experience changes in other areas of physical functioning. For example, neurofibrillary tangles and amyloid plaques, commonly found in the brains of Alzheimer's disease patients, are also thought to be part of the normal aging process. Similarly, there are reported decreases of the neurotransmitters acetylcholine in the hippocampus and dopamine in the substantia nigra–basal ganglia pathway, but these changes are most pronounced in association with the progression of Alzheimer's disease and Parkinson's disease. There are emerging investigations using measures of brain structure and function in living individuals that offer significant new information on how aging affects the brain. In studies using magnetic resonance imaging (MRI) techniques, it has been found that a certain amount of brain atrophy is common in old age, but it has also been noted that individuals varied widely both in patterns of cortical atrophy and in ventricular enlargement. In studies of the frontal lobes using both MRI and positron-emission tomography scans, age reductions appear to be more conclusively demonstrated than in studies of other cortical areas (Whitbourne, 1998).

Aging of the CNS has direct effects on a variety of sensory, motor, and cognitive capacities and behaviors, including perception, short-term memory, fine motor coordination, and large muscle control. It is essential that those working with older people are knowledgeable about and sensitive to the symptoms of normal decline and those symptoms that are indicative of Alzheimer's disease and other dementias so that appropriate referrals for assessment and treatment can be made when indicated.

DRUG CLASS VERSUS DIAGNOSIS

In planning this chapter we considered the advantages and disadvantages of organizing the material into specific classes of drugs versus the various diagnoses and symptoms for which the drugs may be used. We decided to focus on drug classes primarily because information about similar drugs can be presented in a more concise and accessible manner. Keep in mind that some psychotropic medications are helpful for different types of diagnoses and symptoms. For example, many antidepressants are helpful in controlling anxiety. This is important to know because depression and anxiety very commonly occur simultaneously, especially in older people, and antidepressants are typically safer for long-term use than other anxiety medications. In the sections that follow, we present both the primary and the alternate uses of the different drugs.

The specific information on psychotropic medications in this chapter is referenced in many sources, including *Explicit Criteria for Determining Potentially Inappropriate Medication Use by the Elderly* (Beers, 1997), *Geriatric Pharmaceutical Care Guidelines* (Philadelphia College of Pharmacy and American Geriatrics Society, 1999) and *Treatment Of Agitation In Older Persons With Dementia* (Alexopoulous, Carpenter, Frances, Kahn, & Silver, 1998).

This chapter does not contain a comprehensive list of all of the drugs that could be classified within each category. This is a selection, or sets of examples, of some of the most commonly used drugs. New therapies and medications are being developed continually, and it is important for the professionals working with older persons to remain current with these developments.

Interdisciplinary teams have become vital to the care of older persons. With all of the new developments in assessment, treatment, and education of this patient population, it is impossible for one professional to comprehensively and effectively provide the best care for the differing needs of each patient. Physicians, psychiatrists, nurses, psychologists, social workers, rehabilitation therapists, administrators, caregivers (including resident family members), pharmacists, and the resident are all important members of a wellness team. Geriatric consultant pharmacists, practicing a relatively new specialization in pharmacy, are making a tremendous impact on safer and more effective drug regimens for elderly patients, particularly in residential settings. These pharmacists can provide valuable information for the care of individual residents. The following are general guidelines for geriatric medicine.

ANTIDEPRESSANTS

Of all the psychotropic medications, antidepressants stand out as the only class that are underused in geriatric residential care facilities. Research has shown that among the elderly who have serious health problems (such as those in nursing homes), depression is prevalent but underdiagnosed and undertreated. This situation leads to tremendous increases in disability and mortality. Depression in the elderly is often unrecognized due to atypical symptoms such as irritability, aggression, angry outbursts, verbal abuse, agitation, sleep disorders, and eating disorders. Regarding anxiolytic (antianxiety) properties, it has been suggested that both antidepressants and benzodiazepines produce some similar effects. There is a strong relationship between depression and anxiety in the older population. For example, anxiety is often associated with comorbid depression and dementia (Kasl-Godley, Gatz, and Fiske, 1998). Certain antidepressants have been found to be useful in treating neuropathies, obsessive–compulsive behaviors, anxiety, aggression, sleep disorders, and eating disorders. In many cases, the side-effect profile is safer with an antidepressant than with the alternative medications developed to treat these conditions. It is important to note, however, that a few antidepressants have severe, even dangerous, side effects for the elderly, which are outlined later in this section. The antidepressants described in this section are characterized within the following categories: selective serotonin reuptake inhibitors (SSRIs), tricyclic antidepressants (TCAs), heterocyclic antidepressants, and monoamine oxidase inhibitors.

Selective Serotonin Reuptake Inhibitors

SSRIs provide more serotonin (a neurotransmitter that enhances mood) action to the central nervous system by stopping reuptake of serotonin at nerve terminals. SSRIs are the most commonly used antidepressants in older persons.

The SSRIs are useful medications for treating depression in the elderly. They are equally effective as the older antidepressants but with fewer and less severe side effects. In addition to treating depression, many practitioners are using them as the preferred choice for anxiety, aggression, angry outbursts, agitation, verbal abuse, and obsessive–compulsive behaviors. In addition, the SSRIs currently are typically the best option for treating chronic anxiety with or without depression. As reported in *Treatment of Agitation in Older Persons With Dementia* (Alexopoulous et al., 1998), SSRIs are the experts' first-line preference for depression that also involves secondary symptoms, including balance and orientation problems, very poor memory, lethargy, constipation, concern with weight gain, prostatic hypertrophy, congestive heart failure, orthostatic hypotension, cardiac disease, angina, renal insufficiency, chronic obstructive pulmonary disease (COPD) and overall safety. With respect to specific medications, the experts' first-line choice to treat depression with secondary symptoms of dementia and agitation is sertaline (an SSRI), followed by paroxetine (an SSRI), nortriptyline, venlafaxine, fluoxetine (an SSRI), nefazodone, desipramine, trazodone, and bupropion. There are significant differences in specific SSRI medications. The half-life of a medication describes how long it will have an effect, desirable or adverse, on the patient. Fluoxetine has a much longer half-life and may be useful in noncompliant patients. Paroxetine has the shortest half-life and may be problematic in noncompliant patients. Flu-like symptoms have been reported as early as the first missed dose. Sertaline and citalopram have intermediate half-lives in all populations. The elimination half-life of fluoxetine averages 4 days, and that of its active metabolite, norfluoxetine, averages 7 days. Sertaline has an average elimination half-life of between 26 and 32 hours. Paroxetine has a average elimination of 24 hours.

The pharmacokinetics of sertraline are not altered in the elderly, but plasma levels of fluoxetine, norfluoxetine, and paroxetine are higher in the elderly when they are given the same dose as a younger patient.

Anticholinergic side effects include increased confusion, sedation, decreased cognition, increased constipation, balance and orientation problems, urinary retention, dry mouth, and dry eyes. Paroxetine is significantly more anticholinergic than the other SSRIs. Its anticholinergic effects are more similar to imipramine, a tricyclic antidepressant. This issue should be considered when treating an older patient with paroxetine due to the increased risk of these side effects. Paroxetine is less likely to cause insomnia.

When prescribing any new medication for an older person, its interactions with other drugs should be closely evaluated because of the effect on liver enzymes. Sertraline and citalopram have less effect on liver enzymes and are less likely to interact with other medications.

It may be beneficial to use lower doses of SSRIs initially and for a longer period of time in older versus younger patients to avoid an initial increase in anxiety or agitation. Common side effects of SSRIs include insomnia, anxiety, nausea, diarrhea, sexual dysfunction, and headaches. With the possible exception of paroxetine, SSRIs are best dosed in the morning to help avoid insomnia.

TCAs

TCAs are one of the oldest classes of antidepressants. TCAs block the neuronal uptake of the neurotransmitters norepinephrine, serotonin, and dopamine to various degrees depending on the specific medication. This is thought to potentiate the actions of biogenic amines in the CNS. TCAs may be helpful in treating depression with neuropathy and decreased appetite in the elderly. They also are used in older persons who have trouble sleeping.

Tricyclic antidepressants, with the exceptions of nortriptyline and desipramine, should generally be avoided in the elderly. However, they are still commonly used in the older population, because they are dramatically less expensive than other medications for treating depression. Because of the severe side-effect profiles of these medications, the cost of treating these adverse events generally makes this a less cost-effective treatment for depression in the elderly than the safer, but more expensive, antidepressants.

Nortriptyline and desipramine have low anticholinergic activity and fewer cardiac side effects than other TCAs. Nortriptyline also causes less orthostatic hypotension. Nortriptyline and desipramine are often used in treating neuropathies and other peripheral pain. They are considered to be a relatively safe and inexpensive treatment for depression. Desipramine is generally not as sedating as other TCAs and, at times, causes insomnia.

Amitriptyline, doxepin, and imipramine are best avoided in the elderly. Frequent side effects include sedation, orthostatic hypotension, and anticholinergic effects, which are of particular concern. TCAs may cause a negative inotropic effect as well as delayed intraventricular conduction. It is common to see these agents impair cognition and greatly increase fall risk. Constipation and dry eyes, nose, and mouth are all part of the anticholinergic effect. At times, use of one of these medications is necessary for an older patient. In these instances, the risk versus benefit of using one of these agents must be evaluated and closely monitored.

Heterocyclic Antidepressants

Heterocyclic antidepressants, with the exception of trazodone, are relatively new antidepressants. In addition to treating depression, these drugs are helpful in treating secondary symptoms including anxiety, insomnia, and poor appetite. Heterocyclic antidepressants are being prescribed with more frequency as practitioners become more familiar and comfortable with these agents. Trazadone, as the oldest of these agents, is most commonly used in older persons. The mechanism of action of the heterocyclic antidepressants varies greatly from agent to agent.

Bupropion is considered a weak blocker of dopamine reuptake. Mirtazapine blocks alpha-2-adrenergic inhibitory receptors to increase the release of norepinephrine and serotonin. Trazodone blocks serotonin reuptake. Nefazodone inhibits neuronal uptake of serotonin and norepinephrine.

For primary treatment of depression, trazodone generally is not the medication of choice because the effective dose (200 mg) is rarely tolerated in older persons because of the sedation. Trazodone is very effective when combined with other antidepressants, providing a possible synergistic effect. It is very useful in older persons with depression who have a difficult time sleeping. Trazodone can be used in small (25 mg) divided doses to help relieve symptoms of anxiety, agitation, and aggression. Trazodone can be a very effective medication in treating demented elderly patients with insomnia, disorientation, and agitation at night (sundowning).

Nefazodone and mirtazapine are particularly helpful for patients who are both depressed and anxious. Mirtazapine is often helpful with patients who have difficulty sleeping and has been useful in stimulating appetite.

Bupropion is a popular treatment choice because it has a low risk of causing cognitive impairment. It does not increase serotonin levels as much as other antidepressants, and therefore there may be less risk of causing "serotonin syndrome."

Bupropion's adverse effects include restlessness, activation, tremors, insomnia, and nausea. Seizures have been reported rarely with higher doses of bupropion and should not be used in patients with seizure disorders.

The most common adverse effects of trazodone include sedation (which in some patients can be beneficial) and cognitive slowing. The most common side effects of nefazodone are nausea, drowsiness, dizziness, constipation, dry mouth, and asthenia. These side effects tend to decrease over the first few weeks of therapy. Agranulocytosis has been reported with mirtazapine and should be closely monitored. Mirtazapine may also cause drowsiness, dry mouth, increased appetite, weight gain, dizziness, and constipation. Buproprion may cause restlessness, tremors, insomnia, or nausea.

Serotonin–Norepinephrine Reuptake Inhibitors

Serotonin–norepinephrine reuptake inhibitors are a newer category of antidepressants. Venlafaxine is currently the only medication that is available in this class. It is a potent inhibitor of both serotonin and norepinephrine reuptake. It is commonly used in treating depression in older persons. Some practitioners feel it is useful in treating depressed patients with anxiety.

The most common side effects attributed to venlafaxine are nausea, drowsiness, dry mouth, dizziness, and nervousness. No dosage adjustments are needed for elderly patients on the basis of age; however, starting doses lower and increasing them slowly may help in avoiding nervousness and dizziness. The long-acting form of venlafaxine is convenient and just as effective as the short-acting form. The long-acting form should not be crushed and should be swallowed whole.

General Guidelines for the Treatment of Depression

No single antidepressant is clearly more effective than any other; no single antidepressant results in remission in all patients; and the choice of an antidepressant agent should be based on factors such as adverse effects, prior response, concurrent nonpsychiatric medical illnesses, and concomitant use of other medications that may interact negatively with the antidepressant agent. Patients started on an antidepressant should be assessed within 6 weeks for response to therapy. For those with full symptomatic response, medication should be continued for 4 to 9 months, and then maintenance treatment should be considered.

For those patients who have not responded or who exhibit a partial response to the antidepressant of choice, five possible options should be considered:

- continue current medication with increased dosage;
- switch to another antidepressant;
- augment current therapy with a second medication;
- add psychotherapy to the initial medication; or
- obtain a consultation or referral.

In many cases, it is a good idea to refer for psychotherapeutic evaluation and treatment concurrently with the commencement of antidepressant therapy.

ANTI-ANXIETY AGENTS (ANXIOLYTICS)

Nationally, approximately one out of every five patients in residential care facilities are being treated with anxiolytics. This does not include residents who are being treated with antidepressants for their anxiety. In the elderly, traditional anxiolytics are being replaced by antidepressants such as SSRIs, trazodone, bupropion, nefazodone, and mirtazapine. These agents are often effective at controlling anxiety and with fewer side effects than traditional anxiolytics. Antihistamines, such as hydoxyzine and diphenhydramine, are occasionally used but generally should be avoided in the elderly due to their highly anticholinergic side effects.

When considering use of an anxiolytic, especially the benzodiazepines, it is critical to first rule out other medical conditions that may be contributing to the patient's anxiety, such as pain, infection, depression, insomnia, or cognitive impairment. Medications such as decongestants, oral albuterol, and theophylline may also cause anxiety.

Benzodiazepines

Benzodiazepines are the most commonly used anxiolytics. They are not only used for anxiety, but also for seizures, as muscle relaxants, and for insomnia. The effects of benzodiazepines appear to be mediated through the inhibitory neurotransmitter, gamma amino butyric acid (GABA).

The benzodiazepines are separated into two categories: short-acting and long-acting.

The short-acting benzodiazepines include oxazepam, alprazolam, and lorazepam. The long-acting benzodiazepines include chlordiazepoxide, clonazepam, clorazepate, diazepam, and halazepam. Long-acting benzodiazepines have the increased risk of accumulation that may prolong the sedative effects. They have also been associated with an increased risk of falls in elderly patients. When treating anxiety in a geriatric patient, long-acting benzodiazepines generally should be avoided. The long-acting benzodiazepines may be necessary in treating other conditions, such as seizures or severe muscle disorders.

Clordiazepoxide, diazepam, and halazepam have active metabolites. Lorazepam and oxazepam have inactive metabolites. The short-acting benzodiazepines are generally safer for use in the elderly. However, they still pose an increased risk for falls, cognitive impairment, psychomotor impairment, and sedation. Many practitioners prefer lorazepam or oxazepam over alprazolam for use with geriatric patients. Alprazolam seems to have harsh effects in older adults. When using a short-acting benzodiazepine for the elderly, the smallest effective dose should be used. Doses above 30 mg per day of oxazepam, 0.75 mg per day of alprazolam, and 2 mg per day of lorazepam should be used with extreme caution in the elderly.

Buspirone

Buspirone is a newer medication developed to treat anxiety. It is popular with many prescribers as a safer alternative for older patients than the benzodiazepines. It is an azapirone and is not chemically related to the benzodiazepines. It has many advantages over the benzodiazepines when treating anxiety. Its side effect profile is much safer as it does not cause significant sedation, cognitive impairment, or psychomotor impairment. Buspirone has low potential for abuse and for withdrawal symptoms. There is also less risk of serious overdose.

The disadvantages of buspirone include cost and delayed efficacy. It normally takes 1 to 3 weeks before a patient experiences a reduction in anxiety symptoms. Because of to its delayed action, it is not indicated for "as needed" usage. Doses of 15 mg three times per day are often required for full benefit. Unfortunately, the common starting dose of 5 mg three times a day is frequently never increased to reach this dose, and full therapeutic effectiveness is therefore never achieved. In some individuals, 60 mg per day in divided doses is needed. When starting buspirone, a low dose of lorazepam or oxazepam may be necessary for short-term use. It is important to remember that buspirone increases serotonin levels. This may be significant when used with antidepressants, tramadol, amphetamines, melatonin, St. Johns Wort, dextromethorphan, l-tryptophan, or lithium, because a negative serotonin overload effect can occur.

Antihistamines

Hydroxyzine was originally developed to treat anxiety, but its antihistaminic effects proved to be more valuable. Hydroxyzine and diphenhydramine are primarily used to treat allergic reactions. However, they are occasionally used to treat anxiety. Because of the severe anticholinergic side effects and the lack of evidence that they really help to reduce anxiety in the elderly, they should generally be avoided in this population.

ANTICONVULSANTS AND LITHIUM

Patients with Alzheimer's disease, frontal lobe dementias, Parkinson's disease, vascular dementia, and other neurological conditions may develop varied behavioral disturbances. Such behaviors may include physical aggression, intermittent excessive anger, hitting, scratching, biting, slapping, verbal aggression, disruptive yelling, territorialism, rejecting food, refusing to get out of bed, refusing to bathe, sexual hyperactivity, sleep cycle reversal, and excessive motor activity. These disturbances can cause concerns to the patient, the family, professional caregivers, and other residents.

Such behaviors are often treated with antipsychotic or anti-anxiety medications with varied and minimally effective outcomes. At times, these medications worsen these symptoms. Occasionally prescribers turn to antipsychotics or anxiolytics before carefully evaluating the patient for acute conditions that may be causing the disturbing behavior.

As cognitive function decreases in a patient, the ability to identify and communicate physical discomfort also decreases. Many horror stories have been told about patients who were treated with a psychotropic medication for disturbing behaviors that were actually caused by an undiagnosed and untreated urinary tract infection, stroke, respiratory infection, electrolyte disturbance, dehydration, congestive heart failure, chronic obstructive pulmonary disease, diabetes, bone fracture, hypothyroidism, head trauma, orthostatic hypotension, constipation, or general pain. Physical, verbal, or emotional abuse by caregivers, neighbors, or relatives is another example of a situation that may precipitate behavioral disturbances. A host of environmental conditions may also be a factor in negative behaviors, and the possibilities should be considered carefully.

In fact, adverse effects of certain medications are the most common cause of agitation in the elderly. These medications include antihistamines, muscle relaxants, anti-Parkinsonian agents, alpha-1-adrenergic blockers, centrally and peripherally acting anti-adrenergic agents, certain beta blockers, TCAs, phenothiazine, antipsychotics, opiates, nonsteroidal anti-inflammatory drugs (NSAIDs), benzodiazepines, digoxin, theophylline, and cimetidine.

The use of some of these medications is at times unavoidable, but a risk versus benefit evaluation should always be done and caution should be used. When all of these considerations have been evaluated and it is determined that a medication is needed, anticonvulsant agents have become a valuable tool for prescribers.

Anticonvulsant Agents

Anticonvulsant Agents have a long history of use in treating adverse behaviors in all populations. They were originally developed to prevent seizures, but they were found to be effective treatment for aggression and agitation. It has been suggested that anticonvulsant agents exert their effect on these behaviors by stimulating GABA. Animal studies indicate that there is GABA modulation of some aggressive conditions.

Divalproex sodium is the most commonly prescribed anticonvulsant agent for behavior problems. It is often the drug of choice in treating bipolar disorders. Prescribers are using it first-line for physical aggression, intermittent excessive anger, hitting, scratching, biting, slapping, verbal aggression, disruptive yelling, and other problematic behavior with favorable outcomes. Its side effect profile is much safer than the antipsychotics and benzodiazepines with more frequency of decreasing disruptive behaviors. Divalproex sodium is particularly effective in treating manic behaviors, angry outbursts, and explosive episodes. The most common side effects include gastrointestinal upset, sedation, thrombocytopenia, leukopenia, and decreased liver function. To avoid these adverse effects, researchers recommend low doses in the initial stage of treatment, with progressive dosage increases every 3 to 7 days. Increasing the bedtime dose more rapidly than the daytime dose may help to avoid daytime sedation. Liver Function Tests (LFTs), Complete Blood Count (CBC), and platelet count should be drawn before initiating divalproex sodium and after 1 month, then repeated every 6 months. Valproate levels are only needed to identify a toxic level or patient compliance. Increases in the medication dosage should be made to decrease symptoms, not to reach a therapeutic blood level. Increases in LFTs are not a concern until they are three times normal LFTs. More frequent LFTs may be needed if they are steadily or rapidly rising. The disadvantage to divalproex is that it may take several weeks to see a response because of the fact that blood and tissue levels must reach therapeutic levels. Ongoing evaluation on the part of caregivers and prescribers is necessary.

Carbamazepine is also used for behavioral disturbances, but less frequently than divalproex. Carbamazepine is an anti-epileptic that has psychotropic properties similar to lithium, but with less neurotoxicity. It has more interactions with other medications than divalproex. Its most common adverse effects include blurred vision, nystagmus, dizziness, headache, nausea, drowsiness, and neutropenia. Carbamazepine carries a "black box" warning regarding its propensity to produce drug-induced bone marrow suppression. Only a few cases of aplastic anemia have been reported, but periodic hematological blood testing is recommended. As with divalproex, doses should be started low and increased slowly. Drug levels need only be assessed to avoid toxicity and to verify compliance.

Gabapentin is one of the newer medications developed as an anticonvulsant agent. It is increasingly being used for behavior problems. Gabapentin has a low incidence of CNS side effects. Its side effects include drowsiness, dizziness, fatigue, and cognitive impairment. Sedation seems to be the limiting factor in increasing doses and in tolerability by older persons.

Lithium

Lithium is a soft silver-white element of the alkali metal group that is the lightest metal known and that is used in treatment of manic depressive psychosis. It affects the synthesis, storage, release, and reuptake of central monoamine neurotransmitters including NE, 5-HT, DA, Ach, and GABA. It's antimanic effects may be the result of increases in norepinephrine reuptake and increased serotonin receptor sensitivity. For many years, lithium was the primary treatment for bipolar disorder. Increasingly, alternatives have been used as lithium's toxic dose is very close to its therapeutic dose. Toxicity is very common in the elderly. Symptoms of toxicity may include confusional states, induction or exacerbation of extrapyramidal signs, ataxia, and other CNS or neuromuscular toxicity at levels considered therapeutic in younger patients. It is difficult to justify using lithium in the elderly patient without a clear diagnosis of bipolar disorder. Monitoring of lithium levels should be done at least every 2 to 3 months.

ANTIPSYCHOTICS

Antipsychotic agents are thought to exert their pharmacologic effect via blockade of postsynaptic mesolimbic dopaminergic receptors in the brain, although the exact mechanism of action is unknown. Schizophrenia, schizoaffective disorder, delusional disorder, psychotic mood disorders (including mania and depression with psychotic features), acute psychotic episodes, brief reactive psychosis, schizophreniform disorder, atypical psychosis, Huntington's disease, organic mental syndromes (including dementia) with associated psychotic features, and Tourette's syndrome are examples of conditions where antipsychotics may be appropriate. With a physically aggressive resident, antipsychotics may be necessary, depending on the severity of the behavior as well as the other approaches or medications that have been tried or considered. In severe cases where the resident or others are in immediate danger, intramuscular injections of haloperidol may be appropriate.

Antipsychotics are often used for other behavioral disturbances with limited success, making them the most overused psychotropic drug classification in older persons (followed closely by benzodiazepines). Even with the development of the atypical antipsychotics, these medications can have severe side effects.

Many conditions that were formerly treated on a routine basis with antipsychotics are now being successfully treated with antidepressants and anticonvulsants. These conditions include physical aggression, anger outbursts, continuous yelling, inappropriate sexual behaviors, agitation, self-inflicted harm, and rapid pacing.

Antipsychotics are at times used for continuous yelling, generally without much success. The risk versus benefit in using antipsychotics for other conditions should be evaluated and closely monitored. It may be appropriate to use an antipsychotic if the problem behaviors are persistent, if the patient poses a risk to themselves or others, or if there is substantial impairment of functioning. Antipsychotics are equally effective when equivalent doses are used, but antipsychotic classes differ greatly in safety and toxicity profiles. These differences are magnified in the elderly, thus doses generally should be started at the lowest possible level and increased only if needed. In severe acute psychotic episodes, when a higher dose may be needed, the dose should generally be decreased when possible and maintained at the lowest effective dose to manage psychotic symptoms. PRN doses of antipsychotics may be needed when titrating a routine dose up or tapering a routine dose down. Because of the history of misuse of PRN antipsychotic medications, regulations in nursing homes encourage discontinuing the PRN dose as soon as the patient is stable.

It is extremely important to evaluate all medical and environmental conditions of the patient before prescribing an antipsychotic. Infections, pain, electrolyte imbalances, dehydration, stroke, hypothyroidism, and nutritional deficiencies can all lead to psychotic symptoms. When these conditions are properly diagnosed and treated, the psychotic features are often relieved. Agitation may be decreased by altering a resident's environment, such as providing a predictable routine for residents, separating disruptive and noisy residents from quieter residents, identifying specific precipitants, providing reassurance, and allowing residents to pace if they want. These methods are discussed in greater detail elsewhere in this book.

Many medications can induce psychotic symptoms, particularly medications with anticholinergic side effects. Hallucinations manifested by spiders or bugs crawling on the walls or by worms in the food are often due to an anticholinergic side effect of a medication. Many of these medications can be discontinued to help resolve or avoid these symptoms. Diphenhydramine, hydroxyzine, carisoprodol, cyclobenzaprine, methocarbamol, amitriptyline, doxepin, imipramine, chlorpheniramine, promethazine, meclizine, cyproheptadine, meperidine, belladonna, oxybutynin, and hyoscyamine are all examples of medications with anticholinergic side effects. In some cases, medications with anticholinergic side effects cannot be avoided, such as the anti-Parkinsonian medications. Drugs used for extrapyramidal symptoms, such as benztropine, amantadine, or trihexyphenidyl, are highly anticholinergic. Even some of the antipsychotic drugs themselves have anticholinergic side effects, such as thioridazine and clozapine.

Generally, antipsychotics should not be used for wandering, poor self-care, restlessness, impaired memory, confusion, anxiety, depression, insomnia, unsociability, indifference to surroundings, fidgeting, nervousness, uncooperative attitude, or confusion.

There are many different classes of antipsychotics, but for the purposes of this chapter, they are separated into two categories: Conventional (typical) antipsychotics and the newer atypical antipsychotics.

Conventional (Typical) Antipsychotics

Conventional antipsychotics have been in use for many years. Their overall side effect profile is much higher than atypical antipsychotics.

Chlorpromazine, mesoridazine, and thioridazine are the most sedating typical antipsychotics. Haloperidol, pimozide, thiothixene, trifluoperazine, and fluphenazine have high incidence of extrapyramidal symptoms, including acute dystonias, akathisia, pseudo-Parkinsonism, and tardive dyskinesia, which occur more frequently in older patients compared with younger patients. Patients on antipsychotics seen with tremors, shuffling gate, tongue thrusts, or other such symptoms may be experiencing these extrapyramidal side effects. Anticholinergic adverse effects are seen in many of the antipsychotics and are more prominent with thioridazine and chlorpromazine; these medications should generally be avoided in the elderly when possible. The low potency agents (such as chlorpromazine, mesoridazine, and thioridazine) commonly cause sedation and orthostatic hypotension but induce extrapyramidal side effects less frequently. High potency agents (such as fluphenazine, haloperidol, loxapine, molindone, trifluoperazine, and thiothixene) have a high incidence of extrapyramidal symptoms and less sedation and orthostatic hypotension. Sedating medications often increase confusion, which may cause problematic behaviors. Orthostatic hypotension has been associated with increased falls that may have serious results in the elderly. The high-potency antipsychotics are better tolerated in the elderly, because they cause less sedation, confusion, and orthostatic hypotension. However, the elderly are more likely to develop extrapyramidal side effects associated with their use.

The decision to use specific antipsychotic medications is based on safety profiles, such as incidence of extrapyramidal symptoms, anticholinergic side effects, sedation, confusion, and orthostatic hypotension. The typical antipsychotics have higher incidence of adverse effects then the newer atypical antipsychotics. Tardive dyskinesia is of particular concern because it may be irreversible. The decreased cost in using the typical antipsychotics is more than lost in treating the adverse effects of these medications. When starting a patient on an antipsychotic, the older

conventional medications should be reserved as second-line agents. When changing a conventional antipsychotic to an atypical antipsychotic, it is important to reduce the dose slowly over a period of time while increasing the dose of the new
medication just as slowly. This is especially important if the conventional
antipsychotic has been used for a long period.

Atypical Antipsychotics

As has been previously noted, the newer atypical antipsychotic medications have a
significantly lower incidence of serious side effects compared with conventional
antipsychotic medications. Clozapine was the first of these agents available, but
because clozapine has been associated with decreased white blood counts, its use
is generally not recommended in the elderly. There are several differences in the
atypical antipsychotics that should be considered when choosing one of these
medications—even cost can vary greatly between these agents. Local pharmacies
can provide information on their respective costs.

In residents with Parkinson's disease, especially those with drug-induced psychosis, clozapine has been the drug of choice for many practitioners. Currently,
many specialists prefer quetiapine because of its low incidence of extrapyramidal
symptoms. Olanzapine and clozapine have the highest affinity for the muscarinic
receptors, which may cause an increase in memory dysfunction and cause more
anticholinergic side effects, but may also mitigate extrapyramidal symptoms.
Risperidone has the least affect on histamine H1 receptors; therefore, it generally
causes less sedation and prevents weight gain.

Quetiapine has the most effect on alpha-1 receptors, which may cause more
hypotension, dizziness, and reflex tachycardia. Clozapine, risperidone, and
olanzapine have effects on alpha-1 receptors similar to each other.

Starting doses should be much lower in the elderly. Risperidone is now available in a 0.25 mg strength, which may be a good starting point. Olanzapine is available in a 2.5 mg tablet. Quetiapine's lowest dose is 25 mg. Studies show that doses
above about 1.5 mg of risperidone greatly increase the incidence of
extrapyramidal effects in the elderly without greatly increasing efficacy.

Unfortunately, there is no single agent that is equally effective for all patients. It
almost becomes an art rather than a science when determining which agent will
work best for an individual.

SLEEP AGENTS

Sedative–Hypnotics

As many as 50% of the elderly residents in long-term care have altered sleep cycles. It is difficult to change these patterns. In all cases of sleep disorder, it is important to determine the underlying cause of the condition. Medications may help in

the short term; however, it is typically more beneficial to make provisions for the patients with altered sleep cycles than to use a medication as the sole remedy.

Medications are most helpful during transitions or in acutely stressful times. There are a variety of medications to address sleep concerns. It is important to consider the efficacy and side effects of the prescribed medication in relation to the specific cause of the sleep disorder as well as the age and overall condition of the patient.

The following section is a summary of advantages, disadvantages, and considerations for specific classes of sleep medication.

Benzodiazepines

Benzodiazepines were previously discussed in the anti-anxiety portion of this chapter. The mechanism of action and scope of use were presented early. Use of benzodiazepines as sleep aids generally should be limited to short term use, as tolerance to the sedative effect develops quickly. Benzodiazepines may also increase the fall risk and decrease the patient's ability to function the next day. This risk is reduced in the shorter acting benzodiazepines and increased in the longer acting benzodiazepines.

Temazepam is the most commonly used benzodiazepine for sleep. It is helpful for early morning awakenings, but less effective for inducing sleep. Doses above 7.5 mg are discouraged for the elderly, and use should be limited to short term use. It may be necessary to taper dosage when discontinuing use. An alternative hypnotic is recommended for patients who are taking a separate benzodiazepine for anxiety. Triazolam is more helpful in falling asleep but will not likely help with morning awakenings. It is indicated only for short-term use, with doses not exceeding 0.125 mg in the elderly.

Because of their long half-lives, flurazepam and quazepam generally should not be used in the elderly. The risk of falls and cognitive impairment are severe. Dosage should be tapered when discontinuing use.

Lorazepam, alprazolam, oxazepam, diazepam, clonazepam, chlordiazepoxide, clorazepate, halazepam, and prazepam generally should not be used as sleep aids. Lorazepam may induce sleep, but interferes with REM and Stage 4 sleep. Benzodiazepines are not recommended when sleep apnea is present.

Antihistamines

Antihistamines are commonly used as hypnotics. However, they are very anticholinergic and generally should not be used in the elderly. This is of special concern as they are available without a prescription. Patients and health care workers often mistakenly view antihistamines as safer medications because they are not addicting and do not require a prescription.

Diphenhydramine is the most commonly used antihistamine for sleep. Diphenhydramine is not safe for the elderly: in fact, it can be dangerous. The severe anticholinergic side effects make it a poor choice for frail older adults.

Barbiturates

Barbiturates are also used for seizures in addition as sleep aids. They can produce CNS mood alterations, such as excitation, mild sedation, hypnosis and coma. Barbiturates depress the sensory cortex, decrease motor activity, alter cerebellar function, and produce drowsiness, sedation, and hypnosis. Over time, barbiturates lose their efficacy for both induction and maintenance of sleep. They impair cognition and physical coordination. They also increase fall risk. Amobarbital, aprobarbital, butabarbital, mephobarbital, pentobarbital, and secobarbital generally should be avoided in geriatric settings. With patients already using a barbiturate, the dose should be tapered to discontinue use to avoid the risk of seizures.

Antidepressants

The antidepressants' uses and actions were discussed early in this chapter. In this section the intent is to discuss those antidepressants that may be used as a sleep aid. Trazodone can be very helpful for residents with long-term insomnia. It is one of the best first-line sleep agents. Not only is it sedating, but it may also help with anxious features and may serve as an adjunct for depression. Orthostatic hypotension should be monitored closely when trazodone is started.

Mirtazapine may be a good choice in patients with insomnia and decreased appetite, depression, or anxiety. CBCs should be monitored for agranulocytosis. Mirtazapine is more expensive than trazodone.

Nortriptyline may help with depression and neuropathic pain as well as providing a sedating effect. Tricyclic antidepressants should be avoided (other than nortriptyline) as sleep aids because of the severe anticholinergic side effects. Amitriptyline is the most anticholinergic TCA, followed by doxepin. Amitriptyline and doxepin should be avoided in older adults.

Zolpidem and Zaleplon

Zolpidem and zaleplon are nonbenzodiazepine hypnotics. Zolpidem binds to the omega-1 subclass of benzodiazepine receptors in the brain. The tolerance that develops with the benzodiazepines does not seem to occur with zolpidem. It is a safer and more effective long-term alternative. However, it is not indicated for long-term use. Zolpidem is also more expensive than some of the available alternatives. Zolpidem and zaleplon have relatively short half-lives and may not help with morning awakenings.

CHOLINESTERASE INHIBITORS

Cholinesterase inhibitors are indicated for mild-to-moderate dementia of the Alzheimer's type. It is very important to note that these agents do not reverse the symptoms of Alzheimer's disease; however, they slow the progression of the disease. Family members and caregivers often expect an improvement in the patients' condition as a result of the cholinesterase inhibitors and become frustrated. Patients will not have improved cognition when these medications are started, but studies show they do allow the patient to remain independent longer than if not treated with a cholinesterase inhibitor. The cholinesterase inhibitors are generally not effective or indicated for severe Alzheimer's disease.

Tacrine was the first cholinesterase inhibitor. It is rarely used at present because of the newer agents that are available. Tacrine requires a dose titration on initiation, must be given in divided doses during the day, and requires monitoring of liver function during treatment.

Donepezil and rivastigmine are the newer cholinesterase inhibitors that have recently become available. Donepezil is dosed once daily. Rivastigmine is dosed twice a day. Neither donepezil nor rivastigmine require liver function monitoring. Rivastigmine does require an initial dose titration to avoid adverse effects such as nausea, vomiting, abdominal pain, or loss of appetite.

Adverse side effects for tacrine include nausea, vomiting, diarrhea, dyspepsia, myalgia, anorexia, and ataxia. The most common side effects for donepezil include nausea, diarrhea, headache, and insomnia. Rivastigmine has side effects that may include nausea, vomiting, anorexia, and diarrhea.

MEDICATIONS THAT MAY CONTRIBUTE TO BEHAVIORAL PROBLEMS, PSYCHOLOGICAL PROBLEMS, OR BOTH

Adverse effects of medications are a leading cause of behavior disturbances in the elderly. Anticholinergic side effects are of particular concern. Medications that act on the central nervous system often have negative effects on behaviors or moods.

Common medications that have anticholinergic effects are gastrointestinal antispasmodics such as hyoscyamine, dicyclomine, propantheline, and belladonna alkaloids. Older antihistamines such as chlorpheniramine, diphenhydramine, hydroxyzine, cyproheptadine, promethazine, tripelennamine, and dexchlorpheniramine may cause severe adverse anticholinergic effects in the elderly and are generally best reserved for short-term use to treat acute allergic reactions. Most of the tricyclic antidepressants have potent anticholinergic side effects. Amitriptyline and doxepin are of most concern, with nortriptyline and desipramine being the safest tricyclic antidepressants. Most muscle relaxants and antispasmodic drugs are poorly tolerated by the elderly and have anticholinergic side effects. Methocarbamol, carisoprodol, oxybutynin, chlorzoxazone, metaxalone, and cyclobenzaprine are seldom effective at doses tolerated by the elderly. It is important to remember that some of the antipsychotics also have anticholinergic side effects, especially clozapines, thioridazine, and chlorpromazine. Olanzapine also has a high affinity for the muscarinic receptors. Anti-Parkinsonian agents are necessary in controlling Parkinson's disease. These medications are anticholinergic and may induce psychosis or behavior problems. Medications used to treat extrapyramidal symptoms such as benztropine, amantadine, or trihexyphenidyl are also anticholinergic.

NSAIDs may have CNS side effects. This is of particular concern with indomethacin. Pentazocine is a narcotic analgesic that causes confusion and hallucinations more commonly than any other narcotic drugs. Methyldopa may exacerbate depression in the elderly, as may reserpine. Alternative medications generally should be considered when using or starting any of these medications.

SUMMARY

This chapter has highlighted some of the more prominent drugs that are used in treating older adults who present with medical issues, psychiatric issues, or both, that require pharmacological intervention. The classes of drugs addressed in this chapter underscore the great variety of drug options available for any given medical or psychiatric problem. As the field of geriatric pharmacology has evolved, drugs specific to older adult physiology have emerged. It is important to note, however, that drugs are a treatment adjunct and should be combined with psychological, medical, or social interventions in order to comprehensively treat any given problem. The overreliance of drug therapy to address problems of aging may work against long-term quality of life. It is important for specialists from different areas of health care to come together to form a cooperative interdisciplinary team for each patient. Medication management for older persons can be extremely challenging, and the services of a geriatric consultant pharmacist with ongoing training in the emerging therapies is vital to the effort of providing the best possible care.

REFERENCES

Alexopoulous, G. S., Carpenter, D., Frances, A., Kahn, D. A., & Silver, J. M. (1998). Treatment of agitation in older persons with dementia. *The expert consensus guideline series*. William O. Roberts, Ed., Minneapolis, MN: McGraw-Hill Healthcare Information Programs.

Beers, M. H. (1997). Explicit criteria for determining potentially inappropriate medication use by the elderly. *Archives of Internal Medicine, 157,* 1532–1536.

Kasl-Godley, J. E., Gatz, M., & Fiske, A. (1998). Depression and depressive symptoms in old age. In I. H. Nordhus, G. R. VandenBos, S. Berg, & P. Fromholt (Eds.), *Clinical geropsychology*. Washington, DC: American Psychological Association.

Levy, M. L. & Uncapher, H. (2000). Basic psychopharmacology in the nursing home. In V. Molinari (Ed.), *Professional psychology in long term care* (pp. 279–297). New York: Hatherleigh Press.

Ogland-Hand, S. M., & Zeiss, A. M. (2000). Interprofessional health care teams. In V. Molinari (Ed.), *Professional psychology in long term care* (pp. 257–277). New York: Hatherleigh Press.

Philadelphia College of Pharmacy and American Geriatrics Society (1999). *Geriatric pharmaceutical care guidelines, 1999 edition*. Covington, KY: Omnicare.

Whitbourne, S. K. (1998). Physical changes in the aging individual: Clinical implications. In I. H. Nordhus, G. R. VandenBos, S. Berg, & P. Fromholt (Eds.), *Clinical geropsychology*. Washington, DC: American Psychological Association.

IV

The Residential Care
Organization

10

Training Residential Staff in Intervention Execution and Maintenance

Kimberly O. Sieber
Private Practice, Salt Lake City, Utah

INTRODUCTION

Over the past two decades, there has been an increase in awareness of the need for appropriate interventions with residential care patients. The emphasis on improving the quality of life for these patients is evidenced by a growing literature identifying effective intervention strategies for various treatment issues (e.g., Moniz-Cook et al., 1998; Schnelle, Cruise, Rahman, & Ouslander, 1998; Thomas, 1996). Unfortunately, many patients do not have the opportunity to benefit from such interventions because staff do not use them in their care routines. Thus, despite increased knowledge about effective strategies, residential care workers are not using this knowledge to improve the care of their residents (e.g., Moniz-Cook et al., 1998; Schnelle, Ouslander, & Cruise, 1997).

A frequent reason that well-intentioned interventions fail in residential care is that staff are not adequately trained or prepared to carry out the intervention. Without proper training, care providers will avoid using the intervention or, worse, will use it incorrectly. Such misunderstanding may create a domino effect of problems for the residential care patient. For instance, nursing staff who are not adequately trained in assessing the warning signs of a urinary tract infection may misinterpret associated mental status changes and may apply behavioral, rather than medical, interventions. As a result, the infection may go undiagnosed and may abruptly lead to delirium, urosepsis, and even death. Likewise, symptoms of depression (i.e., apathy, fatigue, psychomotor slowing) may remain untreated because of perceptions

185

that they are the result of "normal aging." Without appropriate interventions, such as medication and psychotherapy, the patient's mood and level of functioning could continue to deteriorate. Therefore, intervention strategies are only useful to the extent that staff are adequately trained to apply them.

Clearly, the consequences for inadequate training are multidimensional. In addition to the potential negative effects on residents (e.g., Mullins, Moody, Colquitt, Mattiasson, & Andersson, 1998), a lack of satisfactory training can have consequences for the care providers themselves (e.g., Pearlman, Mahoney, & Callahan, 1991) and the organization as a whole (e.g., Halbur & Fears, 1986). Much has been written about the need for more consistent use of effective interventions (e.g., Schnelle et al., 1997), but staff may hesitate to execute these interventions because of minimal practical training, disinterest in the process, and obstacles within the organization or environment. The unwillingness or inability of care providers to carry out effective interventions may be the direct result of these barriers. Thus, more effective strategies for training and engaging staff must be identified.

The aim of this chapter is to increase the likelihood of successful interventions in residential care settings. Effective interventions require effective execution; as such, this chapter addresses the following three issues: (a) potential consequences of inadequate training, (b) common barriers to staff participation in intervention, and (c) strategies for overcoming these barriers through effective training. Throughout this discussion, an attempt will be made to address concerns about the impact on residents, staff, and the organization. It is hoped that the information provided herein will serve as a resource to facilitate staff's ability to execute interventions within the practical limits of their care routines.

CONSEQUENCES OF INADEQUATE TRAINING

The care facility environment presents multiple challenges. Problems with residents range from minimal environmental stimulation and inactivity (Stones, Dornan, & Kozma, 1989) to outright physical and emotional abuse (Foner, 1994). Staff may exhibit low morale and job dissatisfaction (Helmer, Olson, & Heim, 1993), resulting in high turnover within the organization (Price, 1977). A number of causes for these problems have been proposed (e.g., Waxman, Carner, & Berkenstock, 1984), but many argue that staff shortages and inconsistent care are the result of limited, ineffective training (e.g., Mercer, Heacock, & Beck, 1993; Wagnild, 1988). This section outlines the consequences of inadequate training on residents, staff, and the organization as a whole.

Effects on Residents

Traditionally, the primary aim of nursing and certified nursing assistant (CNA) training programs has been to address physical needs of patients. For example, the nursing staff is responsible for monitoring and recording vital signs, administering medications, assisting with activities of daily living, and encouraging adequate nutrition. Clearly, when caregivers are not properly trained in these areas, there are serious consequences for residents. The inaccurate assessment of vital signs, for instance, can lead to untreated infections, heart failure, and other potentially fatal conditions. Unfortunately, given the high rate of turnover in residential care facilities (Pearlman et al., 1991; Phillips, 1987; Price, 1977; Stryker, 1981), these basic needs may remain unmet. Without a stable, consistent staff, some conditions may go unnoticed or unreported (Halbur & Fears, 1986), and physical care deteriorates as a result (Helmer et al., 1993; Stryker, 1981). Because consistent caregivers may have knowledge of patients' idiosyncratic backgrounds, habits, and medical conditions (Waxman et al., 1984), their absence can have serious consequences for the patient's physical health. Thus, training and consistency are essential for meeting basic physical needs.

Although psychological–emotional health is a key contributor to quality of life in the elderly (Atchley, 1991), most nursing and CNA programs do not address these needs. Without proper training, caregivers may not acknowledge patients' needs to retain fundamental human rights, such as privacy, dignity, and respect. Stereotypes about patients' helplessness and inability to participate in decisions may result in intrusions on personal freedom and self-regulation (Mullins et al., 1998), as well as the lack of opportunity for autonomy and choice (Wetle, 1991). It is not uncommon for nursing staff to misperceive or make assumptions about what is best for the resident or what the resident is capable of (Mullins et al., 1998). The belief that residents are helpless and incompetent can lead to a loss of dignity and self-respect (Atchley, 1991; O'Conner & Rigby, 1996). Moreover, these losses are exacerbated when unnecessary care is being provided (i.e., choosing clothes when residents are capable of dressing themselves) or when the individual is uncomfortable with certain cares (i.e., male CNAs giving showers to female residents).

Dr. William H. Thomas, author of "Life Worth Living" (1996) and advocate for the Eden Alternative, argues that the bulk of the suffering in nursing homes is due to feelings of loneliness, helplessness, and boredom. Unfortunately, there are no traditional medical interventions for these feelings; thus, they may go unnoticed and "untreated." In addition, the circumstances leading to a patient's admission to a care facility may heighten feelings of loneliness, helplessness, and boredom by threatening the individual's sense of self-identity and self-worth (Atchley, 1991). For example, patients entering care facilities are often coping with multiple physical and psychological losses, including limited mobility, decreased independence and autonomy, and reduced spousal or family contact. In addition, leaving the home environment can be particularly difficult when the individual is forced to sort through a lifetime of accumulations, and may be mourning the losses of treasured possessions, family pets, and a sense of "home."

Natural reactions to experiencing multiple losses include feelings of grief, sadness, and anger. Without supportive intervention, these emotional responses may manifest themselves behaviorally. For example, consider the resident who was admitted to a facility following the death of his wife, who was his primary caregiver. He is probably mourning (a) the loss of his wife, (b) the loss of his home and belongings, and (c) the loss of independence. He could be exhibiting a range of behavioral responses to these losses, including isolation, demandingness, and verbal or physical aggression. Without understanding the emotional basis for these behaviors, caregivers may misinterpret the meaning of his responses and may react in ways that are unhelpful and even damaging. For instance, responding to this man's demanding behavior by telling him "You are taking too much of my time" will only increase feelings of loneliness that are the basis for his behavior. Because the emotional need is not met (reducing loneliness), his undesirable behavior (demandingness) will continue to increase.

An even more damaging response to behavioral problems occurs when caregivers are emotionally and physically abusive toward residents. In a recent qualitative study examining the characteristics of care providers in nursing homes, Foner (1994) found that 92.5% of staff participating in the study were aware of the abuse, neglect, or mistreatment of one or more residents. Dr. Foner spent eight months "immersing" herself in a care facility environment by working alongside the nursing aides as a volunteer. She found that emotional–verbal abuse is more common than physical abuse, but that both are occurring more frequently than one would hope. For example, she observed several instances of yelling, insulting, and teasing residents, particularly in response to the aide's frustration and inability to control his or her temper. More passive forms of emotional abuse included ignoring residents' calls for help, being insensitive to their needs for privacy, and participating in cares with indifference and apathy. Physical abuse in care facilities typically comes in the form of "rough handling," particularly during bathing and dressing, and "retaliation" for the resident's aggressive or combative behavior (Mercer et al., 1993). In these instances, caregivers have been known to use excessive restraints, or to push, grab, shove, and even pinch residents (Foner, 1994).

As these examples illustrate, a lack of adequate training in meeting the needs of residents can have deleterious physical, emotional, and behavioral effects and can even lead to mistreatment and abuse. Research suggests that abusive behavior on the part of care providers is typically the result of frustration and feelings of helplessness regarding residents' behavior (Foner, 1994; Mercer et al., 1993). Thus, staff's lack of understanding and access to coping strategies contributes to ineffective treatment and care practices. Clearly, inadequate training has far-reaching consequences for staff that may be the basis for problems with residents.

Effects on Staff

There is little question that caregivers are ill-prepared to manage the range of problems inherent in nursing homes (Mercer, et al., 1993; Schnelle et al., 1998; Waxman et al., 1984). Current training programs focus on meeting physical needs, which, as illustrated earlier, severely limits the quality of care provided. Nursing aides, who provide the majority of care (Friedman, Daub, Cresci, & Keyser, 1999; Mercer et al., 1993), receive less training than any other care provider in the nursing home. One study found that only 25% of those surveyed were satisfied with their training, and those were aides who had been employed for more than five years (Mercer et al., 1993). These findings suggest that nursing staff is providing care for which they are inadequately trained. Certainly, feeling responsible for tasks for which they are unqualified not only negatively affects the residents, but the caregivers themselves.

One consequence that has already been mentioned is that caregivers experience feelings of frustration and helplessness when they are unable to manage a resident's difficult behaviors. There is strong evidence that abusive behavior from caregivers is due to an inability to cope with a resident's behavior. For example, Foner (1994) observed that yelling often occurred after repeated failed attempts to manage a resident's undesirable behavior. Further, she noted that residents who incessantly repeated words, phrases, complaints, and so forth, were eventually ignored by caregivers. These abusive responses from caregivers were presumably means of coping with negative, unmanageable behaviors. It is possible that feelings of anger, helplessness, and apathy arise when caregivers do not have the skills to cope with or manage the behaviors of residents.

In addition to these emotions, caregivers who are undertrained may experience outright fear in response to residents' difficult behaviors. A vast majority of nursing aides have experienced some form of mistreatment from a patient, with one study reporting that 92% surveyed had been the victim of verbal or physical abuse from a care facility resident (Mercer et al., 1993). The unpredictability of residents' behavior is especially likely when they are suffering from a dementia process, whereby confusion and agitation are more common. Staff in these settings consistently complain about their lack of training and supervision, reporting difficulty caring for patients with memory and behavior problems. These caregivers express fear that they will be unable to cope with or manage aggressive outbursts, and that paranoid behavior could lead to repercussions from management (Pearlman et al., 1991). Clearly, without adequate training, supervision, and support, these fears are not unreasonable.

Given the minimal training in managing difficult behavior, it is not surprising that nursing aides receive little to no training in understanding normal behavior within their elderly patients. Common myths and stereotypes about older adults can lead to negative attitudes and poorer quality of care (Thomson & Burke, 1998). An appropriate response to either normal or abnormal behavior requires an awareness of the basis for such behavior as well as skills for coping with it. Without this knowledge, caregivers are likely to make erroneous assumptions about their patients and may provide care that lacks thoughtfulness or empathy (APA, 1998). Unfortunately, the long-term effects of such an approach to patient care can leave residents feeling frustrated, helpless, and dehumanized.

There is little question that nursing aides play a major role in the lives of their patients and therefore have a significant impact on their well-being. Clearly, they interact with residents with higher frequency and intensity than any other caregiver, providing 80%–90% of care received and participating in the most intimate details of care (Mercer et al., 1993). Because of a lack of recognition and respect for their efforts, however, nursing aides may underestimate their importance in patients' lives. Aides in traditional nursing home settings report feeling undertrained, overworked, and underappreciated (Friedman et al., 1999; Mercer et al., 1993), which can contribute to poor morale and a negative attitude toward care (Mercer et al., 1993). Paradoxically, then, the most important care providers do not perceive themselves as such, and this belief is likely to lead to decreased effort and investment in executing interventions.

Overall, the combined effects of (a) having difficulty coping with residents' behavior, (b) being responsible for the majority of care, and (c) feeling unappreciated and unimportant has obvious consequences for staff. CNAs report feelings of resentment over heavy workload (Kiyak, Namazi, & Kahana, 1997) and lack of preparation–training for their job (Phillips, 1987), citing these difficulties as directly linked to poor morale and job dissatisfaction. As mentioned earlier, unhappy workers are less invested in providing good care for their residents. In addition, job dissatisfaction can lead to employee turnover (Helmer et al., 1993; Kiyak et al., 1997; Phillips, 1987), which will create additional strain for the remaining staff and for the organization as a whole.

Effects on the Organization

Inadequate training can have direct and indirect consequences for the organization and management of residential care facilities. A direct consequence of inadequate training can be summed up in one phrase: poor quality of care. Because both residents and staff suffer when there is limited training, the organization will suffer as well. Poor quality of care can lead to a variety of problems for the organization, ranging from dissatisfied residents and families, to fewer referrals to the facility, to failure to meet state licensure regulations. Thus, poor quality of care due to inadequate training may threaten the very survival of the organization.

An indirect consequence of limited training, as previously discussed, is its contribution to job dissatisfaction and employee turnover. Higher rates of turnover have been found to be related to inadequate orientation, lack of knowledge about the job, and lack of recognition (Wagnild, 1988). Estimates of the rate of staff turnover in care facilities range from 40% to 80% (Price, 1977; Stryker, 1981), with the highest rate of turnover found in staff with the least education and training. Halbur and Fears (1986) reported the highest rate of turnover in nursing aides (69%), a more moderate rate of turnover in licensed practical nurses (51%), and the lowest rate of turnover in registered nurses (36%). A turnover rate of 50% is considered problematic for organizational effectiveness (Halbur & Fears, 1986), suggesting that the high rate of turnover in undertrained staff creates significant costs to the care facility.

Three organizational costs of employee turnover have been proposed by Stryker (1981): financial strain, poor morale, and reduced quality of care. Each time an employee is replaced, the organization is responsible for the cost of recruiting, selecting, interviewing, checking references, and training a new employee, which can cost as much as four times the monthly salary involved (Price, 1977). High turnover results in greater demands on permanent staff to train and supervise new workers, which may lead to a snowballing effect of burnout, dissatisfaction, and even more turnover (Pearlman et al., 1991; Stryker, 1981). New and temporary employees may lack knowledge of their patients' backgrounds and conditions (Waxman et al., 1984), placing them at higher risk for errors in judgment regarding care needs. Thus, inadequate training can lead to a vicious cycle of employee dissatisfaction, staff turnover, and poor quality of care.

In summary, the negative effects of inadequate training are multifaceted and multidirectional. There are numerous consequences for residents, staff, and the organization, and these consequences are not mutually exclusive. The following case example illustrates the interaction between resident, staff, and organizational factors:

Ethel B, an 83-year-old widowed woman, has been a resident of Whispering Pines Care Facility since she suffered a hip fracture six months ago. At the time of her admission, she was under the impression that she would return to her home following her rehabilitation. However, after two weeks of rehabilitation therapies, her family determined that she would benefit from long-term care at Whispering Pines. Her only daughter lived in another state and there were no other close relatives to care for her. Mrs. B's family informed her that she would be limited to certain clothing and keepsakes in her "semi-private" room and that it would be necessary to sell her home and furniture to help pay facility costs. Mrs. B complied with these plans, as she believed that her family was acting in her best interests.

Over the weeks that followed, Mrs. B's participation in her rehabilitation therapies became more and more sporadic. She often refused treatment because she was "not feeling well" and was observed to be increasingly fatigued, somnolent, and withdrawn. Nursing staff expressed frustration that Mrs. B was "not motivated to get better," and that she "stayed in bed all the time." Eventually, Mrs. B's rehabilitation therapies were discontinued, and she spent the majority of her time in her bed watching TV and sleeping. She refused to eat her meals in the dining room with the other residents, preferring to eat alone in her room. She rarely ate more than a few bites. Upon the caregiver's return to pick up her tray, Mrs. B would feign sleep so that she would not have to contend with typical comments, such as "You had better eat some more, or you're going to get sick." Caregivers dubbed Mrs. B "Lazy Miss Daisy," and often giggled as they entered her room.

Six months later, Ethel B's daughter returned to visit her mother. She was horrified to find that Mrs. B was no longer participating in any rehabilitation, that she had lost over 30 pounds, and that she was suffering from three decubitus ulcers. Mrs. B told her daughter that the caregivers "ignored" and "made fun of" her, and that she wanted to "go home." Mrs. B's daughter vehemently complained to the Administrator and Director of Nursing that her mother had been neglected and mistreated and threatened to report the facility to the state licensing board. Management, in turn, reprimanded the employees involved, and issued an apology to the family. Three of the employees were so angry about the reprimand that they did not show for work the next day and were then terminated. Mrs. B was placed in another facility.

Although this case example is a fictional depiction of the consequences of inadequate training, it does represent the interplay of residents, staff, and the organization. Mrs. B's apathy, fatigue, withdrawal, and appetite loss were all signs of depression. These symptoms were not surprising in light of the multiple losses she had experienced within a matter of weeks (i.e., physical ability, home, belongings, independence). However, they seem to have been misinterpreted by staff as being typical "difficult" behaviors, such as resistance, laziness, and lack of motivation. As a result, minimal effort was exerted to understand the basis for these behaviors, and she was left to deteriorate. Thus, consequences for this resident (depressive symptoms) created consequences for the staff (frustration due to lack of understanding), which lead to further consequences for the resident (physical and psychological deterioration).

The interplay between the organization and staff is also evident in this example. Nursing staff were not provided with adequate training and support from management regarding "problem" behaviors, which led to the patient's deterioration and, ultimately, her removal from the facility. Following family complaints, the administration responded by reprimanding rather than communicating with the employees involved; as such, three staff members were lost. The end results, therefore, were poor quality of care, dissatisfied staff, and organizational instability.

As this case example illustrates, inadequate training can have deleterious effects on residents, staff, and the organization. Although much has been written about the availability of successful treatment methods (Blair & Eldridge, 1997; Mayers & McBride, 1998; Schnelle et al., 1998), researchers and practitioners have been frustrated with the lack of follow-through in residential care facilities (Moniz-Cook et al., 1998; Schnelle et al., 1998). There is no question that the effectiveness of such treatment protocols is dependent on staff's willingness and ability to participate in interventions. However, there are a number of barriers that interfere with such participation, including inadequate training, lack of investment in interventions, and organizational problems. These barriers are discussed in the following section.

BARRIERS TO STAFF PARTICIPATION IN INTERVENTION

Despite awareness of the need for more effective interventions in residential care facilities, staff in these facilities are notorious for their lack of consistency and follow-through. How do we explain such unwillingness to participate in treatment? Are caregivers cruel and inhumane? Lazy? Incompetent? In reality, staff in care facilities face a number of barriers that interfere with their participation in interventions. For example, caregivers who are not adequately trained in specific interventions will be unable to participate in their execution. In addition, unclear treatment protocols and excessive workloads can interfere with the caregiver's investment in participating. Finally, problems within the organization itself can present barriers for staff participation.

Inadequate Training

Staff in care facilities are faced with numerous challenges for which they are inadequately trained. Although CNA training programs address factors pertaining to physical needs, there is little emphasis on the psychological and emotional needs of residents in long-term care. For example, caregivers may be trained to recognize when a patient needs his or her brief changed, but they may not be trained to approach this issue with emotional sensitivity. Further, although caregivers are trained to assist with activities of daily living (i.e., dressing, bathing), they are inadequately trained regarding the importance of autonomy–choice (Wetle, 1991). Without awareness of a patient's need for dignity, respect, and privacy, caregivers are likely to complete their physical cares in ways that can result in emotional and psychological damage (Atchley, 1991; O'Connor & Rigby, 1996).

Another psychological–emotional issue for which caregivers are inadequately trained is the process of adjustment to a care facility. Patients entering care facilities are often grieving multiple losses, including health and physical ability, home environment, and personal belongings. Although some individuals adjust to these losses with ease, grief can result in vastly different responses, with one set of patients experiencing sadness, another set experiencing anxiety, and a third set experiencing anger and hostility. Without training in these areas, caregivers do not possess the tools to respond to these emotions appropriately, which could lead to exacerbation of behavior problems. Thomas (1996) argued that the majority of behavior problems in nursing homes are the result of ineffectively "treating" loneliness, helplessness, and boredom. Unfortunately, none of these emotional needs are addressed in traditional CNA training programs, which may explain caregivers' difficulties coping with behavior problems (Pearlman et al., 1991).

In addition to poor training regarding the link between emotional needs and behavior, CNAs receive minimal training concerning behavioral ramifications of common physical illnesses and disabilities. For instance, patients with organic brain impairment (i.e., dementia, cerebral vascular accident, traumatic brain injury) may present with disinhibited behavior, aggression, or memory deficits that, without adequate training, could be misinterpreted as volitional. Patients with chronic obstructive pulmonary disease (COPD) often exhibit symptoms of anxiety, including shortness of breath, fear of suffocation, and panic attacks, because of the oxygen deprivation that occurs with the illness. Finally, patients who develop infections, such as pneumonia or urinary tract infections, can exhibit altered mental status, hallucinations, and delusions due to delirium. In each of these cases and more, the accurate assessment of the problem will drive the direction of the intervention. However, traditional CNA training programs have failed to address these important issues.

In general, caregivers are provided with little training regarding the assessment and management of behavior. For example, because of common myths and stereotypes about older adults (i.e., "they're more difficulty and rigid"), caregivers may become easily frustrated with normal behavior (Moniz-Cook et al., 1998). In addition, problematic behavior, such as noncompliance, perseveration, and aggression, may seem uncontrollable to caregivers who have not been trained in appropriate behavioral management techniques. Thus, training regarding emotional, physical, and behavioral issues is essential for the execution of interventions.

Lack of Investment in Interventions

Research suggests that even when caregivers are provided with necessary training opportunities, they are not likely to use new interventions (Moniz-Cook et al., 1998; Schnelle et al., 1998). This finding suggests that there are other factors, such as interest, motivation, and self-perceptions, that interfere with the consistent execution of interventions.

For example, although caregivers attend mandatory inservices, they may not be interested in the material presented and thus will not incorporate new interventions into their care routines. Aides have described inservices as "boring and repetitious," with an emphasis on rudimentary skills such as hand washing and participation in fire drills (Mercer et al., 1993). Further, much of the material is presented in a lecture format. Lectures can be tedious and may not be effective for the majority of nursing aides, who have limited formal education and may not be fluent in English (Schnelle et al., 1998). Finally, there is often a punitive focus to inservices, as they are usually held on payday and caregivers are told that they will be reprimanded if they do not attend (Mercer et al., 1993). This focus may result in feelings of resentment and a lack of interest in material presented. Traditional training formats, therefore, do not communicate the information in a manner that can be understood and applied, and may decrease the likelihood that interventions will be used.

A second reason caregivers may not use interventions in their care routines is that treatment protocols are unclear and unreasonable. Although the Omnibus Budget Reconciliation Act (OBRA, 1987, cited in Schnelle et al., 1997) regulations provide guidelines on several conditions found in care facilities (i.e., pressure ulcers, urinary incontinence, depression), outcomes of these guidelines are not well-documented (Schnelle et al., 1997). In addition, interventions, though effective, may be too complex to maintain and may be poorly received by staff (Schnelle et al., 1998). There are multiple physical and emotional demands on caregivers that may interfere with their willingness to accept additional responsibilities, as illustrated in the following description:

> There is the sheer physical effort of lifting and bathing fragile and often immobile patients. Many patients are bitter and hostile, often because they are so confused. Patients may yell and scream while aides try to wash and dress them or help them eat. Some actively resist, while others, usually through no fault of their own, undo work aides have already completed. Throughout the day, residents understandably make constant demands, and patients suffering from dementia frequently cry, plead, and moan. On top of this, there is abuse from residents, ranging from angry comments to actual physical violence. "Curse you, scratch you, bite you," is how one aide ... summed it up. There are insults, name-calling, swearing, and even threats of blackmail. (Foner, 1994, p. 247)

Given these demands, caregivers may be more invested in making their job easier than in executing new interventions. For instance, although there are effective treatment protocols designed to decrease incontinence, it takes more time to assist with toileting than to change a brief. Because of sheer time and effort demands, therefore, caregivers tend to revert to old practices regardless of training received (Schnelle et al., 1997).

In general, despite their heavy workload and obvious necessity, caregivers may not participate in interventions because they do not recognize their own importance. Although nursing aides perform the majority of care in a facility (Mercer et al., 1993), they repeatedly receive the message that they are not important. Concrete evidence comes in the form of low wages, limited benefits, and little opportunity for career advancement. In addition, aides receive minimal appreciation of work performed and are not likely to be recognized for extra effort. Finally, nursing aides have minimal autonomy to make decisions about their patients; despite their frequent contact with residents, they are rarely asked their opinions about care practices (Pearlman et al., 1991). Overall, these experiences may lead to caregivers' beliefs that their contributions are insignificant, resulting in apathy and unwillingness to use suggested interventions.

Finally, given the lack of appreciation and recognition for their efforts, nursing staff may harbor feelings of resentment and distrust of administration–management. Job dissatisfaction and poor relationships with superiors can result in hostility toward the organization. Angry employees will certainly exert minimal effort, and use of new interventions is unlikely. Thus, problems within the organization itself can present a barrier to staff participation in interventions.

Organizational Problems

With a 40% to 80% rate of turnover (Price, 1977; Stryker, 1981), it is clear that the organizational effectiveness of the majority of care facilities is limited (Halbur & Fears, 1986). The challenge of hiring, training, and retaining employees creates significant financial and emotional strain for management and for remaining staff (Pearlman et al., 1991; Stryker, 1981). These strains can lead to poor morale and resentment (Mercer et al., 1993), which contributes to a vicious cycle of job dissatisfaction, employee turnover, and poor quality of care.

In addition to these organizational problems, high employee turnover makes continuity of care nearly impossible. Consider the following scenario:

> Jackie, a new nurse's aide at Whispering Pines Care Facility, was hired on October 12th. She attended an employee orientation on October 14th and began on-the-job training on the 15th. On the 15th, 16th, and 17th, she was trained in three different sections of the facility by three different aides. On completion of her training, she had met all of the residents and had begun to develop an understanding of their care routines. Jackie began working independently on October 20th.

> Over the course of the next two weeks, Jackie worked a total of eight shifts. In an effort to increase continuity of care, the majority of her shifts were scheduled in one section. Residents began to recognize her and know her name. Jackie, however, was having difficulty coping with the erratic behavior of some residents and became frustrated with the low pay and heavy work demands. She failed to show for work on November 3rd, choosing instead to work at a fast food restaurant. She was replaced on November 4th.

As this example illustrates, a significant amount of time and effort were invested in orienting and training Jackie that ultimately resulted in greater cost than benefit to the organization. First, Jackie was paid for her participation in orientation and three training sessions. Second, three permanent aides, who may have neglected resident needs in the process, invested energy into training her. Finally, despite attempts to increase the likelihood of continuity of care, Jackie left the facility after only two weeks; residents were then forced to adjust to a new caregiver. Unfortunately, this scenario is not uncommon in care facilities. Given the 69% rate of turnover in nursing aides (Halbur & Fears, 1986), Jackie's replacement is likely to exhibit a similar pattern of hiring, training, and quitting. Continuity of care, when employees invest only three weeks into the process, is difficult for the organization to attain.

Another barrier related to organizational problems is a lack of mission or philosophy surrounding patient care. In many facilities, the general approach to patient care is to avoid untoward effects (Kane, 1995) rather than to provide good care and enhance quality of life. In addition, paper compliance tends to be emphasized over actual care because of state survey issues, so that care received is typically inferior to what is documented (Schnelle et al., 1997). Frighteningly, then, patients may not actually receive care that is noted in their chart. Facilities have also been known to "prepare" for yearly state surveys by improving their residents' appearances (i.e., improving grooming and hygiene) and the physical surroundings (i.e., painting and redecorating). This general philosophy emphasizing the importance of appearance, rather than the importance of high-quality care, certainly interferes with staff's motivation to participate in interventions.

Finally, communication problems and lack of follow-through from management may present a barrier for effective execution of interventions. Communication between aides, nurses, and management in care facilities is notoriously poor, and the majority of such communication is negative. In a recent survey of nursing aides, 70% reported that they were not treated with respect from their superiors (Helmer et al., 1993). In addition, interviews with nursing aides suggest that superiors do not follow through with intervention programs after starting them. The perception that "no one seems to care about" the new intervention results in a lack of motivation for the caregiver to continue (Schnelle et al., 1998). If there is a lack of engagement or modeling by management to participate in intervention strategies, caregivers are not likely to maintain them over time (Moniz-Cook et al., 1998). Thus, poor communication and lack of follow-through from the administration is likely to lead to apathetic workers and underutilized interventions.

In summary, staff's ability and willingness to participate in interventions can be obstructed by several factors. When not provided with adequate training, they do not have access to techniques and strategies and therefore are unable to use effective interventions. In addition, caregivers may not be invested in interventions because of ineffective training formats, unreasonable treatment protocols, and the belief that their actions are unimportant. Finally, organizational instability, lack of a positive mission or philosophy, and poor communication and follow-through can interfere with staff's willingness to participate in interventions. The following section addresses each of these barriers and identifies strategies for effectively training and motivating staff.

STRATEGIES FOR TRAINING STAFF:
OVERCOMING BARRIERS

Thus far, this chapter has identified potential consequences of inadequate training, as well as factors that interfere with staff's participation in interventions. This final section focuses on strategies for addressing these barriers through (a) emphasizing essential areas of training, (b) increasing investment in interventions, and (c) enacting organizational changes.

Essential Areas of Training

As previously mentioned, most CNA training programs focus almost exclusively on meeting the physical needs of residents. Certainly, this issue remains a fundamental aspect of CNA training. However, to more effectively treat and care for residents in long-term care, a generalized shift in training philosophy is necessary. Training must not only focus on physical needs, but on understanding the individual as a whole (Kiyak et al., 1991). Fully understanding a patient requires knowledge of his or her physical, psychosocial, and behavioral issues, as well as recognizing how these factors interact.

Physical Needs

It is clear that caregivers require training in providing basic physical care, and traditional CNA training programs effectively accomplish this goal. However, caregivers should also be provided with training regarding common physical illnesses and disorders as well as the behaviors that may accompany these disorders. As an illustration, patients suffering from dementia or other forms of brain injury may present with various symptoms of frontal lobe impairment, including impulsivity, social and sexual disinhibition, and aggression. Recognizing and understanding these behaviors in light of their physical basis can increase the possibility of an appropriate response. Caregivers with such knowledge are less likely to become offended by the behavior, for example, and may be more likely to respond with such appropriate strategies as distraction and redirection.

Other common physical illnesses and disorders (and their behavioral ramifications) that should be addressed in caregiver training include (a) any form of organic brain impairment (i.e., cerebral vascular accident, traumatic brain injury, dementia), (b) other neurological illnesses (i.e., Parkinson's disease, Multiple Sclerosis), (c) COPD and other illnesses causing hypoxia, (d) hypertension–heart disease, (e) rheumatoid arthritis and osteoarthritis, and (f) adult-onset diabetes. In addition, caregivers should be trained to recognize the physical and behavioral signs of an infection (i.e., urinary tract infection, pneumonia, cellulitis), including changes in vital signs and mental status.

Finally, training regarding physical issues should also include information about normal changes in late life. For example, caregivers should know that many older adults suffer from hearing loss and that it is necessary to speak slowly and clearly to such patients without yelling. In addition, patients with visual impairment should be provided with glasses in an effort to increase engagement in activities and social interaction. Normal physical and cognitive changes, such as slowed movement and mild memory decline (APA, 1998), should also be addressed as patients may require increased assistance in these areas.

Psychosocial Needs

Certainly, patients in long-term care present with a range of emotional, psychological, and communication issues that should be addressed in caregiver training. Emotional issues that may be triggered by admission into a care facility include the needs for privacy, dignity, and respect, as well as the need to feel emotionally connected to others. Training, therefore, should focus on (a) understanding why these needs are triggered by placement in long-term care, (b) recognizing how these needs are manifested, and (c) identifying responses that are sensitive to these needs. The following case example illustrates these points:

> George N, a 75-year-old retired dentist, was admitted to Whispering Pines Care Facility as a result of multiple health problems, including frequent urinary tract infections, arthritis, and poorly managed diabetes. Prior to admission, his wife of 52 years was caring for him at home. Because of urinary incontinence, Mr. N was forced to wear briefs. In addition, he required assistance with transfers–mobility as well as monitoring of blood glucose levels. On admission, Mr. N was shocked to learn that caregivers as young as his granddaughter would be changing his briefs, bathing him, and dressing him. He would often refuse these interventions, stating that he was "not dirty," and he would become hostile when caregivers insisted on completing these tasks. When his wife visited him in the facility, he complained that he was not receiving adequate care and he begged to return home.

Mr. N's emotional needs for privacy, dignity, respect, and emotional connection are evident in this example. Receiving intimate care from young, female caregivers triggered feelings of shame and embarrassment. As a result, he frequently refused care and became hostile when he was forced to allow such care. In addition, his expressions of dissatisfaction were masking the need for emotional connection to his wife. He desired to return home, not due to inadequate care, but because he missed his wife. A caregiver trained to recognize the basis for these behaviors is more likely to respond appropriately to underlying needs. Ultimately, these abilities will make the caregiver's job easier, as noncompliant behaviors and hostility may subside when the patient is provided with empathy and validation.

Psychologically, a patient who is adjusting to long-term care faces changes that can result in threats to sense of self, independence, and worth. Placement in a care facility may trigger changes in an individual's self-identity that are brought about by failing health, disability, and impending death (Atchley, 1991; Compton, 1989). In addition, patients may be struggling with needs for autonomy–choice in an environment whose purpose is inherently paradoxical to these needs (Wetle, 1991). As a result, some patients struggle with self-denigration and reduced feelings of competence and worth (Atchley, 1991). Mr. N's psychological struggle was characterized by a change in identity from a successful health care professional to a nursing home patient. The shift from providing care to receiving care left him feeling dependent and incompetent, which lead to resistant, hostile behavior. Caregivers, therefore, should be aware of the importance of allowing patients to maintain their sense of self, independence, and worth, despite multiple losses and decreased control over life (Atchley, 1989; Compton, 1989).

Another psychosocial need that should be addressed in caregiver training concerns communication strategies. Human beings communicate directly and indirectly, through verbal and nonverbal means. Because there are so many forms of communication, residents may express their needs in manners that are difficult for staff to comprehend. As a result, the communication may be inconsistent with the response, leading to further behavioral problems. Mr. N, for example, indirectly communicated his needs for dignity and respect by being hostile to his caregivers. Caregivers interpreted his behavior as being due to a stubborn disposition, and responded by providing care against his will. Thus, the response ("You will do as you are told") was directly opposed to Mr. N's underlying communication ("I need dignity"). Further, staff's forcible behavior communicated to Mr. N that he had no rights to dignity and respect, resulting in an exacerbation of his resistance and hostility.

When addressing psychosocial needs in training, it is important to emphasize that these needs are more difficult to recognize than are physical needs. Residents may struggle with emotional and psychological needs without knowing how to communicate them to their caregivers. As such, caregivers should be educated about (a) common emotional–psychological needs in residents (i.e., dignity, self-preservation), (b) ways these needs may be communicated (i.e., nonverbal, behavioral), and (c) effective means of responding to these needs (i.e., empathy, validation). Finally, caregivers should be provided with specific strategies for responding to needs when behavior becomes unmanageable.

Behavioral Management

A consistent finding in the literature is that staff in care facilities need more training in behavioral management strategies (Blair & Eldridge, 1997; Foner, 1994; Mercer et al., 1993; Schnelle et al., 1998). One study found that the most frequent requests for additional training were for (a) managing the behavior of residents with depression, dementia, and aggressive behavior; (b) enhancing knowledge of diagnostic issues; and (c) improving communication skills (Mercer et al., 1993). As highlighted earlier, when physical and psychosocial needs are addressed, behavioral management "strategies" may not be necessary. Addressing symptoms of loneliness, helplessness, and boredom, for example, should lead to a reduction in problematic behaviors (Thomas, 1996), theoretically eliminating the need for behavioral management.

Practically speaking, however, behavioral management strategies are necessary for the successful operation of care facilities. There are numerous behavioral issues that arise in this environment because of the prevalence of physical and cognitive disorders with behavioral correlates. Caregivers, therefore, should be trained regarding basic principles of behavioral management as well as practical guidelines for their use in this setting.

For example, a general principle of behavioral management is that reinforcing (rewarding) a behavior will increase its frequency and intensity. If a patient is making socially inappropriate or offensive comments to a caregiver, and the caregiver responds by laughing, the comments are likely to persist because they are being reinforced. With a goal of decreasing this undesirable behavior (offensive comments) and replacing it with desirable behavior (socially appropriate interactions), caregivers would ignore the offensive comments and respond only to appropriate interactions. The reinforcement, therefore, only occurs when the patient is exhibiting desirable behavior, which will lead to an increase in that behavior and a decrease in the undesirable behavior. Accordingly, this patient may learn to interact more appropriately with staff. These basic principles can be applied to a variety of problematic behaviors, including those associated with dementia, psychiatric disorders, and noncompliance.

Overall, training focused on addressing physical, psychosocial, and behavioral issues, as well as the interplay among these factors, will have positive effects for residents, staff, and the organization as a whole. Residents will have their needs met, staff will feel competent in meeting those needs, and the organization may experience decreased turnover as a result. For these effects to occur, however, the information provided in training must be presented in a manner in which it can be understood and applied. Furthermore, staff must be invested in participating in training and in implementing interventions in their care routines.

Increasing Investment in Interventions

Effective training will provide caregivers with skills to meet the various needs of their residents. For caregivers to develop these skills, they must be interested in the information provided and invested in using interventions. This section discusses several strategies for increasing the investment in training, thereby increasing the likelihood that interventions will be used consistently.

Traditional inservice trainings typically use a lecture format, which has limited use within the care facility setting. Nursing aides often experience this training strategy as "boring" (Mercer et al., 1993) and therefore may assume the information provided is not worthwhile. Because of limitations in language and formal education, caregivers may not understand material presented and may stop listening altogether. An alternative to the lecture-based format is the use of active, nonverbal training strategies. Caregivers may be more interested in information that is presented in the form of role-plays, modeling, and personal illustrations. The experience of actively participating in training will promote understanding of resident needs and will increase skills for using intervention strategies. For these reasons, nonverbal learning strategies have been found to be more effective in maintaining interventions than traditional lecturing and inservices (Schnelle et al., 1998).

Training programs that include both theoretical and experiential strategies can effectively improve staff attitudes and increase investment in interventions (Mayers & McBride, 1998; Moniz-Cook et al.,1998; Thomson & Burke, 1998). One example of such a training program attempts to increase empathy for residents through both didactic and participative formats. The four phases of this training program (Thomson & Burke,1998) include the following:

1. Brief introduction to training: Facilitator discusses the theoretical basis for information to be discussed.
2. Self-examination exercise: Participants identify important aspects of their life and then identify how these same issues are important to their residents.
3. Game eliciting empathy: Participants assume the role of an older, dependent individual, which leads to examination of attitudes and perspectives.
4. Debriefing and self-reflection: Facilitator encourages participants to consider the emotional and practical outcome of the training experience.

This training format has been found to increase understanding of specific age-related issues (Mayers & McBride, 1998), increase feelings of competency to participate in interventions (Moniz-Cook et al., 1998), and improve attitudes toward the elderly in general (Thomson & Burke, 1998). Thus, providing both theoretical and experiential training will increase staff's investment in using interventions and will therefore result in improved quality of care.

The training program discussed earlier emphasizes the importance of enhancing empathy for residents. This issue should be an essential aspect of training, as caregivers who understand and have good relationships with their residents will generally provide better care for them. Studies suggest that empathy for residents and their families results in positive relationships and increased job satisfaction (Friedman et al., 1999; White, 1980), thereby improving quality of care.

Empathy can be elicited through participation in exercises that promote an understanding of the interplay between physical, emotional, and psychological needs. For example, understanding the need for autonomy–choice can be enhanced by reading vignettes that illustrate this need in personal, meaningful terms (Mullins et al., 1998). In addition, caregivers encouraged to understand the personal attributes and rights of their patients are more likely to experience empathy (Kihlgren & Thorsen, 1996), which may result in more respectful treatment.

In addition to promoting overall empathy for residents, training programs should emphasize development of basic skills for using interventions. When new interventions are introduced, caregivers should be provided with simple, meaningful explanations regarding their purpose and application. Specific guidelines for carrying out interventions should be outlined, and staff should be encouraged to voice concerns about the practicality of such interventions. For example, a training session focused on meeting residents' need for dignity and respect might apply the following strategies:

1. Identify the purpose of the inservice.
2. Caregivers participate in an exercise eliciting empathy for dignity and respect needs.
3. Highlight the need for changes in care routines to enhance dignity and respect.
4. Outline specific intervention strategies (i.e., respectful communication, private dressing and bathing, opportunities for autonomy–choice).
5. Practice strategies through role-plays, and discuss personal experiences using these strategies.
6. Discuss benefits and potential barriers to carrying out interventions (i.e., time and effort demands, resident behavioral issues).

Providing practical guidelines in an active, empathy-enhancing format should result in increased use of intervention strategies, as caregivers are more likely to value, understand, and feel committed to the process.

   Following formal training experiences, caregivers may be more invested in maintaining intervention strategies when a mentoring system is used. In this system, a new employee is matched with a senior staff member, who provides on-the-job training and facilitates friendships within the workplace (Crowley, 1993). Success of training efforts is dependent on ongoing feedback and follow-up (Moniz-Cook et al., 1998; Schnelle et al., 1997); thus, new employees in particular will require frequent contact with those who are more experienced. Mentors, rather than management personnel, have the unique characteristic of being peer-advisors. They can provide immediate feedback in ways that are empathetic and non-threatening, thereby increasing the likelihood that the feedback will be used.

   In summary, staff will be more invested in participating in interventions when (a) information is presented in a manner that is interesting and meaningful, (b) relationships with residents are improved through increased empathy, (c) practical guidelines are outlined, and (d) feedback is provided from non-threatening co-workers. The long-term success and maintenance of these interventions may be further enhanced by improvements within the organization itself.

Organizational Changes

Given the problems inherent in most care facilities, it is clear that many changes are necessary for improving the care of residents. In addition to problems with training content and format, organizational issues may interfere with the motivation to provide good care. This section recommends changes in overall philosophy and activity that will benefit residents, staff, and the organization as a whole.

A major concern in most care facilities is that those who are providing the majority of the care do not feel important or appreciated (Friedman et al., 1999; Helmer et al., 1993; Mercer et al., 1993). As a result, caregivers exert decreased effort and are less invested in providing good care (Mercer et al., 1993). Therefore, a significant shift in management philosophy is necessary. Most importantly, staff members need to feel valued and respected by their superiors. Management must make concerted efforts to instill pride in caregivers regarding their job responsibilities. Organizational commitment can range from verbally acknowledging employees for their efforts, to recognizing them in a staff meeting, to offering them pay raises or bonuses. Management's behavior can improve self-perceptions of caregivers, thereby improving the quality of their work.

Another way to improve quality of care is to instill pride in caregivers through their efforts with residents. Foner (1994) found that caregivers were more invested in their work when they were proud of how they cared for their residents, when they believed they were needed and valued, and when they felt emotionally connected to a "family" environment (Foner, 1994). Creative mechanisms that acknowledge nursing assistants who have the best cared-for (groomed, healthy, functioning) residents can result in increased pride and effort and may also decrease negative resident behaviors.

Along with improving the overall status of caregivers, management should provide opportunities for staff to offer their opinions and participate in decisions surrounding the care of their residents. Despite their frequent contact with residents, CNAs have little control over their care routines, and they rarely participate in treatment decisions. In addition to increasing caregivers' perceptions of their value–worth, providing them with autonomy and respect for their opinions is likely to result in improved quality of care. Studies have repeatedly found that organizations promoting autonomy retain employees who are more satisfied and exert more effort in their work (Friedman et al., 1999; Helmer et al., 1993; Kiyak et al., 1997; Sargent & Terry, 1998; White, 1980). In addition, having control over decision-making can result in increased investment in positive outcomes (Helmer et al., 1993; White, 1980).

For training and interventions to be effective over the long term, the organization must demonstrate its commitment through consistency, modeling, and follow-through. Without such commitment, training effects will not be maintained (Moniz-Cook et al., 1998; Schnelle et al., 1997). Because staff will mirror the behavior of their superiors, management personnel must consistently model appropriate interventions, and must participate actively in follow-through and the evaluation of outcome. For example, staff trained in behavioral management principles are more likely to use these interventions when they observe their superiors effectively using them. In addition, management personnel should monitor resident behavioral changes to determine the effectiveness of the intervention.

The training and intervention strategies presented in this section have addressed many of the barriers found in the care facility environment. Providing education about physical and psychosocial needs, as well as training regarding behavioral management principles, creates a more holistic picture of the individual. This information must be presented in a manner that can be understood and applied, with practical, experiential strategies being more effective than the traditional lecture format. Finally, effective organizations must change their philosophy to emphasize the importance of the caregiver role and to evaluate outcomes of training and intervention.

SUMMARY

In summary, the likelihood of successful interventions in care facilities may be increased through (a) heightened awareness of the consequences associated with inadequate training, (b) recognition of barriers that interfere with staff participation in interventions, and (c) identification of strategies for overcoming these barriers. The interaction between residents, staff, and the organization plays a significant role in training and interventions. Information must be communicated in a respectful and validating manner at all levels of an organization. Caregivers need to be educated about both physical and psychosocial needs, and facilities must move from treating medical needs in a compartmentalized fashion to treating the whole person through interdisciplinary cooperation. This paradigm shift includes changes in care approaches, management strategies, and organizational philosophy. The ultimate result of such a shift will be increased use of successful interventions, yielding positive outcomes for all: residents, staff, and the organization.

REFERENCES

American Psychological Association. (1998). What practitioners should know about working with older adults. *Professional Psychology: Research and Practice, 29*, 413–427.

Atchley, R. C. (1989). A continuity theory of normal aging. *The Gerontologist, 29*, 183–190.

Atchley, R. C. (1991). The influence of aging or frailty on perceptions and expressions of the self: Theoretical and methodological issues. In J. E. Birren, J. E. Lubben, J. C. Rowe, & D. E. Deutchman (Eds.), *The concept and measurement of quality of life in the frail elderly* (pp. 207–225). San Diego, CA: Academic Press.

Blair, C. E., & Eldridge, E. F. (1997). An instrument for measuring staff's knowledge of behavior management principles (KBMQ) as applied to geropsychiatric clients in long–term care settings. *Journal of Behavior Therapy and Experimental Psychiatry, 28*, 213–220.

Compton, B. R. (1989). Psychological aspects of aging in residential care. *Residential Care Journal, 3*, 221–230.

Crowley, C. H. (1993). The human factor: Unmasking staff potential. *Provider, 19*, 22–27.

Foner, N. (1994). Nursing home aides: Saints or monsters? *The Gerontologist, 34,* 245–250.

Friedman, S. M., Daub, C., Cresci, K., & Keyser, R. (1999). A comparison of job satisfaction among nursing assistants in nursing homes and the Program of All-Inclusive Care for the Elderly (PACE). *The Gerontologist, 39,* 434–439.

Halbur, B. T., & Fears, N. (1986). Nursing personnel turnover rates turned over: Potential positive effects on resident outcomes in nursing homes. *The Gerontologist, 26,* 70–76.

Helmer, T., Olson, S. F., & Heim, R. I. (1993). Strategies for nurse aide job satisfaction. *The Journal of Long-Term Care Administration, 21,* 10–14.

Kane, R. L. (1995). Improving the quality of long-term care. *JAMA, 273,* 1376–1380.

Kihlgren, M., & Thorsen, K. (1996). Violation of the patient's integrity, seen by staff in long-term care. *Scandinavian Journal of Caring Sciences, 10,* 103–107.

Kiyak, J. A., Namazi, K. H., & Kahana, E. F. (1997). Job commitment and turnover among women working in facilities serving older persons. *Research on Aging, 19,* 223–246.

Mayers, K. S., & McBride, D. (1998). Sexuality training for caretakers of geriatric residents in long term care facilities. *Sexuality and Disability, 16,* 227–236.

Mercer, S. O., Heacock, P., & Beck, C. (1993). Nurse's aides in nursing homes: Perceptions of training, work loads, racism, and abuse issues. *Journal of Gerontological Social Work, 21,* 95–112.

Moniz-Cook, E., Agar, S., Silver, M., Woods, R., Wang, M., Elston, C., & Win, T. (1998). Can staff training reduce behavioural problems in residential care for the elderly mentally ill? *International Journal of Geriatric Psychiatry, 13,* 149–158.

Mullins, L. C., Moody, L., Colquitt, R. L., Mattiasson, A., & Andersson, L. (1998). An examination of nursing home personnel's perceptions of residents' autonomy. *The Journal of Applied Gerontology, 17,* 442–461.

O'Connor, B. P., & Rigby, H. (1996). Perceptions of baby talk, frequency of receiving baby talk, and self-esteem among community and nursing home residents. *Psychology and Aging, 11,* 147–154.

Pearlman, D. N., Mahoney, D. F., & Callahan, J. J. (1991). A shortage of long-term care workers: Effects on clients with dementia. *The American Journal of Alzheimer's Care and Related Disorders and Research, 6,* 9–15.

Phillips, C. (1987). Staff turnover in nursing homes for the aged: A review and research proposal. *International Journal of Nursing Studies, 24,* 45–57.

Price, J. L. (1977). *The study of turnover.* Ames, IA: Iowa State University Press.

Sargent, L. D., & Terry, D. J. (1998). The effects of work control and job demands on employee adjustment and work performance. *Journal of Occupational and Organizational Psychology, 71,* 219–236.

Schnelle, J. F., Cruise, P. A., Rahman, A., & Ouslander, J. G. (1998). Developing rehabilitative behavioral interventions for long-term care: Technology transfer, acceptance, and maintenance issues. *Journal of the American Geriatrics Society, 46,* 771–777.

Schnelle, J. F., Ouslander, J. G., & Cruise, P. A. (1997). Policy without technology: A barrier to improving nursing home care. *The Gerontologist, 37,* 527–532.

Stones, M. J., Dornan, B., & Kozma, A. (1989). The prediction of mortality in elderly institution residents. *Journal of Gerontology: Psychological Sciences, 3,* P72–P79.

Stryker, R. (1981). *How to reduce employee turnover in nursing homes and other health care organizations.* Springfield, IL: Thomas.

Thomas, W. H. (1996). *Life worth living: How someone you love can still enjoy life in a nursing home.* Acton, MA: Vanderwyk & Burnham.

Thomson, M., & Burke, K. (1998). A nursing assistant program in a long term care setting. *Gerontology & Geriatrics Education, 19,* 23–35.

Wagnild, G. (1988). A descriptive study of nurse's aide turnover in long-term care facilities. *Journal of Long-Term Care Administration, 16,* 19–23

Waxman, H. M., Carner, E. A., & Berkenstock, G. (1984). Job turnover and job satisfaction among nursing home aides. *The Gerontologist, 24,* 503–509.

Wetle, T. (1991). Resident decision making and quality of life in the frail elderly. In J. E. Birren, J. E. Lubben, J. C. Rowe, & D. E. Deutchman (Eds.), *The concept and measurement of quality of life in the frail elderly* (pp. 279–296). San Diego, CA: Academic Press.

White, K. (1980). Nurse recruitment and retention in long-term care. *Journal of Long Term Care Administration, 7,* 25–36.

11

Designing Therapeutic Environments for Residential Care Facilities

Nancy A. Pachana
University of Queensland

Physical as well as psychological aspects of residential care environments for older adults can facilitate cognitive functioning, enhance social interaction, and promote emotional well-being. Research has shown that such environmental manipulations can result in positive therapeutic outcomes across a range of geriatric populations and presenting problems, including dementia. Design and intervention strategies to be examined in this chapter include (a) physical aspects of the environment (e.g., architectural design and layout); (b) psychological, emotional and social aspects of the environment (e.g., erecting interpersonal frameworks of respect, trust, and safety, which are echoed and reinforced in the residential care context); and (c) environmental enhancements (e.g., therapeutic gardens and pet-assisted therapy programs).

PSYCHOSOCIAL CHARACTERISTICS OF NURSING HOME RESIDENTS

Approximately 5% of adults over age 65 in the U.S. reside in nursing homes. Persons residing in nursing care facilities often have a range of physical, psychological, and behavioral disturbances. Data from the 1997 National Nursing Home Survey (Gabrel & Jones, 2000) show that approximately 75%–94% of nursing home residents have a diagnosable mental disorder, with a significant number affected with depression. A significant number of residents have some form of dementia, often with attendant behavioral disturbances (Fisher, Harsin, & Hayden, 2000). Other neurological conditions may also be present.

Each of these types of disabilities may affect several aspects of life, including mobility, functional capacity, interpersonal interactions, and psychological well-being. Approximately 85% of residents of nursing facilities receive assistance with personal care activities (e.g. bathing), and over two thirds receive help with three or more activities of daily living (Gabrel & Jones, 2000). Emotional and psychological disturbances decrease quality of life and may interact with health issues to increase morbidity and mortality (Zeiss, Lewinsohn, Rohde, & Seeley, 1996). Comorbid depression may be difficult to diagnose in frail, cognitively impaired nursing home populations (Goodwin & Smyer, 1999). Behavioral disturbances represent a significant management problem for caregivers and may require significant amounts of nursing time. Zimmer, Watson, and Treat (1984) found that 66% of nursing home residents had at least one significant behavioral problem such as physical resistance to care or agitation and aggression.

The structure and environment of many nursing homes conspire to have a negative impact on their residents, as discussed by Corson and Corson (1987). Being an essentially closed social system limits opportunities for interpersonal interaction. Low staff-to-resident ratios and high degrees of regimentation can limit individualized attention and treatment, decrease a sense of privacy and autonomy, and stifle individual initiative. According to Corson and Corson, the environment provided is not "conducive to the maintenance and development of positive affective states [or] a feeling of being needed and respected." (p.18). However, increased research into developing nursing home environments that are therapeutic has suggested a host of design elements that can improve functioning for older adults. In this chapter, physical, emotional, and social aspects of the environment are discussed with respect to their therapeutic value. Specific interventions, such as therapeutic gardens and animal-assisted therapy, are also discussed.

PHYSICAL ASPECTS OF THE ENVIRONMENT

Many aspects of the physical environment in nursing home facilities can affect residents' psychological well-being and facilitate functional ability. A useful framework for conceptualizing the effect of the environment on older adults is the competence-press model of Lawton and Nahemmow (1973). In this model, the individual and the environment form a sensory feedback system. The ways in which individuals react to environmental pressures is both consistent with and dependent on the individual's physical and mental capacity. Furthermore, in a corollary to this model, Lawton, Altman, and Wohlwill (1984) describe an "environmental docility hypothesis" which posits that as functional competence decreases, there is an increased dependence on external pressures (i.e. the environment) to structure behavior. Hall and Buckwalter (1987) described a "lowered stress threshold theory," which holds that cognitively impaired persons may develop lowered stress thresholds that make them vulnerable to noxious environmental stimuli. Thus, an ecological view of aging holds that aging is a process that continues in and is affected by one's environment.

Environmental Prostheses

Such models lead directly to the conception of the environment as a prosthetic device. This involves viewing the person and his or her environment as a dynamic system, each taking cues from and being changed by the other, rather than seeing the person existing against a passive and static background environment. In the active person–environment dynamic, not only can the environment be manipulated to facilitate functioning, but the patient's effect on and interaction with the environment can be anticipated and possibly used as well.

Environmental prostheses may be designed to help facilitate a range of cognitive and functional activities. Large residential facilities with extensive identical corridors can provoke disorientation. A common feature of such large institutions is extensive use of signage or arrows to assist with wayfinding. However, for older adults, especially those with cognitive disturbance, architectural features such as potted plants, murals, and artwork are more useful for orientation (Weisman, 1987). Similarly, strange shadows, harsh glare, and large objects such as trees that suddenly loom into view are inadvertent design features that go largely unnoticed by cognitively intact individuals but may adversely affect the behaviors of dementia patients.

Architectural features have also been shown to affect behaviors more directly. In one controlled study (Hussian & Brown, 1987), black lines were painted onto flooring directly in front of doors through which dementia patients were not supposed to go. The effect of painted horizontal bars on the floor was compared with the effect of similar but vertical lines placed before the same door. The behavior of crossing the painted lines to go through the door was greatly reduced in the horizontal but not the vertical condition. Unfortunately, a later study (Chafetz, 1990) failed to replicate the findings of the earlier study, but still provided support for the use of ambiguous visual barriers to combat wandering in dementia patients.

Environmental features to assist with functioning may be conceived on a macro or micro scale. Use of background white noise has been shown to decrease disruptive vocalizations (Burgio, Scilley, Hardin, Hsu, and Yancey, 1996), and use of natural sounds such as birdsong decreased patient agitation and was associated with positive affective response (Whall et al., 1997). Structured administration of bright lighting has been demonstrated to reduce sleep–wake cycle disturbance and sundowning (Mishima, Okawa, Hishikawa, Hori, & Takahashi, 1994; Satlin, Volicer, Ross, Herz, & Campbell, 1992). Architectural features to assist with functionality can also operate in the microenvironment; examples include the use of lever-action handles instead of door knobs or pressure-plate light controls rather than ordinary switches (Cohen & Day, 1993).

Increasing the salience of environmental features (such as installing a flashing light fixture over restrooms) have been shown to reduce problematic behaviors (such as inappropriate soiling). In one study, corridors within a nursing facility were decorated in different themes, which both improved orientation for residents and as a by-product improved staff morale (Bignall, 1996). In a similar fashion, decreasing the salience of environmental features can assist with management of behaviors. Disguising the function of objects, such as camouflaging door handles, will allow for the dementia patient to avoid danger without radical restructuring of the environment or physical restraint. Avoiding frequent rearrangement of furnishing helps maintain orientation and keeps the environmental context more constant.

Research has also been conducted comparing the behavior and affect of residents living in general purpose care facilities with those in special care units (SCUs), where organizational, architectural and social efforts are aimed at improving functioning of dementia patients. Kovach, Weisman, Chaudhury, and Calkins (1997) conducted behavioral observations of dementia patients before moving into an SCU and then two months postrelocation. After admission to the SCU, significant numbers of residents increased their use of activity spaces and their social participation as well as improved their interactions with staff regarding self-cares and assistive behavior. Such purpose-built designs are generally acknowledged to have superior therapeutic effects to general purpose settings, although further empirical research on variables and dimensions of the SCU environment is required (Weisman, Calkins, & Sloane, 1994).

Reducing Excess Disability

Functional changes that may occur with aging, including physical limitations such as decreased strength, as well as disease states such as arthritis, directly affect accessibility and functionality. When such limitations are overlaid onto impaired cognitive functioning, individuals may find it impossible to function at the level of their physical capacity. The additional cognitive impairment contributes to excess disability, which in turn may lead to declines in motivation and depression (Regnier & Pynoos, 1992). For example, although an individual may have the physical capacity to bathe him or herself, dementia may remove motivation for maintaining hygiene or the capacity to remember when he or she last had a bath. Finding ways around the sequelae of the cognitive impairment can require much creativity. Allowing residents to attempt to take part in such activities as bathing and eating can be enhanced by environmental modifications such as hand rails in bathrooms and utensils for patients with arthritis or poor grip strength. Allowing patients to continue to participate in the activities of daily living reduces dependence and can increase autonomy and self-esteem. The addition of passive devices that do not rely on direct input from the cognitively impaired patient may work best (e.g. automatic temperature controls in baths, automatic lighting controls).

PSYCHOLOGICAL, EMOTIONAL, AND SOCIAL ASPECTS OF THE ENVIRONMENT

The need to develop individual design modifications to suit unique cognitive and behavioral demands may be easier to achieve when dementia patients are cared for at home or in smaller assisted-living facilities. Unfortunately, in larger institutions the overall style may be forced onto all residents. The same can sometimes occur with the interpersonal environment in larger facilities. An institutional culture may be dominant and may create an environment that does not facilitate functionality.

Psychological Aspects of the Environment

Often behaviors labeled as "problems" are provoked by the environment, are of concern only to certain individuals, and may be an outgrowth of the resident's past history or personality. All people may be said to have traits that others find irritating, but in residential settings such "problems" can quickly become the focus of management strategies (which may include medications) without the approval or involvement of the resident (Rader, 1995). Oftentimes the regimentation and high nursing load can exacerbate the use of overly restrictive controls. Silverman (1987) pointed out that at times the behavior problems of residents can be traced to long-standing practices of caregivers. For example, a single fall or instance of wandering can lock controls such as restraints into place for the duration of the resident's stay.

An understanding of the underlying cognitive processes that influence residents' behaviors within environments can be invaluable for designing therapeutic strategies and anticipating problems. For example, background noises can be quite distracting to persons who have diminished attentional capacity, leading to confusion or agitation. Perceptual difficulties in Alzheimer's patients can make shadows into threatening objects. Decreased cognitive processing and frustration can combine to create anger that the resident can no longer reliably vent in appropriate ways; other avenues such as pillows that need fluffing or an outdoor space just for digging may have to be provided (Silverman, 1987). Indifference and withdrawal may be the resultant coping strategies used by patients with dementia when faced with an environment that has become too complex to manage (Lovering, 1990). Conversely, simple, familiar tasks have been shown to increase concentration and engagement in Alzheimer's patients (Namazi & Johnson, 1992).

Erecting Interpersonal Frameworks of Respect

Privacy looms large as an issue in nursing home care. How privacy issues are handled can have a direct bearing on a patient's self-esteem as well as the emotional care environment. For example, if patients can expect caregivers to consistently fail to knock on doors to announce their presence, residents will feel as though their right to privacy and personal dignity is not respected (Blazer, 1990). When varying gradients of privacy are available to nursing home residents, they are able to control the amount of stimulation and social interaction they are exposed to (Cohen & Day, 1993).

Technology can assist in enhancing nursing care while helping to maintain residents' privacy. Marshall (1996) described how infrared devices and computer-controlled monitoring systems can be programmed to track residents' movements and actions. Once a baseline of usual behaviors is established, the computer can be programmed to alert staff if a patient's actions deviate from their usual patterns. Thus, patients can be afforded a level of privacy while safety is monitored. Thoughtful use of technology can increase the time staff spend interacting with patients and decrease routine surveillance or other mundane tasks.

Another important issue in the nursing home is the balance between an individual's right to independence and autonomy and the desire to provide optimal care. The process of assessing risks and benefits of increased individual autonomy should be shared by caregivers, family members and, to the extent possible, the patient. If all parties can recognize and accept some risk taking as essential to maintain personal dignity and self-respect, and a safety plan is put in place that all parties feel comfortable with, then autonomy can be preserved (Rader, 1995).

Managing Difficult Behaviors

Stimulus control procedures and behavioral approaches undoubtedly have an important role to play in providing a theoretical framework in which to conceptualize managing difficult behaviors. However, it is unlikely that such broad principles will be able to afford help in managing specific disturbances of behavior. The history of the patient, his or her interactions with caregivers, and the environment in which behaviors occur all conspire to make intervention challenging. Careful observation, creative attempts to ferret out antecedents to behaviors, and flexible application of management strategies applied in individually tailored ways to manage unique problems have the best chance of success. The testing out of hypotheses is a critical tool in the care of nursing home patients.

Examples of individualized management strategies abound. They may be more generalized, as in affording patients a fixed choice of when cares will take place, rather than relying on forcing compliance in the moment. Some may work for particular patients, as in the observation in one home that a resident with particular aggressive behaviors during bathing could have her hair washed without incident in a salon-type chair and basin (Bird, 2000).

Management of difficult behaviors can be enhanced by qualities in the environment as well as characteristics of staff themselves. Good, ergonomic designs throughout, the proper tools to do the task and good administrative support can assist staff with their jobs. Flexibility and imagination; good interpersonal, problem-solving, and communication skills; and an ability to manage people individually as well as in groups are all helpful attributes for staff in nursing facilities (Regnier, Hamilton, & Yatabe, 1995).

Provision of Safety

Physical restraints are often used with cognitively impaired residents to restrict movement, generally for the purpose of decreasing unsafe behaviors such as wandering or falls, or to avoid disruption of medical treatment (e.g., pulling out of catheters or intravenous lines). However, the benefits of restraints have been questioned in a number of studies. Folmar and Wilson (1989) found that decreased appropriate social interactions increase the chances of a resident being placed in restraints, while simultaneously the resident's ability to engage in appropriate prosocial interactions is decreased by restraint use. Agitated patients in one study were found to display similar or increased levels of disturbance while in restraints, suggesting that the use of restraints may increase agitation (Werner, Cohen-Mansfield, Braun, & Marx, 1989).

Werner et al. (1989) suggested that many negative consequences follow use of restraints, including physical consequences such as increased muscle atrophy, osteoporosis, and constipation, as well as adverse psychological effects including loss of dignity and increased agitation. Numerous deaths related to restraint use have also been recorded (Miles & Irvine, 1992).

Considered from the viewpoint of the cognitive effects of dementia, restraint use becomes especially problematic. The patient with dementia is most likely unaware of the nature or purpose of the restraints and cannot understand why they are being applied or comprehend that this confinement is only temporary. The caregiver applying the restraints may not even be recognized. Any attempt to explain or reassure the patient, particularly if they are in an increasingly agitated state when being restrained, falls onto uncomprehending ears. When the cycle of restraint use is repeated, it is possible that the only portion of the experience that remains over time is growing aversion and confusion.

Although the reasons cited for the use of restraints generally involve safety (particularly falls), decreased use of physical and chemical restraints in nursing facilities has not resulted in an increase of falls (Brawley, 1994).

Staff Training and Family Involvement

Proper training of staff and caregivers is important not only in ensuring quality of care but also in preventing staff burnout and increasing therapeutic efficacy. Staff in residential care facilities for older adults often suffer low morale, burnout, and stress (Baillon, Scothern, Neville, & Boyle, 1996). Successful programs initiated

on geriatric nursing wards and in long-term care facilities include frequent interdisciplinary staff meetings to optimally plan for the multiple needs of patients and
provision of staff support groups to ensure well-being of staff (Rheaume et al.,
1988). In one study, a one-year support and education program for nurses improved attitudes toward patients, reduced staff stress, improved the quality of care
of patients, and decreased difficult-to-manage patient behaviors (Edberg,
Hallberg, & Gustafson, 1996).

Using a team approach offers an opportunity to combine the collective training,
experience, and perspectives of multiple disciplines as well as serving as a support
mechanism for its members. Generally, interdisciplinary team approaches result
in improved quality of care and better functional outcomes (Abraham et al., 1991).
Teams can facilitate collegiality as well as communication, leading to better patient outcomes (Lichtenberg, Strzepek, & Zeiss, 1990). However, teams must be
thoughtfully assembled and managed to function most effectively. Some empirically based recommendations to optimize interdisciplinary team functioning include good team leader support and long-term commitment in administrative
support (Liebowitz & DeMuse, 1982) combined with unambiguous roles and locus of responsibilities for team members.

Nursing home facilities that actively involve family in care plans also see benefits. In one facility, care plans were the combined effort of staff and family working
together; the notes on the plan were kept in resident's rooms so as to be available to
relatives (Benson, 1996). Family can sometimes be brought into participation of
activities or caregiving routines, so family members can have a role in daily life as
well as take part in the social networks within the facility.

Finally, the aesthetics and atmosphere of nursing facilities can have a positive
impact of staff morale and efficacy, which in turn can make a tangible difference to
patient care. A carefully designed environment that promotes resident well-being
can in turn facilitate team cohesion and help to promote a calm and relaxed atmosphere (Benson, 1996)

Increasing Socialization

In larger institutions the same homogenous features that lead to disorientation and
way-finding difficulties may also indirectly discourage appropriate social interactions, both between residents and between staff and residents. Long hallways without chairs discourage socialization and may increase isolation. Provision of
alcoves and comfortable seating in such facilities can facilitate social exchange
(Regnier & Pynoos, 1992). Features of interest such as aquariums and aviaries can
provide stimulation as well as focal points for conversation. Potentially overstimu-
lating features such as loud televisions can lead to negative social outbursts and
should be avoided.

Social interactions between residents are often structured around group activities. Yet frequently the resident's history of hobbies and interests is not inquired

into, and a cognitively impaired resident's dislike of engagement in an activity may be labeled "resistance." At times confused patients may react poorly to group situations, and one-to-one activities may be more appropriate. Social interactions may also be hampered by sensory impairments such as hearing loss, which makes conversation difficult.

ENVIRONMENTAL ENHANCEMENTS

Whereas the impact of the structure of the environment on patients has been discussed, there are also interactions between environments or environmental features and the caregiving approach, both for caregivers and patients. Ways in which therapeutic gardens and companion animals can enhance the physical, psychological, and social environments of nursing facilities are now discussed.

Therapeutic Gardens and Gardening Activities

There is a long history of the therapeutic use of plants and gardens in the care of patients with both physical and psychological illness. As far back as the 18th century, the process of working in gardens as well as their aesthetic properties were thought to have curative effects (Warner & Baron, 1993). More recently, research into the benefits of both active and passive participation in a range of horticultural activities has pointed to their value on a range of populations, including older institutionalized adults.

Passive gardening activities can include looking at plants, wandering through gardens, and participating in group discussion activities with gardening or plants as a focus. In perhaps the most well-known study of the therapeutic benefits of merely viewing outdoor scenes, Ulrich (1984) found that length of stay in the hospital for a group of gall bladder surgery patients with a window view of a grove of trees was shorter than for a comparable patient group whose windows looked onto brick walls.

Exposure to sunlight has been linked with health benefits such as increased bone density (a result of increased Vitamin D absorption; Glerup et al., 2000). Hypovitaminosis has been found in inpatient nursing homes (Ley, Horwath, & Stewart, 1999) and in elderly women with Alzheimer's disease (Sato, Asoh, & Oizumi, 1998). Turner et al., using information from the U.S. National Health and Nutrition Examination, compared various forms of exercise, including gardening, cycling, aerobics, walking, and weight training in women over age 50. Only gardening and weight training were associated with higher bone density. Exposure to sunlight has also been linked to circadian rhythms and sleep cycles (Refinetti, 1999; O'Connor & Youngstedt, 1997). By allowing patients increased exposure to sunlight, outdoor gardens may well have a positive influence on both uptake of Vitamin D and circadian rhythm cycles.

Outdoor gardens have been suggested as a means of improving morale, self-confidence, cooperation, social interaction, and physical functioning for residents of a geriatric facility (Hill & Relf, 1982). Ideally, such gardens incorporate a variety of plants to stimulate the senses (Vellas & Sedeuilh, 1991). Simple exposure to plants and outdoor gardens has been shown to facilitate the coping strategies of older adults, including caregivers of frail elders (Smith & McCallion, 1997).

The importance of regular physical activity in maintaining good health later in life has been recognized (Galloway & Jokl, 2000). Regular participation in common physical tasks such as gardening can help prevent age-related declines in musculoskeletal function (Galloway & Jokl, 2000), increase bone mineral density, and reduce risk of primary cardiac arrest (Lemaitre et al., 1999). Again, having access to a garden or small gardening activities on in-patient wards could have positive health benefits, particularly for older adults.

Active participation in gardening activities in in-patient settings usually includes the actual planting or propagating of plants. Various patient groups have been successfully involved in active horticultural therapy programs. Participation in plant-based activities has been shown to increase autonomy in older residents in long-term care (Catlin, Milliorn, & Milliorn, 1992) and to provide patients with a mode of self-expression (Burgess, 1990). In terms of older residents with psychiatric diagnoses, gardening activities can provide both physical and mental stimulation, offering a pleasant engaging activity that can be incorporated into therapeutic programs addressing depression (Riordan & Williams, 1988) and help offer stimulation to those in long-term care settings (Stein, 1997).

An enclosed, safe garden area for patients with Alzheimer's disease to wander in has been cited in several studies and texts on the care of dementia patients (Regnier & Pynoos, 1992). Gardens attached to dementia care wards or nursing facilities can provide safe places for mental, visual, and auditory stimulation, along with a pleasant place for exercise (Burgess, 1990). Gardens can provide a means of interaction between patients that requires a minimum of verbal skills (Bryan, 1991).

Architectural considerations come into play in gardens designed for dementia patients, and elements such as the height of walls, and the presence of comfortable benches in both sunlight and shade should be considered, along with even, slip-resistant, glare-reducing paving surfaces. As dementia patients, especially those in later stages of the disease, often place objects in the environment into their mouths, nontoxic plantings should be used as a rule. Way-finding issues should also be considered in the planning and layout of gardens; distinctive landmarks and looping path systems can assist with orientation.

Confused dementia patients have been shown to be able to derive benefits from gardening therapies in terms of increasing social connections (Bryant, 1991). Dementia patients on a day care ward were able to participate in a range of gardening activities, including growing vegetables and visiting a nursery (Pachana, 1995). In this study the caregivers of the dementia patients reported positive benefits of the study, such as more restful sleep. When older frail patients are involved in such gardening activities, there are many garden design features (e.g., wheelchair height planters, tools designed for arthritic persons) that take into account the specific needs of older individuals and can help increase participation and enjoyment (Rothert & Daubert, 1981).

Although participation in the active components of gardening generally involve growing plants, other activities associated with gardens include flower arranging and producing nature crafts such as decorative objects, pressed and dried flowers, and potpourri. Gardens and gardening projects can be the focal point for remembrance therapy, wherein aspects of the garden are designed to reflect stages of human development (Hoover, 1995). Ancillary activities such as movement therapy groups may also have gardens as their settings.

Both observation and participation in gardening activities can help to foster a sense of community. The introduction of a garden conservatory not only improved the rated pleasantness of a geriatric inpatient ward but was also "adopted" by the community of the ward, whose members contributed their own plants and made it their own (Pachana, McWha, & Arathoon, in press). Gardening activities can help to create a sense of community from the shared activity, as well as serving as a source of stimulation (Lewis, 1992). Gardens in a community provide both a place and an activity that encourages socialization.

In an account of a horticultural therapy program in a 150-bed nursing home in upstate New York, Stein (1997) commented on the residents' sense of satisfaction as a community with their gardening endeavours. Flower borders created by the residents resembled flower borders in other parts of the town and thus reflected a normal part of town life rather than reflecting their unique living situation. The fact that visitors and staff alike deeply admired the flowers, vegetables, and herbs, many of which had been grown from seed by residents, were a source of pride. These activities and creations helped to create new, pleasant memories associated with this new community and living space in which the residents found themselves.

Pet-Assisted Therapy Programs in Nursing Homes

Like gardens, animals have been associated with care of institutionalized patients for centuries. The first recorded setting in which animals were used therapeutically was at the York Retreat, a psychiatric hospital in England, in 1792 (Netting, Wilson, & New, 1987). While working with animals in farming situations has been considered a therapeutic activity, more recently the value of interactions with the animals themselves in promoting well-being and emotional health is being explored. Physical, psychological, and social effects of person–animal interactions have been examined in the literature for a wide variety of populations, among them older adults in general and nursing home residents in particular.

Companion animals usually interact with nursing home residents in one of two ways. Some nursing care facilities have resident companion animals on the premises; these can include tropical fish, small animals such as hamsters, dogs, cats, as well as birds. Other facilities have animals as visitors, either informally through family or volunteers, or more formally through an animal-assisted therapy (AAT) program. AAT programs go beyond casual interactions between pets and people and seek to cause a prescribed effect on specific patients in accordance with professional standards (Delta Society, 1996). Animal-assisted activities (AAA) designed for entertainment or to simply allow residents to interact with animals also garner largely anecdotal evidence of benefits such as increased socialization, mental stimulation, and relaxation (Hines & Fredrickson, 1998). Research-based studies have begun to confirm the benefits of AAA on several populations, including residents of long-term care facilities (Ptak, 1995).

Physical benefits most often associated with pets and their interaction with people include moderating blood pressure changes (Friedmann, 1995). Animal companions have also been shown to affect survival after heart attack (Friedmann, Katcher, Lynch, & Thomas, 1980), and pet owners have been shown to be at decreased risk of cardiovascular disease compared with those who do not own pets (Anderson, Reid, & Jennings, 1992). AAT has been shown to improve aspects of mobility, including wheelchair skills and standing balance (Allen & Blascovich, 1996).

Siegal (1990) found that for older adults who did not own a pet, stressful life events resulted in more physician visits compared with pet-owners. In a study of community-dwelling older adults, Raina, Waltner-Toews, Bonnett, Woodward, & Abernathy (1999) found that ADL levels in respondents who did not currently own pets deteriorated more on average over a one year period than those of respondents who currently owned pets, after adjusting for other variables such as age and health.

Various aspects of psychological functioning have been associated with contact with animals in older adults. Alzheimer's patients exposed to pets were rated by caregivers as less anxious than a control group (Fritz, Farver, Kass, & Hart, 1995). A sample of residents from three nursing homes in Australia showed decreased tension, stress, and depression in an 18-month time period (including three month follow-up) following introduction of a visiting or resident therapy dog (Crowley-Robinson, Fenwick, & Blackshaw, 1996).

In a study of patients with Alzheimer's disease residing in a special care unit, communicative behaviors were increased in the presence of a dog (Kongable, Buckwalter, & Stolley, 1989). Similarly, socialization behaviors were shown to increase among older hospitalized psychiatric patients (Haughie, Milne, & Elliott, 1992) and institutionalized patients with Alzheimer's disease (Batson, McCabe, Baun, & Wilson, 1998) in the presence of a therapy dog. Alzheimer's patients residing at home with companion animals experienced fewer episodes of verbal aggression and anxiety than those living without pets (Fritz et al., 1995). Time spent with animals has also been used as a component of a token system, used as a reward in a behavior modification program (Corson & Corson, 1987).

There are many theories as to how companion animals influence well-being (e.g., attachment theories such as that by West & Sheldon-Keller, 1994). In older adults, particularly those in long-term care, critical features of interactions with pets may include giving tactile comfort, providing distraction from worries, and representing a familiar feature from past living experiences. The role of animals in facilitating socialization and thus providing social support (McNicholas & Collis, 1995) could play an important role in forming individual and community bonds among older adults in residential settings. Social competency and verbal skills are not required for animal–person interactions, and thus companion animals can interact with patients at varying levels of physical, cognitive, and emotional functioning. Pets may improve self-esteem by simultaneously being perceived as caring about their owners and also needing them, regardless of the owner's status as perceived by self or others (Collis & McNicholas, 1998). Netting et al., 1987 hypothesize that pets may allow older adults scope to take on a variety of roles such as caregiver, confidant, or companion, which otherwise might not be possible.

Like gardens, the presence of companion animals in the nursing home can reflect a normal part of life not only associated with the particular assisted-care living environment. Over half of all U.S. households have a companion animal (NIH, 1988); for older adults, a move to a nursing home very likely will involve giving up their pet. This represents additional loss. However, even if a pet was not owned by the resident immediately prior to living in a nursing facility, the presence of animals nevertheless can contribute to a decrease in institutional atmosphere for both residents and staff.

However, other aspects of the therapeutic effects of companion animals in nursing facilities and other residential settings may be linked to the nature of facilities that allow animals. Hartrick and Pachana (in press) have suggested that the additional flexibility which characterizes institutions that permit resident or visiting pets may contribute to the emotional well-being and satisfaction of residents. Corson and Corson (1981) proposed that animals serve as catalysts for social interactions among residents and staff of nursing facilities, which in turn lead to an improved social atmosphere. Carmack and Fila (1989) report benefits to nursing staff of companion animals on wards as including breaking down of patient–carer barriers and providing stress-relief for nursing staff.

Although the literature on person-animal interactions continues to expand, several factors limit the generalizability of the results found so far. Many studies use small sample sizes, lack reliable assessment measures, fail to operationalize procedures and quantify results, and are rarely replicated. In one overview of the literature, Garrity and Stallones (1998) stated that while tangible benefits to quality of life and well-being have been demonstrated in the literature, to date these benefits have been reliably demonstrated only in select situations and under certain circumstances. Nevertheless, the findings of the NIH Technology Assessment Workshop (NIH, 1988) suggested that attachment to animals might be an important variable for study, particularly among those groups who may have decreased social support networks, such as older adults.

FUTURE RESEARCH DIRECTIONS

A great deal of territory remains to be explored with respect to the many effects of environments on physical, psychological, and social functioning for nursing home residents and particularly dementia patients. Such research has continued to grow with the number of nursing home facilities in use and the increase in older populations wishing to age in place.

Such research could take advantage of new research findings. For example, research on the use of environmental spaces for recreation and exercise activities is relatively sparse (Regnier & Pynoos, 1992). More empirically based research on the efficacy of SCUs, alternate strategies to restraints, and improved environmental prostheses will no doubt help to decrease excess disability and increase well-being and quality of life for older nursing home residents.

REFERENCES

Abraham, I. L., Thompson-Heisterman, A. A., Harrington, D. P., Smullen, D. E., Onega, L. L., Droney, E. G., Westerman, P. S., Manning, C. A., & Lichtenberg, P. A. (1991). Outpatient psychogeriatric nursing services: An integrative model. *Archives of Psychiatric Nursing, 5,* 151–164.

Allen, K., & Blascovich, J. (1996). The value of service dogs for people with severe ambulatory disabilities. *Journal of the American Medical Association, 275,* 1001–1006.

Anderson, W. P., Reid, C. M., & Jennings, G. L. (1992). Pet ownership and risk factors for cardiovascular disease. *Medical Journal of Australia, 157,* 298–301.

Baillon, S., Scothern, G., Neville, P. G., & Boyle, A. (1996). Factors that contribute to stress in care staff in residential homes for the elderly. *International Journal of Geriatric Psychiatry, 11,* 219–226.

Batson, K., McCabe, B., Baun, M. M., & Wilson, C. (1998). The effect of a therapy dog on socialization and physiological indicators of stress in persons diagnosed with Alzheimer's disease. In C. C. Wilson & D. C. Turner (Eds.), *Companion animals in human health* (pp. 203–215). Thousand Oaks: Sage Publications.

Benson, S. (1996). Designer lifestyle. *Journal of Dementia Care, 4,* 16–17.

Bignall, A. (1996). Look and learn: Designs on the care environment. *Journal of Dementia Care, 4,* 12–13.

Bird, M. (2000). Psychosocial rehabilitation for problems arising from cognitive deficits in dementia. In R. D. Hill, L. Backman, & A. S. Neely (Eds.), *Cognitive rehabilitation in old age* (pp. 249–269). New York: Oxford University Press.

Blazer, D. (1990). *Emotional problems in later life.* New York: Springer.

Brawley, E. (1994, July). *Form versus function.* Paper presented at the Alzheimer's Association National Education Conference, Chicago.

Bryan, W. (1991). Creative group work with confused elderly people: A development of sensory integration therapy. *British Journal of Occupational Therapy, 54(5),* 187–192.

Burgess, C. W. (1990). Horticulture and its application to the institutionalized elderly. *Activities, Adaptation & Aging, 14(3),* 51–61.

Burgio, L., Scilley, K., Hardin, J., Hsu, C., & Yancey, J. (1996). Environmental "white noise": An intervention for verbally agitated nursing home residents. *Journal of Gerontology: Psychological Sciences, 51B,* P364–P373.

Carmack, B. J., & Fila, D. (1989). Animal assisted therapy: A nursing intervention. Nursing Management, *20*(5), 96–101.

Catlin, P. A., Milliorn, A. B., & Milliorn, M. R. (1992). Horticulture therapy promotes 'wellness,' autonomy in residents. *Provider, 18*(7), 40.

Chafetz, P. K. (1990). Two-dimensional grid is ineffective against dementia patients exiting through glass doors. *Psychology and Aging, 5,* 146–147.

Cohen, U., & Day, K. (1993). *Contemporary environments for people with dementia.* Baltimore: Johns Hopkins University Press.

Collis, G. M., & McNicholas, J. (1998). A theoretical basis for health benefits of pet ownership. In C. C. Wilson & D. C. Turner (Eds.), *Companion animals in human health* (pp. 105–122). Thousand Oaks, CA: Sage.

Corson, S. A., & Corson, E. O. (1981). Companion animals as bonding catalysts in geriatric institutions. In B. Fogle (Ed.), *Interrelations between people and pets* (pp. 146–174). Springfield, IL: Thomas.

Corson, S. A., & Corson, E. O. (1987). Pet animals as socializing catalysts in geriatrics: An experiment in non-verbal communication therapy. In L. Levi (Ed.), *Society, Stress, and Disease* (pp. 305–322), Vol. 5: Old age. Oxford, England: Oxford Medical Publications.

Crowley-Robinson, P., Fenwick, D. C., & Blackshaw, J. K. (1996). A long-term study of elderly people in nursing homes with visiting and resident dogs. *Applied Animal Behaviour Science, 47,* 137–148.

Delta Society. (1996). *Standards of practice for animal-assisted activities and animal-assisted therapy* (2nd ed.). Renton, WA: Author.

Edberg, A. -K., Hallberg, I. R., & Gustafson, L. (1996). Effects of clinical supervision on nurse-patient cooperative quality. *Clinical Nursing Research, 5,* 127–149.

Fisher, J. E., Harsin, C. W., & Hayden, J. E. (2000). Behavioral interventions for patients with dementia. In V. Molinari, (Ed.) *Professional psychology in long term care: A comprehensive guide* (pp. 179–200). New York: Hatherleigh Press.

Folmar, S., & Wilson, H. (1989). Social behavior and physical restraints. *Gerontologist, 29,* 650–653.

Friedmann, E. (1995). The role of pets in enhancing human well-being: Physiological effects. In I. Robinson (Ed.), *The Waltham book of human–animal interaction: Benefits and responsibilities of pet ownership* (pp. 33–53). Oxford, England: Pergamon.

Friedmann, E., Katcher, A. H., Lynch, J. J., & Thomas, S. A. (1980). Animal companions and one year survival of patients after discharge from a coronary care unit. *Public Health Reports, 95,* 307–312.

Fritz, C. L., Farver, T. B., Kass, P. H., & Hart, L. A. (1995). Association with companion animals and the expression of non-cognitive symptoms in Alzheimer's patients. *Journal of Nervous and Mental Disease, 183,* 459–463.

Gabrel, C., & Jones, A. (2000). The National Nursing Home Survey: 1997 summary. National Center for Health Statistics. *Vital Health Statistics, 13,* 147.

Galloway, M. T., & Jokl, P. (2000). Aging successfully: The importance of physical activity in maintaining health and function. *Journal of the American Academy of Orthopaedic Surgeons, 8,* 37–44.

Garrity, T. F., & Stallones, L. (1998). Effects of pet contact on human well-being. In C. C. Wilson & D. C. Turner (Eds.), *Companion animals in human health* (pp. 3–22). Thousand Oaks, CA: Sage.

Glerup, H., Mikkelsen, K., Poulsen, L., Hass, E., Overbeck, S., Thomsen, J., Charles, P., & Eriksen, E. F. (2000). Commonly recommended daily intake of vitamin D is not sufficient if sunlight exposure is limited. *Journal of Internal Medicine, 247(2),* 260–268.

Goodwin, P. E., & Smyer, M.A. (1999). Accuracy of recognition and diagnosis of comorbid depression in the nursing home. *Aging and Mental Health, 3,* 4, 340–350.

Hall, G. R., & Buckwalter, K. C. (1987). Progressively lowered stress threshold: A conceptual model for care of adults with Alzheimer's disease. *Archives of Psychiatric Nursing, 1,* 399–406.

Hartick, O., & Pachana, N. A. (in press). Companion animals in nursing homes. *Bulletin of the New Zealand Psychological Society.*

Haughie, E., Milne, D., & Elliott, V. (1992). An evaluation of companion pets with elderly paychiatric patients. *Behavioural Psychotherapy, 20,* 367–372.

Hill, C. O., & Relf, P. O. (1982). Gardening as an outdoor activity in geriatric institutions. *Activities, Adaptation and Aging, 3(1),* 47–54.

Hines, L., & Fredrickson, M. (1998). Perspectives on animal-assisted activities and therapy. In C. C. Wilson & D. C. Turner (Eds.), *Companion animals in human health* (pp. 23–39). Thousand Oaks, CA: Sage.

Hoover, R. C. (1995). Healing gardens and Alzheimer's disease. *American Journal of Alzheimer's Disease, 10,* 1–9.

Hussian, R. A., & Brown, D. C. (1987). Use of a two dimensional grid pattern to limit hazardous ambulation in demented patients. *Journal of Gerontology, 5,* 558–560.

Kongable, L., Buckwalter, K. C., & Stolley, J. (1989). The effects of pet therapy on the social behavior of institutionalized Alzheimer's clients. *Archives of Psychiatric Nursing, 3,* 191–198.

Kovach, C., Weisman, G., Chaudhury, H., & Calkins, M. (1997). Impacts of a therapeutic environment for dementia care. *American Journal of Alzheimer's Disease, 12,* 99–110.

Lawton, M. P., Altman, I., & Wohlwill, J. (1984). Dimensions of environmental behavior research. In I. Altman, M. P. Lawton, & J. Wohlwill (Eds.), *Elderly people and the environment* (pp. 1–15). New York: Plenum.

Lawton, M. P., & Nahemow, L. (1973). Ecology and the aging process. In C. Eisdorfer & M. P. Lawton (Eds.), *The psychology of adult development and aging* (pp. 619–674). Washington, DC: American Psychological Association.

Lemaitre, R. N., Siscovick, D. S., Raghunathan, T. E., Weinmann, S., Arbogast, P. & Lin, D. Y. (1999). Leisure-time activity and the risk of primary cardiac arrest. *Archives of Internal Medicine, 159,* 686–690.

Lewis, C. A. (1992). Effects of plants and gardening in creating interpersonal and community well-being. In D. Relf (Ed.), *The role of horticulture in human well-being and social development* (pp. 55–65). Portland, OR: Timber Press.

Ley, S. J., Horwath, C. C., & Stewart, J. M. (1999). Attention is needed to the high prevalence of vitamin D deficiency in our older population. *New Zealand Medical Journal, 112,* 471–472.

Lichtenberg, P., Strezepek, D., & Zeis, A. (1990). Bringing psychiatric aides into the treatment team: An application of the Veterans Administration's ITTG model. *Gerontology and Geriatrics Education, 10,* 63–73.

Liebowitz, S., & DeMuse, K. P. (1982). The application of team building. *Human Relations, 35,* 1–18.

Lovering, M. J. (1990). Alzheimer's disease and outdoor space: Issues in environmental design. *American Journal of Alzheimer's Care and Related Disorders and Research, 5,* 33–40.

Marshall, M. (1996). Into the future: A smart move for dementia care? *Journal of Dementia Care, 4,* 12–13.

McNicholas, J., & Collis, G. M. (1995). The end of a relationship: Coping with pet loss. In I. Robinson (Ed.), *The Waltham book of human–animal interaction: Benefits and responsibilities of pet ownership* (pp. 127–143). Oxford, England: Pergamon.

McNicholas, J., Collis, G. M., Morley, I. E., & Lane, D. R. (1993). Social communication through a companion animal: The dog as social catalyst. In M. Nichelmann, H. K. Wierenga, & S. Braun (Eds.), *Proceedings of the International Congress on Applied Ethology* (pp. 368–370). Berlin, Germany: Humboldt University.

Miles, S. H., & Irvine, P. (1992). Deaths caused by physical restraints. *Gerontologist, 32,* 762–766.

Mishima, K., Okawa, M., Hishikawa, Y., Hori, H., & Takahashi, K. (1994). Morning bright light therapy for sleep and behaviour disorders in elderly patients with dementia. *Acta Psychiatrica Scandanavica, 89,* 1–7.

Namazi, K. H., & Johnson, B. D. (1992). How familiar tasks can enhance concentration in Alzheimer's disease patients. *American Journal of Alzheimer's Care and Related Disorders and Research, 7,* 35–40.

National Institutes of Health. (1988). *National Institutes of Health Technology Assessment workshop: Health benefits of pets* (DHHS Publication No. 88-216-107). Washington, DC: Government Printing Office.

Netting, F., Wilson, C., & New, J. (1987). The human–animal bond: Implications for practice. *Social Work, 32,* 60–64.

O'Connor, P. J., & Youngstedt, S. D. (1997). Sleep quality in older adults: Effects of exercise training and influence of sunlight exposure [letter; comment]. *Journal of the American Medical Association, 277,* 1034–1035.

Pachana, N. A. (1995). Therapeutic gardening. *Psychologists in Long Term Care, 9* (4), 3–4.

Pachana, N. A., McWha, L. & Arathoon, M. (in press). A passive therapeutic garden and its impact on an inpatient geriatric ward. *Journal of Gerontological Nursing.*

Ptak, A. L. (1995). Studies of loneliness: Recent research into the effects of companion animals on lonely people. *InterActions, 13*(1), 7.

Rader, J. (1995). Exploring control and autonomy issues. In J. Rader & E. M. Tornquist (Eds.), *Individualized dementia care: Creative compassionate approaches.* New York: Springer.

Raina, P., Waltner-Toews, D., Bonnett, B., Woodward, C., & Abernathy, T. (1999). Influence of companion animals on the physical and psychological health of older people: An analysis of a one-year longitudinal study. *Journal of the American Geriatrics Society, 47,* 323–329.

Refinetti, R. (1999). *Circadian physiology.* Boca Raton, FL: CRC Press.

Regnier, V., Hamilton, J., & Yatabe, S. (1995). *Assisted living for the aged and frail: Innovations in design, management, and financing.* New York: Columbia University Press.

Regnier, V., & Pynoos, J. (1992). Environmental interventions for cognitively impaired older adults. In J. E. Biren, R. B. Sloane, & G. D. Cohen (Eds), *Handbook of mental health and aging* (2nd ed.; pp. 763–792). San Diego, CA: Academic Press.

Rheaume, Y. L., Fabiszewski, K .J., Brown, J., Innis, P., Glennon, M., Berkley, D., Shea, S., & Volicer, L. (1988). Education and training of interdisciplinary team members caring for Alzheimer patients. In L. Volicer, K. J. Fabiszewski, Y. L. Rheaume, & K. E. Lasch (Eds.), *Clinical management of Alzheimer's disease* (pp. 201–222). Rockville, MD: Aspen.

Riordan, R. J. & Williams, C. S. (1988). Gardening therapeutics for the elderly. *Activities, Adaption and Aging, 11*(½), 103–111.

Rothert, E., & Daubert, J. (1981). *Horticultural therapy for nursing homes, senior centers and retirement living.* Glencoe, IL: Chicago Horticultural Society, Horticultural Therapy Department.

Satlin, A., Volicer, L., Ross, V., Herz, L., & Campbell, S., (1992). Bright light treatment of behavioural and sleep disturbances in patients with Alzheimer's disease. *American Journal of Psychiatry, 148,* 1028–1032.

Sato, Y., Asoh, T., & Oizumi, K. (1998). High prevalence of vitamin D deficiency and reduced bone mass in elderly women with Alzheimer's disease. *Bone, 23,* 555–557.

Siegel, J. M. (1990). Stressful life events and use of physician services among the elderly: The moderating role of pet ownership. *Journal of Personality and Social Psychology, 13,* 1081–1086.

Silverman, C. (1987). The resource of environmental design. In. A. C. Kalicki (Ed.), *Confronting Alzheimer's disease.* Washington, DC: Rynd Communications.

Smith, D. J., & McCallion, P. (1997). Alleviating stress for family caregivers of frail elders using horticultural therapy. *Activities, Adaptation and Aging, 22,* (pp. 93–105).

Stein, L. K. (1997). Horticultural therapy in residential long-term care: Applications from research on health, aging and institutional life. *Activities, Adaptation & Aging, 22*(1–2), 107–124.

Turner, S., & Moss, S. (1996). The health needs of adults with learning disabilities and the health of the nation strategy. *Journal of Intellectual Disability Research, 40,* 438–450.

Ulrich, R. S. (1984). View through a window may influence recovery from surgery. *Science, 224,* 420–421.

Vellas, P. M., & Sedeuilh, M. (1991). Therapeutic gardens. *Facts and Research in Gerontology* [monograph]. Paris: Serdi.

Warner, S. B., & Baron, J. H. (1993). Restorative gardens. *British Medical Journal, 306,* 1080–1081.

Weisman, G. (1987). Improving way-finding and architectural legibility in housing for the elderly. In V. Regnier & J. Pynoos (Eds.), *Housing the aged: Design directives and policy considerations* (pp. 441–464. New York: Elsevier.

Weisman, G. D., Calkins, M., & Sloane, P. (1994). The environmental context of special care. *Alzheimer Disease and Related Disorders, 8,* S308–S320.

Werner, P., Cohen-Mansfield, J., Braun, J., & Marx, M. S. (1989). Physical restraints and agitation in nursing home residents. *Journal of the American Geriatrics Society, 37,* 1122–1126.

West, M. L., & Sheldon-Keller, A. E. (1994). *Patterns of relating: An adult attachment perspective.* New York: Guilford.

Whall, A. L., Black, M. E., Groh, C. J., Yankou, D. J., Kupferschmid, B. J., & Foster, N. L. (1997). The effect of natural environments upon agitation and aggression in late stage dementia patients. *American Journal of Alzheimer's Disease, 12,* 216–220.

Zeiss, A. M., Lewinsohn, P. M., Rohde, P., & Seeley, J. R. (1996). Relationship of physical disease and functional impairment to depression in older people. *Psychology & Aging, 11,* 572–581.

Zimmer, J.G., Watson, N., & Treat, A. (1984). Behavioral problems among patients in skilled nursing facilities. *American Journal of Public Health, 74,* 1118–1121.

12

Creating a Progressive Quality Assurance Culture in Residential Care

John B. Bowling
Silverado Senior Living,
San Juan Capistrano, California

Marilynn Snell
University of Utah

INTRODUCTION

An increase in life expectancy coupled with improved medical care has resulted in a population of almost 35 million people in the United States age 65 or older (Administration on Aging, 2000). This puts senior adults as one of the fastest growing age segments in our society, and the oldest old, those who are at least 85 years of age, as the fastest growing segment of America's senior population. Almost 13 % of the U. S. population comprises people age 65 or older, and that is projected to increase to 70 million older adults by the year 2030, more than double the elderly population today. At that time, this elderly group will comprise approximately 20% of the population, or, in other words, one in five people will be 65 years of age or older. Chapter one in this volume includes a more detailed discussion of the growing elderly segment of our society.

Along with increased age comes the propensity for increased disability. Disability among older adults is often the result of multiple medical diagnoses, frequently leading to many functional limitations in living (Mitchell & Kemp, 2000). In order to compensate for functional limitations and to improve or maintain psychosocial well-being and physical health, senior adults with disabilities are likely to need long-term health care services. Approximately 7 million people age 65 and older needed long-term care services in 1997, and that figure is projected to rise to about 11 million by 2030 (Tucker, Kassner, Mullen, & Coleman, 2000).

Long-term care is the umbrella term for supportive services used by elderly adults who need assistance with daily living tasks. Long-term care has been viewed historically as a social necessity for those too frail to look after themselves, with the prevailing sentiment seeming to be that the less care done the better (Kane, 1995). However, there is the alternative hypothesis suggesting that better care can make a difference, particularly in the quality of life of elderly adults. It is possible for disabled older adults, even some severe enough to be housed in nursing homes, to improve their disability status with better care (Manton, 1988; Sui, Ouslander, Osterweil, Reuben, & Hays, 1993). In addition, quality residential care services can help compensate for declining functional ability, thereby helping the older individual to remain engaged in meaningful life activities (see chap. 2). Long-term care services are very diverse and include nursing care, home health care, personal care, rehabilitation, adult day care, case management, social services, assistive technology, and assisted living services (Tucker et al, 2000). Care is administered in a variety of settings including private homes, supportive housing, and nursing facilities.

Residential care facilities for the elderly (RCFEs) are an important option for elderly adults who need assistance with long-term health care services. RCFE is a broad term that ranges from placement in a skilled nursing facility (SNF) with many disabled adults to two or more single senior adults in foster care in a residential home. Amazingly, RCFEs are known by about 20 different names throughout the United States (American Association of Retired Persons [AARP], 1993; Mollica & Snow, 1996). The definition of residential care settings encompasses facilities that are licensed to provide board and care, 24-hour personal supervision, assistance with activities of daily living (ADLs), medication oversight, and transportation as needed (Mitchell & Kemp, 2000). RCFEs constitute a rapidly growing business, with an approximately 37% increase in number of facilities within the past decade (AARP, 1998). Services in 1998 were provided to approximately 500,000 senior adults across the nation, with California alone providing about 4,090 facilities serving 100,000 residents (AARP, 1993; Mollica & Snow, 1996; Newcomer, Breuer & Zhang, 1994).

Most long-term care of the elderly is provided by unpaid family members and friends, when in-home help is no longer feasible, other care options become important. Confusion over terms for residential long-term care facilities for the elderly exists because of the variety of terms used by various states. Because the field of residential long-term care of the elderly has not yet been able to agree on the same specific terms and definitions for care facilities, this area can be confusing and complex. In order to simplify the terms of this chapter, the remainder of this chapter focuses on residential care facilities for two main categories: assisted living facilities and nursing homes.

Assisted Living Facility Regulation

Assisted living facilities have become an increasingly popular form of long-term care. Marketed toward elderly people who require more care than is usually provided at home, but less care than is traditionally provided in a nursing home, assisted living facilities are not as highly regulated as nursing homes. Assisted living facilities are flourishing in response to the growing need for an intermediate level of structured care for elderly adults requiring assistance to maintain their current level of functioning.

The term "assisted living" is both a designation of an RCFE and a philosophy of residential care (Mitchell & Kemp, 2000). Based on a Scandinavian model of service for the elderly, assisted living began to develop in the United States in the mid-1980s. As many as 29 different terms may be used interchangeably to describe assisted living, including assisted living, residential care, personal care, sheltered care, and boarding homes (Mollica, 1998). A national study of assisted living for the elderly resulted in a general interpretation of the term emphasizing some form of resident independence, autonomy, and privacy (Lewin-VHI, 1996). The objective of assisted living is to maintain or enhance the capabilities of frail older persons and persons with disabilities so that they can remain as independent as possible.

Assisted living facilities endorse "aging in place" (discussed in chap. 2), which refers to providing health and personal care to frail elderly adults in the least restrictive and most home-like environment possible. Although aging in place is espoused as a goal by many assisted living facilities, most states require placement in a skilled nursing facility if care needs become too great. This reality has sparked debate about whether it is misleading to consumers to "promise" that they will not have to be moved as health needs increase. This issue was highlighted during hearings before the Special Committee on Aging, United States Senate, in April of 1999. Testimony suggested that there are frequent inconsistencies between the marketing materials of assisted living facilities and the actual language contained in accompanying contracts. Contracts often outline physical or behavioral criteria that will promote a mandatory move to a more restrictive setting.

Specific definitions of an assisted living facility vary from state to state, with many states still developing and refining their assisted living rules and guidelines (Mollica, 1998). States are developing their own sets of admission and discharge requirements that determine when a resident becomes too dependent to stay in an assisted living environment and other options, such as a nursing home, must be considered. Estimates of the number of assisted living facilities in the United States vary depending on differing state definitions, but it is suggested to be approximately 600,000 adults living in about 28,000 assisted living facilities (National Center for Assisted Living, 1998; Tucker et al, 2000).

Assisted living is the fastest growing type of senior housing in the United States, with an estimated 20% annual growth rate over the past few years (Administration on Aging, 2000). State policymakers searching for alternatives to nursing home care in an effort to slow down increasing Medicaid expenditures are supportive of assisted living facility growth (AARP, 1999). Also facilitating growth of the industry are the desires of older persons to age in place while being, on average, more financially secure than their predecessors with the means to demand and pay for assisted living. Residents typically pay for their own assisted living fees. Although private long-term care insurance is available, it is neither widely purchased nor used by residents to cover assisted living costs. (This situation is changing however as the next generation of long-term care insurance policies typically include coverage of assisted living facilities). Although the number of states providing Medicaid reimbursement for assisted living is growing, public funding for such services remains limited (AARP, 1999). However, Medicaid coverage of assisted living is likely to expand to more states as supply of assisted living facilities grows, competition for tenants increases, and Medicaid coverage broadens. In order to maintain high occupancy levels, assisted living facilities are becoming more interested in serving tenants with higher impairment levels and lower-to-moderate incomes. There is also a growing realization that many elderly individuals with health needs may actually do as well, or better, in an assisted living environment than in a more institutional skilled nursing facility (Pruchno & Rose, 2000).

Assisted living facilities are typically state-licensed and usually include 24-hour protective oversight, food, shelter, and the provision or coordination of a range of services that promote the quality of life and independence of the individual (Mollica, 1998). Oversight of the assisted living industry occurs at the state level, and industry self-regulation has increased as more than half of the states now regulate some aspect of assisted living operation (National Aging Information Center, 2000). The varying laws and regulations affecting these settings are governed by individual states, resulting in a mix of terminology, settings, and available services for elderly adults across the country.

Although assisted living policy for separate states continues to follow multiple paths, states are defining and creating regulatory standards based on current licensure and regulatory mechanisms. Some have classified assisted living as a new, separate type of residential housing with its own licensure category and regulatory standards. Some states are consolidating previous regulatory classifications (e.g., board and care, adult foster care, multi-unit conventional elderly housing) into a new assisted living category. Other states have licensed assisted living as one category within the broad title of residential housing (AARP, 1999). States that have not created new categories or used the term assisted living seem to be updating regulations and stipulating a higher level of care (AARP, 1999).

Nursing Home Regulation

The quality of care provided in nursing homes in the United States has long been a matter of concern to consumers, professionals, and policy makers. Both the federal and state governments continue to struggle with regulation that will eliminate the poor quality care that tenaciously plagues nursing homes caring for the elderly (Harrington & Carrillo, 1999; Harrington & Curtis, 1997).

Nursing homes typically serve residents who have ongoing medical needs and severe functional impairments. Licensed to provide 24-hour medical care and supervision, nursing homes have a registered nurse on duty at all times and follow a medical model of operation. In 1998, about 1.5 million adults received care in over 17,000 certified nursing facilities (Tucker et al, 2000). As presented in chapter two, nursing homes provide a higher level of care (primarily medical care) that targets individuals at an advanced stage of physical decline.

The growth of the nursing home industry began following the passage of the Social Security Act in 1935. The stage was set for nursing home growth with the creation of the Old Age Assistance program for the elderly and the stipulation that these government funds could not be paid to residents of public institutions (Latimer, 1997/1998). A number of government programs and legislative initiatives further supported the growth of nursing homes, while little regulation of the industry was formally mandated. By the 1950s, there were complaints of poor care, inconsistency, and inadequacy of standards (Institute of Medicine [IOM] & National Research Council Staff, 1986). With the enactment of Medicare and Medicaid in 1965, formal federal regulation of nursing homes was strengthened in an effort to ensure that public money for geriatric residential care was being spent appropriately. Although the Medicaid legislation initially placed the responsibility on the states to ensure nursing home quality, in 1967 Congress added amendments to mandate medical review, record-keeping, an organized nursing service, policies and procedures for medical records and pharmaceuticals, and licensing of nursing home administrators for quality assurance (Edelman, 1997/1998). In 1972, amendments created the intermediate level of care; placed responsibility for standards of care on the Department of Health, Education, and Welfare; and authorized federal funding for state survey activities to ensure that standards were being met.

However, the quality of life for nursing home residents continued to be inadequate. Growing consumer awareness of alarming conditions in nursing homes led to congressional pressure on the Health Care Financing Administration, resulting in a 2-year study of nursing home regulations by the IOM. The 1986 IOM study revealed that although there were good nursing home facilities in many parts of the country, in many nursing homes, individuals who were admitted received very inadequate "sometimes shockingly deficient" care likely to hasten the deterioration of their physical, mental, and emotional health. The IOM study called for regulation to ensure the safety and legal rights of residents and to control and account for the large public expenditures, mainly Medicaid, used to pay for nursing home care (IOM, 1986). These recommendations became the backbone of a nursing home reform provision in the Omnibus Budget Reconciliation Act of 1987 (OBRA). The 1987 OBRA reform law was viewed as a model regulatory system that changed all aspects of federal nursing home law. This included the state survey and certification process used by public agencies to determine facilities' compliance with "requirements of participation," or federal standards of care, and the remedies that public agencies must use when facilities fail to meet required standards of care (Edelman, 1993; Hawes, 1990).

OBRA (1987) mandated uniform comprehensive assessments of all nursing home residents immediately following admission and periodically thereafter so that nursing homes would identify and provide care for residents on functional, cognitive, and affective levels (Harrington & Carillo, 1999). In addition, quality indicators were to be developed that were more outcome-oriented, such as health conditions, resident behavior, and functional and mental status of residents. Federal survey procedures changed from simply reviewing the medical records of residents to actual interviews and assessments of residents. In 1995, the Health Care Financing Administration (HCFA) implemented new enforcement procedures, required by OBRA, to issue deficiencies and intermediate sanctions to facilities failing to meet the federal standards. Sanctions include the authority to impose civil money penalties, deny payment of new patient admissions, impose temporary management for the facility, issue a notice for immediate termination of services at the facility, and other actions, including decertification procedures (USDHHS Transmittal No. 273, 1995; transmittal No. 274, 1995). The state survey requirements are classified into 17 major categories: resident rights; admission, transfer, and discharge rights; resident behavior and facility practices; quality of life; resident assessment; quality of care; nursing services; dietary services; physician services; rehabilitation services; dental services; pharmacy services; infection control; physical environment; administration; laboratory; and other (USDHHS Transmittal No. 274, 1995).

State survey agencies are contracted by HCFA to survey nursing home facilities within that state every 9 to 15 months. In addition, they are to conduct surveys of facilities when complaints are made about poor quality of care. State surveyors are trained to follow federal regulations for surveying and issuing deficiencies and are required to give deficiencies or citations whenever a facility fails to meet a specific federal regulation. Although initial hopes were high that the OBRA (1987) regulation would uniformly cure the problems in nursing homes, that has not proven to be the case, with HCFA itself reporting many variations and problems in the process both within and across state agencies (Abt Associates & USDHHS, 1998).

Regulation Problems

The regulation of residential care facilities has been a very contentious issue, with tension occurring between the industry's interest in minimizing federal oversight and regulation and consumers' demand for public oversight by federal and state watchdogs. Within the regulatory agencies, political considerations have been important in determining policy decisions (Edelman, 1997/1998).

Representatives of industry organizations have argued that care in facilities is improving. A review of literature does show that facilities are making innovative efforts to improve care, reduce the use of restraints, and improve incontinence care (Castle and Mor, 1998; Fries et al., 1997; Phillips, Hawes, and Fries 1993). Some debate has occurred as to whether the improvements are due to the new resident assessment system, a better understanding of the federal requirements by the facilities, or state surveyor fatigue in enforcement procedures. A current prevailing opinion is that HCFA and the various state agencies are not adequately enforcing the regulatory standards (Harrington & Carillo, 1999). The latter argument is strengthened by the literature that indicates that many residential care facilities are continuing to provide poor quality of care despite the great amount of regulation that already exists (Pyle, 1999). In California, the state with the most residential care facilities for the elderly, US Congress Special Committee on Aging (1998) reported that residential care facilities "have not been and currently are not sufficiently monitored to guarantee the safety and welfare of their residents" (p. 3). They found that nearly one in three homes were cited by state surveyors for having serious or potentially life-threatening care problems over a 2-year period (Harrington & Carrillo, 1999), and that only 2% of the California facilities had minimal or no deficiencies.

One of the issues that impedes effective federal and state regulation is that many of the most important elements of caregiving are intangible, such as dedication, compassion, respect, and the personal nature of the care provided (Kane, 1995). Objective assessment of these variables is difficult. Simply delivering services according to a preset list of standards will not achieve the broad goal of maintaining a good quality of life for residents. Elderly adults in residential care facilities still retain needs and expectations for all aspects of their lives. The question becomes how to provide technically competent care without sacrificing the aspects of living that residents and their loved ones value most.

Regulation has tended to focus on ways to eliminate or at least substantially reduce substandard care through setting physical standards at a minimum acceptable level, including lack of physical restraints, lack of pressure sores, adequate food sanitation, and accident prevention. Although these are very important measures, the absence of bad events does not necessarily equal quality care. There must be more to residential care than simply providing harm-free care. Exemplary care should make a positive contribution to residents' lives, meaning that residents are able to maximize their life potential given the constraints of their medical condition. Because the typical resident trajectory in a residential living facility is eventual decline toward death, it is a challenge to objectively reflect the impact of good care. Regulatory programs need to be capable of identifying and rewarding facilities achieving better than expected care, as well as censoring those facilities providing substandard care.

The challenge for the future is to create a regulatory climate that will penalize poor outcomes while fairly rewarding positive outcomes, without becoming such a rigid, dogmatic system that facilities are unable to create innovative care environments. What is needed is a future context that will permit, and even encourage, innovation (Kane, 1995). Rather than stifle the innovations of newer forms of long-term residential care by creating stricter oversight, more creativity and better accountability must occur within a framework that allows affordable care for the elderly population. Whereas a major challenge exists in just defining and distinguishing various types of services, a unique challenge and opportunity exists to develop payment approaches for people with differing needs when federal funds do not pay for room and board. Innovation is essential in a care system where collaborative efforts are necessary to preserve, and hopefully improve, quality life functioning for as long as possible.

ORGANIZATIONAL ASSESSMENT BEYOND STATE REGULATORY REQUIREMENTS

Kane (1995) implied that there are multiple "intangible" factors that affect the quality of care provided in residential care settings. These are areas that have traditionally been difficult to quantify or assess by state and federal regulatory agencies. The Nursing Home Reform Act (OBRA, 1987) attempted to address some of these factors and indeed delineated "Quality of Life" as an important area of assessment and regulation. This category was defined as follows (OBRA, 1987): "Facilities must care for residents in a manner and in an environment that promotes, maintains, or enhances the quality of life" (p. 17). Unfortunately, little guidance or specificity is described beyond this imperative. There is scant evidence demonstrating how residents' quality of life is effectively promoted in residential care settings. The remainder of this chapter outlines specific areas for assessment in order to truly affect both quality of care and quality of life.

Quality of Life Measures

When assessing the status of an elderly population, a useful definition of quality of life must involve the concepts of meaning, purpose, and opportunities for engagement. Meaning is derived from attributions about ones' environment and his or her role within that environment. People derive meaning from common roles such as friend, family member, artist, poet, and so forth. All people identify with multiple roles in their lives. Changes in health, environment, and social patterns are common as individuals age. When change occurs, attempts are made to redefine or re-establish identity roles. Continuity theory (Atchley, 1989) hypothesizes that people strive to maintain identity roles throughout their lives. As aging occurs, physical and psychosocial changes disrupt continuity of roles that provide meaning. The new developmental task is to re-find and redefine aspects of self that have provided prior definition and consistency in life. This process can be quite arduous in residential care settings. When it does not occur, people are left feeling lost or without meaning in their lives. Friedman and Ryan (1986) suggested that many problematic behaviors observed in nursing home settings are the result of attempts on the part of the elderly to reorganize attributions of meaning in the face of an ecological crisis. Residential care settings must have an understanding of this process, make attempts to understand behaviors in terms of "discontinuity," and assist with attempts at re-establishing meaning and identity roles.

One way that individuals derive meaning in their lives is by having a sense of purpose. The "need for purpose" is related to a need for meaning but more specifically relates to experiencing a sense of personal utility. Older adults in residential care settings often begin to feel helpless as their opportunities to feel useful are increasingly limited. Sometimes, residential care staff unintentionally collude in this process. A desire by staff to be helpful may in fact send the message to residents that they are incapable of contributing to their own well-being, much less the well-being of others. For example, encouraging residents to take their meals in bed may communicate that they are unable to assist in the process of meeting their own needs. A significant assessment question to ask of residential care providers is; "How are residents encouraged to feel useful?" Helping others, assisting with small tasks, and sharing the skills and wisdom of experience are all ways that older individuals may regain a sense of utility in life.

Lemke and Moos (1980) suggested that opportunities for resident autonomy help provide a sense of purpose in the lives of older adults living in residential care settings. They developed a measure titled *The Policy and Program Information Form*, which assessed the degree of control experienced by individuals in residential care settings. The development of this scale was based on the assumption that the more residents were able to participate in the decision-making process, the better their quality of life. Lemke and Moos (1980) suggested that residents would derive a sense of purpose from participation in social planning, menu selection, decor choices, and welcoming and orienting new residents. It is difficult to maintain a sense of purpose in life without the right to make choices and participate in a decision-making process. Conversely, it is clear that the opportunity to participate in decision-making provides a sense of purpose and positively affects quality of life in residential care settings.

A third variable important for organizations committed to improving quality of life is opportunities for engagement, which describes a measure of social interaction. It is quite common in large residential care settings for individuals to feel isolated and lonely. Opportunities for engagement simply connotes the number of times in a day when an individual is engaged socially or asked whether they would like to participate in a meaningful activity. This may be as simple as a caregiver staff member stopping to say hello or a housekeeping staff member asking an individual if he or she would like to take a short walk. Although the concept is simple, it is alarming to realize that other than at mealtimes, residents in many residential care settings may only receive one or two opportunities for engagement each day. By contrast, most active younger people have countless daily opportunities for engagement. These may occur at the grocery store, at a gymnasium, at church services, or simply interacting with friends or family members. Mitchell and Kemp (2000) studied social interaction in residential care settings. They defined this construct as participation in activities, family proximity to the living setting, and frequency of family contact. Awareness of the these social interaction factors offers opportunities for staff to intervene effectively. Mitchell and Kemp reported that social interaction, often driven by opportunities for engagement, is the second most significant variable in predicting quality of life in residential care settings. If residential care staff make a conscious effort to engage residents, they may make a positive difference for those who are most socially isolated.

According to Mitchell and Kemp (2000), the most significant predictor of life quality in residential care is a construct described as "social climate." Lemke and Moos (1987) developed the *Sheltered Care Environment Scale* to assess the social climate construct. The primary component of a residential care social climate is interaction and support from staff. The types of interactions that occur between staff and residents set the tone for the living environment. Basic strategies such as requiring all staff to learn the names of all residents and saying hello each time they pass can create a much more home-like and livable environment. Thomas (1996) espoused a belief that the ultimate criteria for improvement of quality of life in residential care settings is the degree to which interventions target loneliness, helplessness, and boredom. Assessment tools developed by Lemke and Moos (1980, 1987) help to operationalize measurement of these quality of life indicators.

Assessment of Clinical Outcomes

The demonstration of quality assurance involves provision of evidence that interventions are effective. State regulations require certain types of data collection in residential care settings. These requirements vary according to the type of setting and specific state regulations for that setting. Examples of areas that are frequently tracked include skin condition, continence, activity patterns, and medication use. Although this data is often collected, little is done in the way of monitoring or promoting positive clinical outcomes. One exception to this is the Medicare system. The federal Medicare system demands that progress be demonstrated prior to reimbursement for rehabilitative services. If progress ceases then so does funding. One defect in this system is that with an elderly population, maintenance of current functioning may in fact represent a positive clinical outcome. Despite this, Medicare rehabilitative services would be discontinued. Although this is an unfortunate flaw, Medicare does make an effort to incorporate clinical outcomes into funding criteria.

Beyond the Medicare system, attention given to clinical outcomes varies by state and setting. Effective residential care settings should move beyond "comfort care" and promote an improvement in quality of life. Organizations should be willing to share clinical outcome data with potential residents. Hash (U.S. Congress, Special Committee on Aging, 1998) suggested that state nursing home survey results and violation records be posted on the Internet. Such a step would certainly enhance consumer awareness of differences between long-term care facilities. There are multiple areas that lend themselves to comparative analyses. Patterns of psychotropic medication use may reflect a residential care setting's approach to understanding and managing mood and behavior difficulties (Raskind, 1998). For example, prevalence of depression in the elderly is higher in residential care settings than in the general community (American Psychological Association, 1998). Therefore, the use of antidepressants should appear higher than in the general community, or there should be assurance that incidents of depression are not being underdiagnosed. Other medication classes such as antipsychotics may be misused in attempts to manage behavior. A higher than average use of antipsychotics in a residential care setting may indicate a lack of staff expertise with understanding environmental management of difficult behaviors.

Outcome data should include information about assessment and treatment for psychiatric disorders. Vandecreek, Knapp, and Jackson (1997) have outlined numerous medical conditions that are correlated with psychiatric symptoms. These symptoms may or may not coincide with a full psychiatric diagnosis; however, they do require attention and treatment (chap. 5 provides more detail about the relationship between physical and psychiatric functioning). Kane (1999) examined the relationship between Alzheimer's disease and psychopathology. He asserted that psychopathology is often misdiagnosed or simply overlooked in persons suffering from Alzheimer's disease. This obviously hinders quality treatment because interventions are only effective with accurate understanding of the individual.

Other clinical outcome categories deserving specific attention include weight-loss monitoring, social interaction, cognitive functioning, continence, ambulation, and ability to self-feed. All of these observable variables may be subject to improvement with appropriate environmental supports and intervention. Each of these variables has implications for level of independence. The more independence that individuals maintain, the greater their reported life satisfaction (Lemke & Moos, 1987).

Weight gain or loss provides a measure of both food quality and nutritional status in residential care settings. There are many stories about individuals who have stopped eating in a specific environment only to reinitiate efforts at eating in another setting. The obvious, but often overlooked, explanation is that people tend to eat when quality food is provided and avoid eating when poor quality food is served. The eating experience takes on great importance in residential care. Mealtimes often serve the dual function of providing nutrition and creating social opportunities. In settings where residents meet in a common dining area, mealtimes may account for almost three hours of a day's activity. This fact alone highlights the need for quality dining experiences.

From a nutritional perspective, weight loss or gain potentially communicates important health status information. Morley, Thomas, and Kamel (1998) stated that the majority of individuals with weight loss in a nursing home setting either have protein energy malnutrition or dehydration. Both of these conditions compromise physical functioning and negatively affect mental status. Significantly, both of these conditions are also treatable in a manner that will directly improve quality of life.

A final clinical outcome area to expound on relates to improvement of social interactions. One way to improve social interactions is to provide high quality and age-appropriate activities. OBRA (1987) guidelines state that nursing home settings must provide evidence that activities are provided. Unfortunately, evidence of the provision of activities may say little about the quality of the programs being offered. Mace (1987) outlined principles of activities specifically designed for individuals experiencing dementing illnesses. She emphasized that effective activities should create immediate pleasure, restore dignity, provide meaningful tasks, restore roles, and enable friendships. A high-quality activity will meet some or all of these criteria. One avenue to provide evidence of high-quality activities is through the use of family and resident satisfaction surveys, which are further described in the following section.

Consumer and Family Satisfaction

Most successful corporations use customer satisfaction data to assist with planning and decision-making about company improvement. Unfortunately, this process is far less prevalent in the residential care provider industry. Every organization should have a well-defined and routine method of assessing customer satisfaction. Survey efforts need to address both resident and family satisfaction. This is particularly true when a family member may be the responsible party. The role of a family member designated as the responsible party typically involves assistance with decision-making. To varying degrees, these individuals may make decisions about long-term care options. Their perspective on quality of care needs to be included in organizational assessment of quality. From a consumer's standpoint, satisfaction survey results should be made available to prospective residents of long-term care facilities. Such an approach actually takes some of the quality assurance burden away from state regulation and places it into the hands of the public consumers. If organizations are to compete successfully, they must provide consumers with evidence that they are providing high-quality services.

Zinn, Lavizzo-Mourey, and Taylor (1993) developed the Nursing Home Resident Satisfaction Scale (NHRSS). The NHRSS is an example of an instrument that can be used to collect feedback about quality issues. It provides a model that might be adapted for use with residents in assisted living settings. The NHRSS elicits quality of care ratings about nursing staff responsiveness and competency, social environment, food quality, and physician options. If similar surveys are conducted by independent auditors, they may be used to provide consumers with information about quality of care. Settings that receive poor marks or are unwilling to participate in the process will suffer economically.

Staff Training

Programs designed to assess and improve quality of care in residential care settings, whether they are implemented by regulatory agencies or internal organizational mechanisms, are only effective to the extent that staff understand how to operationalize subsequent interventions. Most states have in-service training requirements that cover physical, safety, and hygiene issues. Although training in these areas is essential, it does not ensure that staff are trained in psychosocial areas that greatly affect quality of life. Because nursing care historically arose from a medical model, training in the "human" elements of care has often been nonexistent. Fortunately, a good percentage of individuals who seek employment in residential care settings have a natural desire to be helpful and understanding. Training must capitalize on this desire and help caregivers develop skills in psychosocial areas. The need for staff training in psychosocial areas is reiterated throughout this volume because of its importance. (Chaps. 7 and 10 provide extensive specific coverage of this area.)

Training must begin with the realization that all employees in a residential care setting have an opportunity to improve the quality of life of residents. Thomas (1996) surmised that the true "treatment" issues for most individuals in residential care settings are loneliness, boredom, and helplessness. This assertion leads to the question of how to effectively address these issues. An essential starting point is promoting individual understanding as discussed in chapter 7. Understanding individual needs and differences provides a guide to how to best promote improvement in residents' quality of life. In order to do this, employees must have a basic understanding of communication principles, emotions, functional diagnostic differentials, common psychiatric disorders, helpful management of challenging behaviors, interpersonal dynamics, and stress and conflict management (see chap. 10). From a quality assurance perspective, residential care settings must demonstrate not only that they have training programs, but that these training programs are relevant and effective.

QUALITY INDICATORS FOR THE THREE RESIDENTIAL CARE "CUSTOMER" GROUPS

All residential care settings are comprised of three "customer" groups: residents, the staff, and the families of the residents. This conceptualization recognizes the reciprocal relationship between these three groups. If one of these groups is routinely dissatisfied with quality of care, it has an impact on the other two groups. For example, if there is high staff turnover, it adversely affects both the lives of the residents and the lives of the family members that may have questions or concerns. If the needs of family members are poorly understood and they are dissatisfied, it has a negative impact on staff and perhaps on the residents.

Residents as Customers

This chapter has previously outlined strategies to help improve quality of life for people living in residential care settings. Three of these strategies are briefly restated. First, monitoring significant clinical outcomes helps to ensure that quality care is provided to residents. The challenge is to make good decisions about what kind of outcomes need to be monitored. Numerous examples were outlined in the previous section on clinical outcomes. Second, involving residents in decision-making processes assists with making sure their needs are being heard and acted on. Third, administering routine customer service questionnaires and evaluations to residents provides direct feedback about enhancing their quality of life.

Kruzich, Clinton, and Kelber (1992) collected data from a sample of 289 residents in 51 different residential care settings to assess organizational influences on resident satisfaction. Results from this study indicated that longevity of personnel, level of staff benefits, wages for nursing assistants, charge nurses' fairness and competence, and personalization of resident rooms all contributed to resident satisfaction. Teresi et al. (1993) found that residents reported higher quality of care and satisfaction when staff were able to develop close relationships with them. This was most possible when permanent caregiver assignments were made. This means that on hiring, staff were assigned to specific residents and were to continue this assignment throughout the duration of their employment. From a customer service perspective, resident satisfaction is directly related to quality of care. In other words, it is not possible to have satisfied residents if the quality of care is deemed to be poor.

Staff as Customers

The notion of viewing staff as customers is unusual in the residential care profession. Taking this perspective acknowledges that the field of residential care is ultimately staff-driven. A satisfied staff is far more likely to be conscientious about quality issues and customer service. There are several variables that provide information about staff satisfaction. These include absenteeism, cultural sensitivity perceptions, and turnover rates.

Absenteeism causes multiple problems in the residential care industry. When caregivers miss work and replacements cannot be found, it negatively affects quality of care. Simply put, there are less people to assist with family, resident, and other staff needs. Keller (1983) examined ways to predict, and then lower, absenteeism rates. He found that prior absenteeism, group cohesiveness, and health locus of control were negatively correlated with absenteeism. From a quality assurance perspective, the group cohesiveness variable offers an opportunity for intervention. Group cohesiveness among caregivers and other employees should be actively promoted with the goal of improving staff satisfaction and positively influencing resident care.

Harvey, Rogers, and Schultze (1982) studied the impact of "well-pay" rather then sick-pay programs on absenteeism. They found that allowing staff to accrue monetary incentives for not missing work decreased absenteeism. In addition to this finding, the "well-pay" program that was reviewed increased employee satisfaction and saved the organization money. This finding offers an example of a pragmatic intervention that may improve staff satisfaction with their work setting.

In addition to absenteeism, perceptions of cultural sensitivity have an effect on employee satisfaction. Booth-Kewley, Rosenfield, and Edwards (1993) examined the relationship between level of acculturation and turnover among Hispanic workers. They found that the turnover rates were highest among the Hispanic population with the lowest level of acculturation. A theory espoused by the authors of the study hypothesized that workers with low levels of acculturation felt more isolated and more poorly understood by coworkers and supervisors. This means that if turnover rates are to be reduced with low acculturated populations, organizations must increase cultural sensitivity and identify ways to help all staff feel like they are a part of the organization.

Staff turnover has a direct impact on quality of care. Effective training of staff and establishment of meaningful relationships take time. High turnover rates interfere with consistency of relationships and development of staff competencies. High turnover also negatively affects staff morale and job satisfaction. Turnover rates provide information about quality of care. They are an important variable related to quality assurance in residential care settings. There is a clear relationship between staff satisfaction and turnover. Exchange theory suggests that employees provide time and effort to an organization in exchange for benefits and other rewards (Grusky, 1966). Whitener and Walz (1993) reported that individuals appear to consider the joint influence of the attractiveness of alternatives and the value of potential losses associated with changing jobs. Organizations must focus on factors that increase the attractiveness of the work setting. Such factors may include developing close teams, providing spontaneous rewards, helping people feel valued, and promoting understanding of how they are making a difference in the lives of others. Bedian, Kemery, and Pizzolatto (1991) further emphasized the importance of opportunities for advancement within organizations. They found that employees with high career aspirations would only stay with an organization if opportunities for growth were readily apparent. George and Jones (1996) discovered that employees were less likely to leave work settings when the settings had values consistent with their own and when positive moods were routinely experienced in the workplace. Residential care settings can make use of these findings by emphasizing the positive relationships that develop between staff and residents. From an organizational perspective, staff satisfaction will be highest in a values-driven organization when those values are made explicit and followed with consistency.

There are many single mothers employed as caregivers in residential care settings. Turnover may be reduced by finding ways to account for childcare needs (Glass & Estes, 1996). Incorporating children into residential care settings has the secondary benefit of creating a more vibrant community for older adults. Thinking of staff as customers highlights the need to remove barriers to staff stability such as childcare demands. Meeting the needs of residential care staff increases the likelihood of meeting the needs of residents and families and ensuring more consistent quality of care.

Resident's Families as Customers

Resident family members are often in a position to make placement decisions about an older family member. Following placement into a residential care setting, family members may be faced with issues of guilt, loss, or anger. Part of improving the quality of residential care includes understanding that meeting family needs is a part of the overall care picture. Satisfied families have more positive interactions with staff, which improves staff morale and correlates with quality care for residents. Cox (1996) found that family members who have been in caregiver roles are more satisfied with residential placements when they are more involved in the decision-making process. An earlier study (Riddick, Cohen-Mansfield, Fleshner, & Kraft, 1992) found that the perception of burden experienced by family caregivers decreased after placement provided that they had positive feelings about the specific placement setting. Satisfaction with the setting was related to social–recreational activities and the social environment. In summary, if families were invited by residential care settings to be a part of the admission and adjustment process, they were more comfortable with their decisions and more satisfied.

As mentioned in a previous section of this chapter, family satisfaction surveys provide information related to effective quality assurance. A more proactive method to increase family satisfaction is to involve them in training opportunities and facility decision-making. "Partners in Caregiving" is an experimental program designed to improve staff–family member interactions in residential care settings (Pillemer, Hegeman, Albright, & Henderson, 1998). This program focuses on development of effective communication techniques and conflict resolution skills. Evaluation data indicated that satisfaction with this program was high, and that positive changes in staff–family interactions occurred.

In summary, the development of an organizational culture focused on quality care must include assessment of resident, staff, and family satisfaction. Historically, focus has only been on assessing quality variables specific to residents.

This perspective fails to acknowledge the dynamic interplay between the three pertinent residential care customer groups. Without satisfaction in all three of these areas, it is difficult to have a high quality of residential care.

ASSESSMENT OF ORGANIZATIONAL VARIABLES THAT RELATE TO QUALITY ASSURANCE

Organizational mission statements and effective corporate leadership provide a road map for quality assurance efforts. Strong leadership related to corporate missions and core organizational values set the tone for philosophies of employee interactions, patterns of organizational communication, and value placed on ongoing education. Each of these areas is important to assess when making determinations about quality of care. It is an old, but still true adage that quality starts at the top.

Improvement of Quality Through Promoting Organizational Leadership

One indication of a residential care organization concerned with quality is whether employees at all levels know the organization's mission. It makes intuitive sense that if employees do not understand their company's mission, they may not provide service in a manner consistent with that mission. Promotion of organizational missions and concurrent focus on quality requires effective leadership from management. Waldman et al. (1998) offered four propositions for management to improve quality in organizations. These propositions have clear applications to residential care organizations. The first proposition states that the more a senior management team is oriented toward quality, the greater the continuing commitment of organizational activities devoted to quality assurance. The second proposition states that continuing organizational commitment will lead to a cultural shift favoring quality assurance, especially when the process is mediated by planned redirections and adjustments. The third proposition posits that quality assurance initiatives must encompass all areas of the organization if they are to remain constant over time. The last proposition suggests that wavering organizational commitment to quality will lead to general cynicism about change. Essentially, these propositions summarize the impact of consistent leadership from the top down as it relates to organizational support for quality assurance. Without this support in residential care settings, it is unlikely that quality care can be maintained over time.

Promoting Quality Assurance Through Ongoing Employee Education

The social climate of a residential care setting is affected by the interactions between residents and staff and by the interactions between staff (Lemke & Moos, 1987). The concept of a "universal employee" has particular relevance in residential care communities. A universal employee is an individual who is willing to fill in wherever they are needed. A simple example of this concept is an administrator of an assisted living facility that picks up litter outside of his or her office rather then calling housekeeping. A second example is a housekeeper who assists a resident to the bathroom rather than stating that it is not his or her job. This sharing of responsibility promotes a higher quality of care because there are more responsive individuals in a particular setting.

Extensive treatment of training issues with residential care staff is provided in chapters 7 and 10 of this volume. One area that deserves further elaboration is training staff to understand the impact of cognitive impairment on older adults in residential care settings. It is estimated that approximately 30%–40% of assisted living residents suffer from at least mild cognitive impairment (American Psychological Association, 1998). This estimate is even higher in traditional nursing home settings (American Psychological Association, 1998). It is important that staff develop skills to assess cognitive functioning levels of residents so that understanding and effective interventions will be promoted. Zimmerman and Sloane (1999) support extensive dementia training efforts for staff in all residential care settings. Assessment of dementia care competencies will shed light on whether quality care driven by individual understanding is present in a particular care setting.

Assessing Systems of Communication

Patterns of communication directly affect the residential care environment. A basic principle of communication avers that a message is only as effective as the receiver's ability to hear and understand it. Caregivers in residential care settings need to understand the kinds of messages they are sending to residents. Often messages are quite different than words being used or not used. If a caregiver walks briskly by a resident without saying hello, the message may be interpreted by the resident as a lack of respect or interest. Conversely, if a caregiver makes a statement to a resident that is incongruent, the message can be confusing. For example, if a caregiver states angrily, "I'm not mad that I have to help you," the message may be heard as "I'm mad at you" because of the angry inflection. Although these concepts are basic, they need to be taught to heighten awareness about potentially destructive patterns of communication in residential care settings.

Communication from residents to caregivers may be equally confusing or challenging. Individuals residing in care settings are faced with multiple life adjustments. These adjustments can cause frustration, sadness, anger, and other difficult emotions. These emotions frequently affect communication. If employees are not trained to understand this process, they may overly personalize messages and respond with their own frustration rather than with the support that is actually desired and needed.

Communication from supervisory staff to subordinates also affects the care environment in residential settings. Miles, Patrick, and King (1996) studied the relationship between supervisory communication and job satisfaction. As might be predicted, the influence of communication from supervisors to subordinates was far greater then the influence of subordinate to supervisor communication. Positive communications from supervisors to subordinates enhanced job satisfaction. Residential care environments are often stressful because of unpredictability of impaired residents. When staff are already under stress, they require more supportive types of communication from supervisors. These types of supportive communication efforts create a warmer environment and decrease the impact of job stressors (Duncan, 1996).

Smither et al. (1995) examined the impact of an upward feedback program over time. This study was facilitated by the belief that quality assurance is affected by employee morale. Employee morale is in turn related to subordinate's perception of supervisory staff. Results from Smither's study indicated that supervisor's behavior improved with systematic feedback from subordinates. Communication patterns in residential care settings are most effective when they allow for upward feedback. Careful assessment of communication patterns can provide information that may ultimately improve quality across different levels of an organization.

CREATING A QUALITY ASSURANCE "CULTURE" IN RESIDENTIAL CARE

Ultimately, the most successful way to regularly assess and assure quality in residential care settings is to create a culture that promotes and honors this process. Clinical outcomes should be routinely shared with staff at all levels of an organization. They should always be presented in a manner that emphasizes the team's accomplishments. Systems of sharing success stories should be implemented so employees take pride in their jobs and in their organization. Employees should be encouraged to "tell on" each other for episodes of helping that exceed regular job expectations. Systems of rewards should be created that facilitate this process. For example, a dishwasher might be given a gift certificate and honored at a staff meeting for taking the time to leave his or her work station and to comfort a distressed resident.

Value should be placed on consistent education and training in areas pertinent to residential care. Moniz-Cook et al. (1998) found that training efforts designed to reduce behavior problems in residential care settings were effective in the short term, but did not maintain their effectiveness without continued training programs. Training must exceed the minimal requirements demanded by state regulatory agencies. Quality of care is improved when staff has an understanding of psychosocial issues significant to an aging population. Training efforts must be creative so that staff desires, rather than dreads, training programs. Education should be celebrated by honoring staff members that achieve higher levels of learning.

Meaningful evaluation processes will promote open feedback at all levels of an organization. This is a reflection of a quality assurance process based on open and accurate feedback. Effective staff evaluations should involve an interactive process that promotes learning, accountability, and realistic plans of correction. In such a process, staff look forward to evaluations as opportunities for growth rather than with fear of criticism. Efforts at staff improvement will correlate with overall quality improvement.

A quality assurance culture in residential care settings will involve decision-making and feedback from all levels of the organization. In addition to regular quality assurance committees, there should be subcommittees comprised of nonmanagement employees. Results from family and resident satisfaction surveys should be incorporated into quality assurance efforts. Incorporating family and resident feedback underscores the fact that quality assurance programs must involve all three customer groups (residents, families, and staff) discussed earlier in this chapter.

CONCLUSION

The effective residential care organization will adopt a quality assurance culture that strives for improvement because it values the individual lives that it is charged with serving. All employees will have a role in enhancing the quality of life of residents and their families. Although state and federal regulatory agencies have a valuable role in setting and monitoring minimum guidelines for residential care settings, organizations must move beyond these guidelines if they desire to promote a better quality of life for elderly residents. The average life expectancy continues to increase. Medical advances are able to prolong life as never before. We must now focus on the development of systems that meet the psychosocial needs of our aging population and assure quality across all types of residential care settings. This will only be accomplished by creating true quality assurance "cultures" in all types of residential care settings including nursing homes, assisted living facilities, and board and care establishments.

REFERENCES

Abt Associates & the United States Department of Health and Human Services. (1998). *Report to Congress: Study of private accreditation (Deeming of nursing homes, regulatory incentives and non-regulatory initiatives, and effectiveness of the survey and certification system* (Vols. 1–4). Washington, DC: Health Care Financing Administration.

Administration on Aging. (2000, May). *The growth of America's older population* [On-line]. Available: www.aoa.dhhs.gov/May2000/FactSheets/Growth.html.

American Association of Retired Persons. (1993). *The regulation of board and care homes: Results of a survey in 50 states.* Washington, DC: AARP, Public Policy Institute.

American Association of Retired Persons. (1998). *Across the states 1998: Profiles of long-term care systems.* Washington, DC: AARP, Public Policy Institute.

American Association of Retired Persons. (1999). *A profile of older Americans: 1999.* Washington, DC: AARP, Program Resource Department.

American Psychological Association. (1998). What practitioners should know about working with older adults. *Professional Psychology: Research and Practice, 29,* 413–427.

Atchley, R. C. (1989). A continuity theory of normal aging. *The Gerontologist, 29,* 183–190.

Bedian, A. G., Kemery, E. R., & Pizzolato, A. B. (1991). Career commitment and expected utility of present job as predictors of turnover intentions and turnover behavior. *Journal of Vocational Behavior, 39,* 331–343.

Booth-Kewley, S., Rosenfield, P., & Edwards, J. E. (1993). Turnover among Hispanic and non-Hispanic blue-collar workers in the U.S. Navy's civilian work force. *The Journal of Social Psychology, 133,* 761–768.

Castle, N. G., & Mor, V. (1998). Physical restraints in nursing homes: A review of the literature since the Nursing Home Reform Act of 1987. *Medical Care Research and Review, 55,* 139–170.

Cox, C. B. (1996). Discharge planning for dementia patients: Factors influencing caregiver decisions and satisfaction. *Health and Social Work, 21,* 97–104.

Duncan, M. H. (1996). The abusive resident: Learning to manage his behavior while managing your own. *Activities, Adaptation, and Aging, 21,* 23–35.

Edelman, T. S. (1993). The nursing home reform law: The federal response. *Clearinghouse Review, 27,* 454–458.

Edelman, T. S. (1997/1998). The politics of long-term care at the federal level and implications for quality. *Generations, 21,* 37–42.

Friedman S., & Ryan, L. S. (1986). A systems perspective on problematic behaviors in the nursing home. *Family Therapy, 13,* 265–273.

Fries, B. E., Hawes, C., Morris, J. N., Phillips, C. D., Mor, V., & Park, P. S. (1997). Effect of the national resident assessment instrument on selected health conditions and problems. *Journal of the American Geriatrics Society, 45,* 994–1001.

George, J. M., & Jones, G. R. (1996). The experience of work and turnover intentions: Interactive effects of value attainment, job satisfaction, and positive mood. *Journal of Applied Psychology, 81,* 318–325.

Glass, J. L., & Estes, S. B. (1996). Workplace support, child care, and turnover intentions among employed mothers of infants. *Journal of Family Issues, 17,* 317–335.

Grusky, O. (1966). Career mobility and organizational commitment. *Administrative Science Quarterly, 10,* 488–503.

Harrington, C., & Carrillo, H. (1999). The regulation and enforcement of federal nursing home standards, 1991–1997. *Medical Care Research & Review, 56,* 471–503.

Harrington, C. A., & Curtis, M. (1997). State regulation of the supply of long-term care providers. *Journal of Applied Gerontology, 16,* 5–31.

Harvey, B. H., Rogers, J. F., & Schultze, J. A. (1982). Sick pay vs. well pay: An analysis of the impact of rewarding employees for being on the job. *Public Personnel Management Journal, 38,* 218–224.

Hawes, C. (1990). The Institute of Medicine Study: Improving quality of care in nursing homes. In P. Katz, R. L. Kane, & M. Mezey, (Eds.), *Advances in long-term care* (pp. 117–141). New York: Springer.

Institute of Medicine & National Research Council Staff. (1986). *Improving the quality of care in nursing homes.* Washington, DC: National Academy Press.

Kane, R. L. (1995). Improving the quality of long-term care. *JAMA, 273,* 1376–1380.

Kane, M. N. (1999). Mental health issues and Alzheimer's disease. *American Journal of Alzheimer's Disease, 14,* 102–110.

Keller, R. T. (1983). Predicting absenteeism from prior absenteeism, attitudinal factors, and nonattitudinal factors. *Journal of Applied Psychology, 68,* 536–540.

Kruzich, J. M., Clinton, J. F., & Kelber, S. T. (1992). Personal and environmental influences on nursing home satisfaction. *The Gerontologist, 32,* 342–350.

Latimer, J. (1997/1998). The essential role of regulation to assure quality in long-term care. *Generations, 21,* 10–15.

Lemke, S., & Moos, R. (1980). Assessing the institutional policies of sheltered care settings. *Journal of Gerontology, 35,* 233–243.

Lemke, S., & Moos, R. (1987). Measuring the social climate of congregate residences for older people: The Sheltered Care Evironment Scale. *Psychology and Aging, 2,* 20–29.

Lewin-VHI, Inc. (1996). *National study of assisted living for the frail elderly: Literature review update.* Durham, NC: Research Triangle Institute.

Mace, N. L. (1987). Principles of activities for persons with dementia. *Physical and Occupational Therapy in Geriatrics, 5,* 13–27.

Manton, K. G. (1988). A longitudinal study of functional change and mortality in the United States. *Journal of Gerontology, 43S,* 153–161.

Miles, E. W., Patrick, S. L., & King, W. C. (1996). Job level as a systemic variable in predicting the relationship between supervisory communication and job satisfaction. *Journal of Occupational and Orginizational Psychology, 69,* 277–292.

Mitchell, J. M., & Kemp, B. J. (2000). Quality of life in assisted living homes: A multidimensional analysis. *Journal of Genontology: Psychological Sciences, 55B,*117–127.

Mollica, R. L. (1998, June). *State assisted living policy: 1998.* National Academy for State Health Policy [On-line]. Available: aspe.os.dhhs.gov/daltcp/reports/98state.htm.

Mollica, R. L., & Snow, K. (1996). *State assisted living policy: 1996.* Durham, NC: National Academy for State Health Policy.

Moniz-Cook, E., Agar, S., Silver, M., Woods, R., Wang, M., Elston, C., & Win, T. (1998). Can staff training reduce behavioural problems in residential care for the elderly mentally ill? *International Journal of Geriatric Psychiatry, 13,* 149–158.

Morley, J. E., Thomas, D. R., & Kamel, H. (1998). Nutritional deficiencies in long-term care: Part I. *Annals of Long-Term Care, 6,* 183–191.

National Aging Information Center. (2000, June). *Internet information notes: Assisted living.* [On-line]. Available: www.aoa.dhhs.gov/NAIC/Notes/assistedliving.html.

National Center for Assisted Living. (1998). *The assisted living sourcebook, 1998.* Washington, DC: American Health Care Association.

Newcomer, R., Breuer, W., & Zhang, X. (1994). *Residents and the appropriateness of placement in residential care for the elderly.* Unpublished manuscript, University of California, San Francisco.

Omnibus Budget Reconciliation Act of 1987. (1987). *Subtitle C: Nursing home reform.* Public law 100–203. Washington, DC: GAO.

Phillips, C. D., Hawes, C., & Fries, B. E. (1993). Reducing the use of physical restraints in nursing homes: Will it increase costs? *American Journal of Public Health, 83,* 342–348.

Pillemer, K., Hegemen, C. R., Albright, B., & Henderson, C. (1998). Building bridges between families and nursing home care staff: The partners in caregiving program. *The Gerontologist, 38,* 499–503.

Pruchno, R. A., & Rose, M. S. (2000). The effect of long-term care environments on health outcomes. *The Gerontologist, 40,* 422–428.

Pyle, A. (1999, May 28). Seeking a remedy for nursing homes' ills. *Los Angeles Times,* pp. A1, A38–A39.

Raskind, M. A. (1998). Psychopharmacology of noncognitive abnormal behaviors in Alzheimer's disease. *Journal of Clinical Psychiatry, 59,* 28–32.

Riddick, C. C., Choen-Mansfield, J., Fleshner, E., & Kraft, G. (1992). Caregiver adaptations to having a relative with dementia admitted to a nursing home. *Journal of Gerontological Social Work, 19,* 51–76.

Smither, J. W., London, M., Vasilopoulos, N. L., Reilly, R. R., Millsap, R. E., & Salvemini, N. (1995) An examination of the effects of an upward feedback program over time. *Personnel Psychology, 48,* 1–33.

Sui, A. L., Ouslander, J. G., Osterweil, D., Reuben, D. B., & Hays, R. D. (1993). *Journal of Clinical Epidemiology, 46,* 1093–1101.

Teresi, J., Holmes, D., Bennesen, E., Monaco, C., Barrett, V., & Koren, M. J. (1992). Evaluation of primary care nursing in long-term care. *Research on Aging, 15,* 414–432.

Thomas, W. H. (1996). *A life worth living: How someone you love can still enjoy life in nursing home.* Acton, MA: Vanderwyk & Burnham.

Tucker, N. G., Kassner, E., Mullen, F., & Coleman, B. (2000, May). Long-term care [On-line]. Available: research.aarp.org.

United States Congress, Special Committee on Aging. (1998). *Betrayal: The quality of care in California nursing homes.* Testimony of Michael Hash. Washington DC: Government Printing Office.

United States Department of Health and Human Services, Health Care Financing Administration. (1995). *State operations manual. Provider certification.* (Transmittal No. 273) Washington, DC: Government Printing Office.

United States Department of Health and Human Services, Health Care Financing Administration. (1995). *State operations manual. Provider certification.* (Transmittal No. 274) Washington, DC: Government Printing Office.

Vandecreek, L., Knapp, S., & Jackson, T. L. (Eds.). (1997). *Innovations in Clinical Practice: A Sourcebook, Vol. 15.* Sarasota, FL: Professional Resource Press

Waldman, D. A., Lituchy, T., Gopalakrisnan, M., Laframboise, K., Galperin, B., & Kaltsounakis, Z. (1998). A qualitative analysis of leadership and quality improvement. *Leadership Quarterly, 9,* 177–201.

Whitener, E. M., & Walz, P. M. (1993). Exchange theory determinants of affective and continuance commitment and turnover. *Journal of Vocational Behavior, 42,* 265–281.

Zimmerman, S. I., & Sloane, P. D. (1999, Fall). Optimum residential care for people with dementia. *Generations,* 62–68.

Zinn, J. S., Lavizzo-Moury, R., & Taylor, L. (1993). Measuring satisfaction in the nursing home setting: The nursing home resident satisfaction scale. *The Journal of Applied Gerontology, 12,* 425–465.

13

The Residential Care
Organization in the 21st Century

Michael Duffy
Texas A&M University

Jo Ann Duffy
Sam Houston State University College of Business

This final chapter proposes an agenda for future change in the geriatric residential care organization in the 21st century. We gather up the major themes and issues of earlier chapters with our own specific agenda items in order to present a blueprint or outline for change for geriatric long-term care. We hope that this will provide a useful template for future planning for an optimal residential care facility. The chapter is organized to cover several major domains of concern within which we discuss specific issues and prescriptive suggestions for change. Although there is some evidence of a lessening of utilization of nursing home care, perhaps with the increase of home- and community-based alternatives, we believe that consistent trends suggest that the need for residential care systems for older adults will be an increasing phenomenon and critical in future planning.

In the past 40 years of social and health policy there has been a distinct tension between community and residential care systems. The community health and mental health movement of the 60s gave a much needed correction to an overemphasis on long-term institutional care that had become the pervasive norm and seemed to stifle concepts of change and rehabilitation. This re-emphasis is also signaled in social and legal policy, which has over the past several years increasingly emphasized "least restrictive alternatives" in providing care to vulnerable members of society. In a parallel manner, the emerging field of gerontology, both as a discipline and profession, has emphasized health rather than illness and community-dwelling elderly rather than nursing home residence. The necessary paradigm shift that gerontology brought to social and health care, emphasizing the normal versus the abnormal, health versus illness, and an unrelenting fight against negative stereotypes of aging, has unfortunately led to an overcorrection in which long-term institutional care of the elderly has been substantially neglected until recent years. Indeed, we have now come to realize that not every older person can live in the community, with the increased rate of survival of old and very old elderly, intensive institutional nursing care is often needed. A brief visit to a nursing home will confirm this.

A brief anecdote reporting our recent experience in England gives a poignant account of this tension within British national policy between community versus institutional care systems. In recent years British social and health policy at the national level has emphasized the increased availability of community and home care for older adults and de-emphasized (and discouraged) nursing home care. Concretely, government social workers began to authorize less admissions and reimbursements for nursing home care, with the result that many smaller nursing facilities (e.g., 15—30 beds) have had to either close or find themselves in serious financial jeopardy. In the past several years, however, there has been a revealing pattern reversal. The very old debilitated elderly are again being allowed to use residential nursing home care in greater numbers, as it transpires that their needs are too intensive medically and socially for less restrictive environments of home and community. Nursing home staff, however (including the first author's sister, a nursing home director–"matron") report that the current condition of these new residents is considerably more deteriorated and that the process of rehabilitation is now more difficult. In other words, the maintenance of these older adults in less restrictive but also less medically comprehensive environments, in home and community, leads to a medically compromised condition at the point of admission to the nursing home. It is now known that families, far from abandoning their parents, often keep older adults at home and in community settings for too long—sometimes beyond the optimal time for rehabilitation. It seems, therefore, beyond doubt that residential care at a variety of levels will continue to exist and be needed to an even greater extent in the 21st century as we encounter the predicted increase in old-old and very old adults. With regard to the United States, there is some evidence between 1985 and 1995 (Bishop, 1999) of a reduction in the number of older adults staying overnight in nursing homes. However, the predicted population trajectory overall seems to imply that this trend will not continue. It seems likely that this trend is related to the needed increase in Medicare and Medicaid home health opportunities during this period of time. The year 2020 projections (Himes, 1992) leave little doubt that despite a laudable increase in home and community alternatives within long-term care, residential nursing home care will become a critical feature of the next century. Indeed data from the 1990s suggests a 48.6% rate of utilization at some point in life of nursing home care (Alecxih, 1997). This means that after age 65, almost half of all Americans will spend some time in a nursing home as well as that three quarters will need some home care services. Therefore, the demand for long-term care increases dramatically with age, emphasizing the need to give special attention to residential care contexts for those people age 85 and older.

INCREASING THE USE OF CONTINUING CARE MODELS IN LONG TERM CARE

The current explosive growth in the number of assisted living facilities reflects more the interest of home developers who may have little appreciation for the developmental needs of older adults over time, especially those with disabilities and need for rehabilitation. Indeed, we have had conversations with managers of assisted living facilities who took pride in the fact that there were no health or social services present within their assisted living or independent living facilities. Such attitudes reveal a lack of understanding of the manner in which older adults "age in place" and move through developmental stages that require greater physical and psychosocial assistance. The gradual development of continuing care retirement community models (Somers & Spears, 1992) projects a more sensitive and accurate view of the developing health and psychosocial needs of older adults and especially those who survive into very old years. Such continuing care models provide for a smoother and more sensitive transition from levels of home health through minimal care, through assisted living, through skilled care, through intermediate care, and finally into intensive care programs for dementia and other intensive care needs. The need for such sensitive and developmentally oriented care programs suggests a closer working relationship between development and health care professionals, a liaison that can both benefit the well being of older adults and serve the interests of investors. All too often in single-level residential programs, for example in assisted living, older adults become more vulnerable and at risk than the health care level is able to accommodate. In a recent example in our experience, a demented and confused resident, living inappropriately in an assisted living facility, died of cold after exiting the facility during the night and being unable to return through a fire door. In many cases older adults who may be admitted appropriately to a minimal level care context will develop a level of disability that is beyond the resources or intent of that level of care. What follows often is a sad and needless process in which family members scour the local community to find a more appropriate residential environment. This may be achieved, but then there is the co-occurrence of another problem, that of relocation stress, which can have significant psychological impact on the older adult. It is true, of course, that such inappropriate referrals to residential facilities is also the result of poor diagnosis of health or psychological problems, but in many cases it results from the development of problems over time (aging in place) that are beyond the service needs of the organization. Many residential facilities (independent living cottages and assisted living facilities) have attempted to bridge this service gap with some laudable solutions, including the contracting with the home health agency to be located within or on call for residents. However, it is clear that an optimal design for residential care includes a well-articulated system of differing levels of care to cope with the progressive health and psychological needs of older residents who have aged in place. This continuing care, or continuum of care as it is sometimes called, can be achieved in a variety of ways, and chapter 2 of this text highlights this issue Obviously, a predesigned continuing care facility that incorporates all levels of care is an optimal solution. However, in the transitional times and resources that we live with, coordinated arrangements for continuing care between existing separate facilities are certainly a possibility. The tragedy of an assisted living resident having to "go and find" another place to live (a nursing home) can be offset by well thought out arrangements between facilities of different levels of care and indeed across different companies. Such arrangements are often informally made, but the concept of continuing care of older adults needs to be systematized in an organized and seamless manner.

Multiple levels of care also involve differing levels of behavioral function of residents who must in some way live together. We are all familiar with the difficulty experienced by "well" residents in their encounters, in dining room and in social conversation, with other residents who are severely impaired medically, cognitively, or both. Such level of functioning hardly enhances the quality of the environment for well residents. However, one can also feel for the sometimes resultant separation of cognitively and medically impaired residents into separate living areas where they experience increasing isolation, which in turn leads them into more severe disengagement than would otherwise be necessary. Such a quandary clearly points to a clash between two values: that of providing an enhanced living environment for relatively well elderly and also for the well-being and continuing engagement of residents who are cognitively impaired. This tension between values is reminiscent of the classical and continuing discussion within public education about "mainstreaming," in which the potential for achievement of able students is weighed against the needs of less able and special need children. Should we choose to emphasize the well-being of the well or the often critical needs of persons with special needs? This problem, both within public education and in long-term care, has been resolved in a series of often unsatisfactory solutions. Should well residents live in segregated residential settings, eating privately or only with more functional residents, or should the needs of impaired residents be considered and be integrated and potentially enhanced by being part of the larger social group. Clearly, the choice of one over the other of these alternatives will have necessary, if unintended, consequences for one or other group. Our belief is that the 21st Century residential care organization will attempt to find a balance for these needs. In the same way that we need to plan for both privacy and social interaction needs of nursing home residents we can provide both for an independent zone for well residents, and also a context in which they mix with and enhance the experience of more impaired residents. We believe that such periodic altruistic behavior will also enhance a sense of well-being in the well elderly. We have been impressed in conducting psychotherapy groups for nursing home residents that, in limited and structured contexts, well residents can have distinct compassion and understand the importance of their continuing involvement with debilitated older adults. In a recent encounter with two nursing home roommates, one of whom was cognitively clear and the other language impaired, the first author was able to demonstrate to the cognitively well older adult that continuing to talk to her "mute" roommate had a very beneficial effect. Over time and with patience it was possible for the aphasic roommate to signal, through smile and gesture and eye contact, that her voluble roommate was indeed much appreciated. The roommate was clearly touched by the realization that she had been important to her language-impaired friend and was thus encouraged to continue her engagement in conversation with her roommate. Therefore it does seem possible to develop integrated systems in which the health status and independence of well residents is respected and maintained, but not at the entire cost of contact with less fortunate residents.

THE PSYCHOLOGICAL AND MENTAL HEALTH DIMENSIONS IN RESIDENTIAL CARE

There is a minimal awareness of the psychological aspects of daily life and health care within any level of the residential care continuum. The staffs of such facilities are largely medically oriented in the case of nursing homes, or development and social care oriented in the case of less restrictive assisted care settings. This situation is parallel to the general situation in medical and health care where there is limited understanding of the psychological forces that affect the development of disorders, their treatment, and prognosis. Nursing homes largely operate on a medical–illness model to disorders and health care. Assisted living settings frequently can have an "anti-medical" perspective, although unfortunately not replaced with a sophisticated understanding of the psychosocial aspects of care. Within the social services department in these settings it is not unusual that social service personnel are not specifically trained in social or psychological services but have general academic training with some subsequent special training in social services. An anecdote will illustrate the limitations of this situation. Recently, in arranging for a practicum for doctoral students in clinical geropsychology, we were discussing with the social services director of a large multilevel nursing facility which residents the practicum students would work with. He, with some assurance, stated that he had not identified any residents who had mental health problems. Note that this was in a very large facility with over 225 residents! Subsequent inquiry by other members of the nursing home staff revealed that indeed there were many residents (as we would expect) who were in quite acute need of mental health assistance and counseling. A parallel occurance can be found with traditionally trained nursing home administrators who, despite many long days of dealing with "difficult residents," are quite likely to be unaware that there are mental health problems in the facility! Despite some general progress of psychology and mental health being understood as a critical dimension of human experience and health care, there is little institutional appreciation of the mental health and psychological experience of nursing home residents.

There are two levels at which an enhanced awareness of psychological dimensions needs to be in place. The first, and more technical level, is a more effective recognition of mental health problems and psychiatric disorders among nursing home residents. Even though we have ostensibly in place (Pre-admission Screening and Annual Resident Review: Omnibus Budget Reconciliation Act, 1987) a procedure for identifying and requiring active treatment for psychologically impaired nursing home residents, this is still largely a neglected area. Nursing home personnel are simply not trained to identify and plan treatment strategies for residents with psychological impairments. Future decades will hopefully include a corps of well-trained clinical geropsychologists, psychiatrists, clinical social workers, and other mental health personnel who will be an integral part of the residential care environment. This is particularly important in light of the negative fallout of the community mental health movement in the 60s mentioned earlier. It is clear that with the demise of public mental health care systems in many areas of the country, nursing homes are increasingly becoming the new psychiatric hospitals (Tariot, Podgorske, & Blazina, 1993) just as the prison system houses many psychiatric patients. Hopefully, in the next decade this situation will ameliorate and there will be again an increased awareness of a legitimate role of intensive residential psychiatric care for impaired elderly. Even so, there will always be psychological distress and a range of normal psychological problems among residents in nursing homes. Good psychological assessment, including differential diagnosis of organic and functional disorders, will become an integral part of the life of facilities. More importantly, there is a need for an increase in active treatment programs, specialized for particular problem areas (e.g., grieving, depression, relocation stress, personality problems) within facilities. A factor that can reduce the need for facilities to provide services directly, might be an increase of the public outpatient mental health service system, which along with public psychiatric hospitals, has been largely dismembered in the past 30 years. It is not uncommon to hear that nursing homes have minimal or no services provided by local community mental health centers. This situation must change in any coherent delivery system for mental health services for older adults who are fast becoming a significant proportion of mental health patients.

The other critical domain of intervention by psychology is at a more subtle and less technical level. Even well-trained psychologists, frequently graduates of a medical model education, may approach mental health in an overly formal and technical fashion, looking to simple symptomatic Diagnostic and Statistical Manual of Mental Disorders (DSM) diagnoses and structured behavioral and cognitive treatment programs to deal with complex and subtle mental health needs of residents. Necessary though this level of technical care is, there is a much larger domain of sensitivity to quality of psychological life of residents (and staff) which is a critical element in overall care (M. Duffy, 1999). Having nursing home staff, especially nurse assistants, recognize that every contact with a resident becomes an opportunity to enhance that resident's experience of life is a simple, difficult, but critical element in an overall mental health strategy. Mental health services cannot be restricted to formal psychological or social services. To operate in this way is to neglect a large portion of residents and more subtle needs for emotional and psychological contact that they experience on a daily basis. Especially in institutions (any institution), there is a need to offset the debilitating effect of daily structures of life that are designed to maintain group and organizational functioning rather than to be sensitive to individual needs. Also, the current emphasis of clinical psychology on DSM Axis 1 (behavior symptoms) has lead, even in general practice, to ignoring more subtle influences of personality functioning (Axis 2). Emphasis has been on discrete treatments for particular symptom profiles (Chambless & Hollon, 1998) at the cost of attention to more subtle interactive aspects of personality styles and their effect on daily interactions with both staff and other residents. Psychologists and mental health workers, therefore, need to be engaged directly in the remediation of mental health problems among residents, but perhaps even more importantly, psychologists have a unique opportunity to influence the overall mental health climate in a facility by, for example, training nurse aides to enhance and appreciate their daily contact with residents. It is noteworthy, perhaps, that research has indicated that one of the most effective antidotes to burnout among health care personnel is an intimate, satisfying connection with patients. This is intriguing, of course, as many would intuitively assume that the more intense the contact with the patient, the more likely would the burnout occur. The opposite is in fact true, and this becomes a critical factor in training front-line nursing and programmatic staff, nurses, social services personnel, dietary personnel, medication aides, and activity directors.

Finally, this attitude of subtle and systemic intervention in the facility also leads naturally to an enhanced awareness of the need for prevention. As one comes to understand the dynamics of psychological impoverishment in institutions, one is better armed to develop systematic prevention programs that will head off predictable crises. An example of this is to have a paraprofessional or volunteer listener be present with new residents or during transition from one level of care to another within a facility. This intervention has been successfully used within our own programs (Crose, Duffy, Warren, & Velasquez, 1986).

INTERPROFESSIONAL COOPERATION AS A STABLE OPERATING SYSTEM

If psychologists and other mental health professionals are to provide direct services and have a sustained influence on the psychological climate in geriatric residential facilities, it will only be because they become a constituent part of a health care team composed of many different professionals. Luckily interprofessional and interdisciplinary cooperation and understanding is perhaps more advanced in the field of gerontology than in any other area. Gerontology, since its inception, has been an interdisciplinary process, witnessed by the existence of the Gerontological Society of America, which is a vibrant gathering of many academic and clinical professions, including clinical medicine, biology, psychology, social work, and the full range of social sciences. This tradition has meant that there is at least a greater openness to interprofessional cooperation in long-term care. However, one is much more likely to find efficient interprofessional treatment teams in large, multidisciplinary hospitals or clinics than in the average nursing home. Many settings rarely see a physician, even more rarely a clinical psychologist, and almost never a psychiatrist. When there is collaboration, it is a limited affair based on the available professionals. Another problem is imprecision in the meaning of teamwork. The current best-case scenario of cooperation, for example, frequently involves "parallel delivery " in which different professionals refer to one another and work sequentially in the management and delivery of care. However, this is a limited version of collaborative care. In parallel delivery, consultation with other professionals usually implies "handing off" the patient to the other provider for treatment or a clinical opinion; collaborative service delivery, however, implies a joint, cooperative, and mutually interacting involvement in care (Sanders, Brockway, Ellis, Cotton, & Bredin, 1999). Consultation, in this scenario, becomes a mutual and reciprocal process in which information and expertise is shared with the purpose of developing a joint coherent understanding and treatment strategy. As more is learned of the psychophysiological complexity of human life, such a collaborative approach seems essential and is likely to be a feature of care in the 21st Century—at least, with certain conditions met. Such collaboration will be difficult without functioning case conferences at which the different professionals are able to provide reciprocal input into patient planning on a routine basis. Realistically, there will always be a great need for flexibility. Just as it is not assumed that the whole family has to be physically present in order to conduct family therapy, so too case conference collaboration can be managed in a flexible way such that in many cases members of the team will only have limited contact with other members on a day-by-day basis. This flexibility can only exist if efforts are made (with sensitive group process skills) enhanced by working relationships that go beyond formal acquaintance to a comfortable level of trust. It is clear that such comfort and trust be best based on a system that is egalitarian with regard to the various health professions. It will be important for each profession to understand the culture embedded in the other system from an empathic point of view. Psychologists both need and can benefit from knowing the biological model that has been dominant in traditional medicine and, in turn, physicians and nurses can become sensitive to the psychological dimensions of care. We assume that this cooperative approach will be helped by greater contact among the professions during training. The very distinct "self-images" of different professions are surely nurtured and maintained during training where, through a lack of interprofessional connection, separateness is solidified. Thus, although interprofessional collaboration is not easily achieved, it becomes one of the greatest benefits of interdisciplinary team practice. It seems inevitable that health care practice in the next decades will be interprofessional, as science points to the intimate connections between different domains of human experience and disorders. It will also be helpful to pay strategic attention to the fiscal and reimbursement systems that maintain, or promote (or limit) current medical and health training and practice. For instance, there is current consideration within the Health Care Financing Administration (HCFA) to extend some Current Procedural Terminology (CPT) codes to include the work of other health professionals. An example of this would be to provide a CPT code for "management" to nonphysicians authorizing and reimburse there by the work of the psychologists who develop and manage behavioral management programs for individual residents. These systematic behavioral programs do not fit well into the modality of individual therapy but are critical in the maintenance of mental health progress for especially debilitated residents. Such changes are strategically important in supporting the work of various professionals who might otherwise not be eligible for service reimbursement and therefore, realistically, not be part of an ongoing health care team. Policy and strategic management specialists are an important part of the health care planning and management team of the future. The key to delivery of meaningful mental health care services often lies in other (e.g., fiscal or political) sectors of the system.

A SUBSTANTIVE ENHANCEMENT OF QUALITY OF CARE

As in the area of public education there has been an active and heated debate in residential care on the nature and evaluation of quality. The similarities are striking. The result of this debate in both domains has been the development of a comprehensive but quite rigid and simplistic set of evaluative criteria and procedures. Relatively little time has been spent in reflecting on the substantive meaning of the quality of life in residential environments (or quality of teaching in schools). Instead, much time and energy are spent in training the technical methods of evaluating compliance with existing regulations for quality of care and quality of life. The result in long-term care, as indeed in schools, is a pronounced tendency to structure programs in order to "teach to the test." In other words, there is a tendency to organize programs and environments to address existing official and very limited quality indicators. Most persons who have spent time in or lived in a nursing home will likely confirm that these elements certainly do not constitute a substantive meaning of quality of life. In a typical scenario, a nursing home is likely to be cited by regulatory agencies for such technical issues as water temperature and cleanliness of kitchen and much less likely to be cited for an overall lack of morale among residents and staff. We have probably ourselves been in facilities that resemble a railway station waiting room, with a booming, buzzing confusion, but have a vibrant sense of community and interaction among residents and staff with frequent conversation and laughter. Alternatively, we may have experienced situations where a facility is in strict compliance with technical regulations and yet there is a pall of sadness over the environment, where residents complain of too much control and where deviance is little tolerated. These contrasting scenarios encourage a more substantive and subtle evaluation of quality of care and quality of life. Simply put, much more is needed from existing nursing home evaluation criteria to ensure the rich and varied human experience that promotes happiness.

This is not to say that current evaluation systems have had no effect on quality of care Indeed, external evaluation criteria, even the imperfect ones currently available, do have a positive effect on critical behavior such as nursing care. New evaluation criteria (Hawryluk, 1999) established by the HCFA do indeed improve on the simpler criteria of earlier decades. However, although they do emphasize some important criteria of medical wellness (e.g., the absence of decubitus ulcers and urinary continence), they do not capture the many more subtle dimensions of quality of life in long-term care contexts. For effectiveness in these dimensions one would look, for example, for more personal and vibrant relationships between nursing home roommates, an adequate and well-balanced arrangement for both privacy and social engagement, and the presence of nurse aides who make each contact with a resident an opportunity for emotional engagement. These indicators provide a clear sign that case management and planning is attentive to integrative aspects of health care including psychological and social aspects.

The next few decades will bring a more satisfactory discussion to the issue of enhancing the quality of life and health care. We believe there will be several features that will characterize this discussion. There will be considerably more attention to psychological and mental health dimensions within the criteria for well-being in standard evaluation protocols. This emphasis will not only be on overt behavior, but will attend much more to those fine-grain emotional and microbehavioral aspects of life that capture the experience of life satisfaction while recognizing the restraints of intensive health care. These dimensions are, of course, notoriously hard to measure , but we anticipate that psychologists, social scientists, and other mental health professionals will, in the emerging postpositivist era, increasingly focus on this microbehavioral level—a domain that reflects the daily experience of all human beings and that is frequently absent in the formal and traditional world of behavioral science.

Finally, a central feature of a new agenda for quality of care in the 21st century will be the provision of adequate resources to deal not only with medical service needs (which are severely underfunded) but also for those other subtle aspects of daily life that constitute and ensure quality. Resources for long-term care are, to say the least, impoverished and certainly not sufficient to meet the needs of long-term care. When an overnight stay (not including medical services) in an acute care hospital can cost up to five times more than full-service (room and board, medical care, social services, nursing care, dietary services) in a nursing home, then we have some measure of the degree of the underresourcing of long-term care. By the same token, when we consider that the allocated Medicaid dollars for nursing home care in some states (e.g., Texas) are as little as one third of Medicaid funds allocated in other states (e.g., New York), then we also have some measure of the inequity of resourcing of long-term care. Realistically, despite much public discourse about private and pro bono contribution to health and public services, any improvement in quality of service must include adequate resources for both medical and overall life quality.

Paradoxically, although long-term care residential environments are seriously underresourced, they are frequently made a scapegoat for social disenchantment with the fate of our very old and ill adults. It has become standard practice in politics and the media, just as in public education, to identify nursing home care as the source of many problems (just as teachers in schools are blamed solely for poor quality education). In a recent public speech ("Better Nursing Home Care," 2000), President Clinton made a unique reversal in this proclivity of blaming long-term care settings. After many examples where the administration has blamed the long-term care industry for poor quality of care (which has some validity) and promoted emphasis on evaluation, surprise visits, and severe punishments in both monetary and legal terms, President Clinton took a new and hopeful approach. He suggested that an important addition to quality of health care policy was to increase resources for nursing homes to the point where every resident in the nursing home would be able to have at least two hours of meaningful contact each day with another human being. This is a powerful example of focusing the quality of care discussion not only on evaluation criteria and methods but also on the more substantive issues of determining more precisely where quality lies in the lives of older adults within long-term care. For example, in a recent study that evaluated the amount of direct contact that residents have with a registered nurse, the average was 7.9 minutes per day. Further, the average amount of daily contact with the nurse assistant (who is clearly the main, if not the only caregiver) was about 76.9 minutes (Friedlob, 1993). When one considers that in many cases residents are without any other meaningful human contact, it becomes quite clear that this revised policy will have a very clear purpose. Although it is important to note that much of this 76.9 minutes is spent in purely technical assistance (medication, meals, blood testing, etc.), this contact provides a golden opportunity for a well-trained staff to incorporate many moments of meaningful contact. Studies have shown that even minimal physical attention and eye contact during the administration of nursing services can have a significant effect in improving life satisfaction of residents.

Another critical element of quality of life and quality of care assurance is the rehabilitative emphasis of the nursing home policy (Galvin and La Buda, 1991). As we highlighted earlier, statistics indicate that although perhaps only 5% of the

65-plus population is in a nursing home at any given time, almost 50% spend some time in an intensive care environment. This suggests that why it is often perceived by residents and staff the "last stop." This scenario may hold true for the very old, but even in this case it is critical that there be a "rehabilitative attitude" toward residents who have chronic disabling disorders. Although it is often in the psychosocial area that such rehabilitative energy can be most meaningfully directed, it is not unusual to see improved physical health status in an older adult who lives a rich, interactive, and meaningful life. In other words, residential care should emphasize strength-based care management. This is equivalent in psychology to the concept of positive mental health, in which assets are emphasized over deficits and where enhancement of well-being is a normative goal. Rehabilitation hospitals, interestingly, are only recently recognizing their geriatric mission. In recent years it is common to find that a majority of patients in the rehabilitation program are older adults. Such a rehabilitative philosophy requires a sensitive understanding of the special circumstances and needs of older adults. For example, the psychological recovery period from a physical trauma may be hampered by both the environment and internal resources of older adults. Younger patients may have greater physical (if not psychological) resilience to bring to bear on the recovery process. This is an important consideration in the development of geriatric after-care procedures and services. It becomes critical to follow patients into the next environment, whether it be back into a nursing home or back into the community. The increasing number of rehabilitative challenges (such as hip replacements) are becoming routine and require organized and systematic response to the psychological impact they invoke.

SERVICE MANAGEMENT

Nursing homes represent a high customer contact service organization. As such, the administration of nursing homes will be shaped in the 21st. Century by the research and theory evolving around the management of services. Administrators will be concerned with a series of managerial issues: managing the customer–employee "satisfaction mirror," building a cycle of capability, developing techniques to improve service delivery process, and ensuring resident–family satisfaction. Furthermore, administration in the future will assume an anticipatory rather than reactionary stance.

Research indicates that consumer satisfaction correlates with employee satisfaction (Schneider & Bowen, 1995). Employees who are satisfied remain on the job; their turnover is low. Long tenure employees are not only knowledgeable of what the service recipient wants, but can also better establish a relationship with the recipient. In our nursing home research (J. A. Duffy & Duffy, 1999), we found evidence of the satisfaction mirror. Namely, residents find encounters with staff satisfying when the staff use their name, remember what special food they like, and seem interested in them; similarly staff find their encounters with residents to be satisfying when the resident acts kindly toward them or appears to recognize their caring efforts. The employees in our study identified their interactions with residents as the source of satisfaction more frequently than pay or other extrinsic rewards. Successful service encounters and interactive relationships were the common source of satisfaction among both residents and employees (and in that sense, they mirror each other). Administrators, conscious of the satisfaction mirror, will build a delivery system that allows time for interactions to take place. Their decisions will be guided by the understanding that their main job is to serve those who serve the residents, as employee satisfaction leads to customer satisfaction.

Administrators will also be interested in supporting a cycle of capability that starts with hiring employees based on their attitudes rather than their skills. Capability is composed of

> 1) the latitude to deliver results to customers, a clear expression of limits within which frontline employees are permitted to act, 3) excellent training to perform the job, 4) well-engineered support systems such as service facilities and information system and, 5) recognition and rewards for doing jobs well. (Heskett, Sasser, & Schlesinger, 1997, p. 114).

These components of service capability are particularly interesting to administrators because they have been found to significantly contribute to employee satisfaction (Schlesinger & Zornitsky, 1995).

Administrators in nursing homes who stress process improvement will find several techniques particularly helpful. Service mapping is a technique that entails charting activities from the point of view of the resident and identifying which activities are most valued by the resident and which activities are subject to failure. From this analysis, the administrator can determine which part of the service delivery system to focus on. Another technique is cause and effect (fishbone) diagramming in which all categories of possible causes of a problem can be identified. Finally, pareto analysis is a way to determine which of the many possible causes of a service breakdown to concentrate on.

Nursing homes reveal two types of cultures: reactive and anticipatory. The anticipatory culture is best suited to enhance satisfaction. In the anticipatory culture, resident needs are addressed before they are articulated and at times even before the residents are conscious of them. In contrast, in the reactive culture, administrators do not respond to employee needs until the employee actually brings the need to the administrator's attention. Similarly, employees do not respond to resident needs until they are asked (or buzzed), perhaps more than once! Examples of behaviors one might observe in an anticipatory culture follow: A resident drops her book or Kleenex, and the staff member picks it up before the resident even realizes she has dropped it; the resident is reminded that her favorite TV program is starting and asked whether she wants the television turned on; a staff member is asked if she wants to come in early rather than late tomorrow because the administrator realizes it is the employee's birthday and she may wish to celebrate with her family. Individuals in an anticipatory culture feel valued because another person takes the initiative and expresses both interest and understanding of their needs.

ENVIRONMENTAL ENHANCEMENT

The environment is no small contributor to the overall quality of life and quality of health care. It is true that not all persons are especially sensitive to their surrounding environment, but it can be asserted that most persons are significantly affected by their surroundings (Lawton, 1999). Overall, long-term care and related interventions have been relatively attentive to the social environment; the tradition of activities programming within long-term care has enshrined a strong sense of the need to provide active and engaging social activities within residential environments. However, there is much less organized attention to the physical environment, which is potentially a powerful mediator of those programs and of the overall quality of life. Residential care facilities of the 21st century, therefore, will have an explicit and strong emphasis on facility design as a vehicle for quality of life and health care. There is a small but growing interest within behavioral sciences and in psychology on what is termed environmental psychology or human ecology. Architecture, of course, reflects environmental design but tends, in the U.S. culture, to focus on aesthetic aspects of design often at the cost of behavioral considerations. In a recent collaborative project involving a site design for a specialized Alzheimer's unit, we were struck by the tenacity with which designers clung to the artistic but clinically naive design plans for dementia patients. The situation in architecture is improving, and architects are more prone to conduct behavior-oriented consumer research prior to the final development of building plans. This is particularly pertinent because health care design is an increasing and specialized interest within the field of architecture, and attention to more than (but not excluding) aesthetic dimensions is critical in providing adequate settings for older adults in a long-term care context. We became specifically interested environmental design on reflection on the situation that exists in long-term care. Although the psychological impact of design, good, bad, or indifferent, is of our limited impact in environments we inhabit for short periods of time (e.g., home, office, work place, out-patient clinic), the situation is different in long-term care. Whatever are the effects of the design of nursing homes on well-being, we can assume that they are pervasive; residents live and are affected by this environment 24 hours a day, 7 days a week, 52 weeks a year! It is not trivial to suggest that the design of long-term residential care facilities is of critical importance and will assume a prime place in the next decade. There is a growing literature on the variety of design features that affect well-being such as light (older adults require three times the illumination level of younger adults), color, corridor design, external environment, and proximity to other residents (M. Duffy & Wilson, 1984).

Another critical psychosocial issue is the way that the physical environment facilitates both privacy and interaction for residents (J. A. Duffy, Bailey, Beck, & Barker, 1986). Administrators and designers are only visitors to the residential environment; it should come as no surprise that their views of an optimal nursing home environment are at odds with those of residents. Although administrators assume that the primary need for nursing home residents is social interaction, it is instructive to realize that for persons who live permanently in a nursing home environment, the feature in most demand is privacy. Therefore the creative design of environments to allow for reasonable privacy as well as encouraging health-giving social interaction is a key agenda for psychosocial design. Implicit in this discussion is the need for researchers both in the behavioral sciences and in the design professions to give serious attention to the perceptions, needs, and opinions of consumers who are the nursing home residents (J. A. Duffy et al., 1986). It is not true that what people prefer is always what they need (isolation may be chosen but not beneficial), but it is critical to understand the mind-set of the resident in order to plan an environment that is perceived as user-friendly and health-enhancing. There are current programmatic attempts to create comprehensive social and physical environments that enhance human well-being in long-term care. An example of this is the Eden Alternative, which has become an important model for residential care (see Chap. 1).

Finally, it is worth pointing out that optimal environmental design of nursing homes is, to some extent, a function of culture and national preference. In a cross-national study of nursing homes (J. A. Duffy, Duffy, & Kilbourne, 1989), higher recorded life satisfaction and satisfaction with residential setting seemed related to a contrasting residential designs. For example, whereas in many purpose-built nursing homes in the United States the emphasis has been on a medical, hospital-like, functional environment, many British nursing homes are transformed large, old houses. This, although perhaps not intentional, has the effect of creating a more home-like environment, which although it creates service provision difficulties (getting residents up old narrow staircases!), is well compensated by a rich, stimulating, and intimate social environment. Within this same culture of long-term care, we found it was quite common for nursing homes to encourage the relatively well elderly to develop an external social life, not excluding an occasional visit to the village pub! Although the United States may not be gifted with as many ancient manor houses, it be possible to extend this model by adapting medically oriented buildings to conform to more user friendly and homelike design.

Environmental enhancement will also invoke the use of many technical improvements that have been developed in other sectors. Health care designers often continue to promote a somewhat austere and barren hospital-like environment for residential care even though modern technology has developed materials that would allow these environments to be more home-like while maintaining a functional capacity for providing services. For example, floor covering that can be easily cleaned and provide relatively easy locomotion for handicapped persons, attractive wall coverings (although impregnated occasionally with unpleasant aromas) are easily cleaned and provide a more pleasant and idiosyncratic environment for older residents. Of course, many nursing homes have encouraged residents (especially private pay residents) to create a home-like environment by bringing personal furniture and personal belongings into the nursing home.

Other aspects of technology that will become routine in the next decades are merit mentioned here. In an era of continuously improving pharmaceuticals, medications will become available to adults that are more effective, have fewer side affects, and have a smaller half life. It seems optimistic at least to hope for improvements in the pharmaceutical care of patients with dementing disorders, although this is far from certain. Improvements in psychoactive medications, specifically, will perhaps provide a more appropriate use than is currently seen. In the period following OBRA (1987), there has been a reticence in using psychoactive medications that must be characterized as an overcorrection. The fear of overmedication leads some care providers to neglect effective medications for elderly who are painfully agitated as the direct result of dementing disorders. New generations of increasingly benign psychoactive medications should allow for a more reasonable balance between the danger of overmedication and a appropriate treatment of distressed older adults. This issue is described in chapter 9 of this text.

There is no doubt that the advent of telehealth–telemedicine intervention will have a significant impact on geriatric residential care in the 21st century. Although there is some understandable concern over an ensuing lack of personal contact (Stone, 2000), the benefits of telehealth clearly outweigh any possible handicaps. In a setting in which it is very difficult to get either physician or psychologist to be physically present in a nursing home, one might argue that any contact is better than nothing! Research in telehealth, in fact, is showing relatively minor differences in interpersonal terms between face-to-face and telemediated interactions. Many persons who have an auditory preference, for example, are able to interact effectively over telephone. Interactive computer and video conferencing, although creating some initial signal delay in interactions, is also showing that participants can very quickly accommodate to the signal delay and engage effectively in conversation. Thus it seems that telecommunication will make a very significant contribution to the long-term care environment, especially if there is a continued shortage of specialists available such as psychiatrists and a variety of medical specialists including neuropsychologists. Telehealth will allow for a series of activities that would otherwise not be possible, at least in current conditions, such as training of professional staff and nurse assistants, consultation with professionals, and supervision of trainees. In this latter instance, the American Psychological Association (APA) plans to increase the number of psychologists who will become proficient in clinical geropsychology. This plan involves some supervised experience, and the advent of telehealth will make that possible to large numbers of new providers.

Improved technology will also bring a continuing series of prosthetic techniques that will help older adults cope with the chronic physical limitations that are inevitable in very old age. As mentioned earlier, hip replacements have become commonplace, and physical therapy procedures allow a person to be active and engaged within a remarkably short time. My own mother, between the ages of 80 and 87, had two successful hip replacements, which allowed her to continue in a reasonably functional manner during the last years of her life.

DEMENTIA CARE

A key issue in the next decades will be sophisticated psychological care of residents with cognitive impairment. As the numbers of older adults surviving into very old age increases, along with an associated high likelihood of cognitive impairment, the issue of high-quality care becomes imperative It is an almost legendary feature of all institutional care that in a context where persons are in the closest physical proximity (i.e., in a nursing home), they may suffer the most pervasive and soul-destroying psychological and social alienation. This situation becomes exacerbated in the case of cognitively impaired residents who may be thought-and-language impaired and are not able to initiate contact with the staff or with other residents.

Psychology, and particularly behavioral psychology, has contributed significantly over the past 20 years to methods of managing "problematic behaviors" of demented residents (Hussian, 1988). These behavior management strategies have been invaluable in addressing such behavioral problems as aggression, inappropriate toileting, exiting behavior, and inappropriate sexual behavior. These insights into managing associative behavior have been helpful not only to nursing home staff but also to families of persons with dementing disorders who continue to live in a home context. However, psychology and mental health professions need to explore additional methods of enhancing the degree of psychological and affective connection between dementia patients and the world around them. The single most pervasive impression in a typical nursing home is the lack of interpersonal engagement of many residents who are cognitively and language-impaired, including stroke victims. The staffing system is simply not adapted to provide the more subtle level of care that would be required to maintain rich and energizing relationships with such debilitated residents. Contact between nursing home roommates, for example, is minimal, and it is routine to discover that roommates know almost nothing about each other, even minimal information including name, geographic origin, or interests. A similar situation exists between residents and staff in which staff have prescribed technical duties with regard to residents including medication, food, toileting, and what is referred to as "bed and body" duties. In a situation where registered nurses have less than 10 minutes of contact with residents in a 24-hour period, and nurse assistants have little more than one hour of accumulated contact time per day, it is not surprising that isolation becomes an indigenous fact of nursing home life. When contact does occur, it is often technical and impersonal, except in the case of unusual staff members who have a natural, but often rare, talent for intimate human contact. These gifted employees are quite influential within the nursing home, but sadly, are quite rare. Our comments are by no means intended to be critical of the nursing home staff. They simply describe a reasonable portrait of persons who are grossly underpaid and overworked due to the large numbers of residents who need care. We know that in many locations nurse assistants are frequently at or near poverty level themselves, may be struggling with their own family difficulties, and are not in an optimal position to form therapeutic connections with residents. Treatment in the 21st century, therefore, will not only focus on the problem of behavior management of demented residents but also on the more subtle aspects of human interactions that dramatically enhance the well-being and morale of older persons who are in residential care settings (Lawton, Van Haitsma, & Klapper, 1996). Training can start by focusing on each employee's naturalistic appreciation of a difference between the relationship that is intimate and engaged versus one that is formal, technical, and business-like. Warm, personal relationships between professionals and clients, far from inducing burnout, actually have the reverse affect. Nurse aides, for example, who blend warm relationships with technical service in the course of their daily work are more satisfied with their work (Schneider & Bowen, 1995).

When this type of interaction becomes normative, there will be greater capacity to address the cognitive and effective life of demented residents (Feil, 1999). We realize that we become so language-dependent in our interactions with other persons that we do not recognize the degree of subverbal communication that occurs. It is a truism that a relationship can be judged as intimate precisely where language becomes less important between resident and caregiver. In those relationships with demented older adults where language and cognition becomes impaired, staff needs to be trained to maintain interpersonal and affective contact with older adults so that the residual capacities, often substantial, can be enhanced and broadened. Thus it is more likely that the systemic problem of comorbid depression that frequently occurs in demented elderly residents will be able to be offset. Staffs will discover that the loss of cognition and language does not involve the loss of experienced emotion and that in all human relationships the emotional dimension is perhaps the most fundamental to intimacy. To express this metaphorically, we might say that in intimate human relationships (and hopefully in connections with demented elderly), we frequently speak more commonly to the amygdala than the cortex! Training for nursing home staff and indeed other professionals will in the future focus on subtle and naturalistic psychological approaches in addition to behavior management. A primary professional area will be to train staff in how not to react to provocation when caring for older adults, how not to switch off emotional connection when a resident loses language communication, how to stay "present" and validate an older adult who loses language (Feil, 1999), and how to recognize patient aggression as frequently the result of a reciprocal reactive behavior rather than the outcome of organic impairment itself.

It must be said finally however, as in most areas, that these changes can only be brought about systematically if more appropriate resources are devoted to long-term care. As mentioned earlier, when Medicaid reimbursement in many states is so inadequate, it is not reasonable to expect high-level and sufficient care from nursing home staff. When caregivers are themselves underpaid and under-trained, it is not surprising that difficulties emerge.

INCREASED FAMILY INVOLVEMENT IN GERIATRIC RESIDENTIAL CARE

The relationship between families and nursing homes has been traditionally diffi-cult and even conflictual. This is not entirely surprising when one considers that families experience some of the highest levels of stress around issues of admitting an older relative into long-term residential care. Indeed it is important for family therapists to recognize that such "disorder" in families is less psychologically seri-ous than it may seem. The decision to admit a family member to a nursing home, as discussed earlier, is made with great difficulty and after considerable agonizing on multiple care alternatives. This degree of ambivalence often finds expression in other emotions such as anger within the family, and some of this anger may spill over to nursing homes. Nursing home administrators, in turn, may handle these in-teractions poorly and set up a relationship that is beneficial neither to the residents nor the nursing home itself. The situation is such that instead of the family becom-ing an advocate in a patient's care, they frequently become an adversary (M. Duffy 1996). While sometimes nursing home administrators become reciprocally ag-gressive with families, the more common reaction to family stress and intrusion is for the nursing home to become overly compliant with regard to the families wishes, rather than treating them as a necessary partner in care. In the 21st century it will be helpful if residential care facilities gain a greater sense of entitlement and authority in their care of residents and in dealings with family members. It is our experience that when nursing homes clearly establish policy and guidelines for continuing family involvement that are flexible but clear, family members will fre-quently not only become reassured and calmer, but also more collaborative with patient care. This kind of collaborative but firm relationship is more likely to be a platform for the discussion and negotiation of a division of labor for family and nursing home. With this kind of collaboration in place, facility and family can clearly understand who is responsible for differential aspects of care such as mate-rial possessions, clothes, visiting, financial payments, and the more subtle aspects of nurturance of residents.

With this atmosphere established, the nursing home has provided the opportu-nity to enhance the resident–family relationships. Frequently, despite popular neg-ative misconception, the nursing home becomes the last and best venue in which family relationships can be enhanced. In the case of the very old patients, it indeed may be the last residence, and family members sense that "a clock is running" with regard to dealing with unfinished and unresolved issues in family relationships. Earlier detachment from family intimacy often brings loneliness to residents, and it can be a significant contribution of the nursing home to provide a platform in which such relationships can be corrected and enhanced. It will be helpful here also for nursing homes to become aware and use the services of family therapists, especially family therapists who are sensitive and skilled in dealing with complex issues of intergenerational family relationships (Long & Martin, 2000).

Family members are also vulnerable to the affects of language deprivation in their relationships with their relatives. They may have the same need for instruction and training in how to continue emotionally important relationships when their relative is struck by a dementing and language-depriving disorder. Nursing homes can help families with simple skills in how to make a visit to their relative–a task that becomes difficult for family members and can even result in pervasive avoidance of visitation. To help someone understand how to stay with their older relative even despite loss of their language becomes an important task. In a recent situation in which we provided psychological therapy to an older man who had terminal bone cancer and eventually became comatose and noncommunicative, it became an important part of family therapy to stay with and model for the family how to remain connected with their father under these conditions. In a touching note after their father's death, a family member expressed gratitude for our advice to stay with and keep talking to their father even beyond the point when they were sure that he was able to understand. This not only ensured the well-being of the dying father but also provided great comfort to the family in their grief.

WORK FORCE DEVELOPMENT

This final section addresses the plans and problems in providing trained workers in geriatric residential care, both in the paraprofessional workforce (e.g. nurse aides) and also in the professional workforce (physicians, nurses, psychologists, social workers, etc.).

The recent Milbank Memorial Fund report (Stone, 2000) estimates that the shortage of paraprofessional workers, certified nursing aides in nursing homes, and home care aides is currently at a crisis level for long-term care. Paraprofessionals are among the worst paid workers in the service sector and have many unattractive job features including low wages, frequently few or absent benefits, a lack of career development, a fairly high potential for work-related injury, and exposure to much emotional stress. The median hourly wage for nurse assistants is $7.46, and we recognize that it is frequently at the minimum wage level. About 30% of nurse aides have no health insurance and yet, as the result of back injuries resulting from inappropriate lifting and transferring patients, they often seek worker's compensation only to find that this is often a tortuous process and frequently results in failure. Although a reasonable workload for a nurse aide is around 12 patients on an 8-hour shift, it is not at all unusual for understaffing to lead a nurse aide to be responsible for two wings (30–40 residents) in a long-term care facility. The remedy for these problems will depend on the political climates in the next decades. It must be hoped that younger cohorts of workers will become increasingly aware of legitimate long-term care needs and support increased public funding (Binstock, 1998).

Another future variable will be increases in private or public long-term care insurance. Even though there has been a modest increase in such programs during the last decades of the 20th century, the increased availability of such insurance programs have been dogged by poor risk-assessment methodologies (Stone, 2000). Future availability of workers in residential care setting will also, depend on future immigration policies. Current policies largely discourage the infusion of foreign workers into the U.S. workforce. It should be noted, however, that ethnic minority and foreign workers make up a large proportion of nurse assistant staff in many states. Other "graying nations" have found it necessary to allow integration for long-term care settings: Italy, for example, admits many geriatric workers from Peru, and Japan admits workers from the Philippines (Stone, 2000). This trend will be affected by the future wage structure for long-term care settings, as it has in other U.S. industries. If wage structures become more appropriate to the task definition in nursing homes, then issues of workforce immigration may become moot.

Another possible source of paraprofessional staff for nursing homes can be found in volunteer programs, especially those that train volunteers to a paraprofessional level (Crose et al., 1986). Project OASIS, for example, was specifically designed to bring intensive interpersonal assistance to very old and neglected residents, and this concept can be seen as a viable element in staffing of long-term care. It certainly was viable at a period when there was no formal mental health or social service dimension in medical long-term care. However, it is important to comment that it is an alluring but inappropriate proposal to suggest that all psychosocial care should be provided on a volunteer or religiously oriented basis. Such a position clearly avoids shared public responsibility for the oldest members of the community.

The needs for increased support for professionals in long-term care remains acute, especially for mental health professionals. In 1987, the National Institute on Aging estimated that there are currently 2,425 board-certified geriatric psychiatrists and only 200–700 geropsychologists. They estimated that each profession would need 5,000 specialists within the next two decades to meet projected needs. The mental health professions clearly have a long way to go to meet the mental health needs of older adults, especially in residential care settings where such providers are even more rare.

There are optimistic signs of serious attempts to remedy the situation. The APA recently recognized a new proficiency of clinical geropsychology, and the APA College of Professional Psychology is currently considering the possibility of a certificate in geropsychology that establishes basic parameters for clinical practice with older adults. Also, APA Division 20, Adult Development and Aging, has created Section 2, Clinical Geropsychology, which provides a professional forum for psychologists seeking support and continuing education in this relatively new area. Similarly, many of the divisions of the APA have established special committees on aging with a variety of interests and programs. There are, however, relatively few graduate programs in clinical, counseling, or health psychology that provide supervised clinical training in working with older adults. Clearly this area needs dramatic expansion. The Veteran's Administration has been a leader within psychology for several decades, establishing and supporting both predoctoral and, more recently, postdoctoral training in geropsychology. Perhaps the most promising avenue for increases of professionals in geriatric residential care will come from already established professionals in psychology, social work, and psychiatry who seek continuing education training to develop a proficiency in working in geriatric contexts. This can relatively easily be supported through professional associations and by extensions of existing continuing education systems to include organized sequences of training in academic and clinical work. This has been the intent of the APA's Interdivisional Task Force on Clinical Geropsychology in providing a model of content and methods for the continued training of experienced professionals for the field of geriatric residential care.

Finally, as mentioned earlier, it is difficult to be completely optimistic about such efforts without the necessary resources being designated for this purpose. As it is well known, funding for behavioral science in general is relatively limited and although there is much political attention on the well being of older adult, there are relatively few public resources committed to this area. If this situation can change, and we must assume it will, then the professionalization of mental health in residential care can be accomplished.

Some examples of future directions would be to extend graduate medical education to the support of mental health professionals in addition to physicians and to enable mental health professionals to provide training programs in mental health and aging. At this time there is a proposal in Congress to ammend the Older Americans Act to include the training resources for mental health in long-term care. Such initiative not only provides support for training but would also send a strong political message throughout the health care system and political community of the importance of the mental health services in residential care. It will also be a great help if the HCFA would provide parity in mental health services such that mental health services were reimbursed at the same rate as general health services (50% vs. 80%) and also that the HCFA methodology used to calculate the monetary value of mental health services would provide a more sensitive measure of mental health services.

CONCLUSION

This final chapter has reviewed the status of geriatric residential care as a guide for future planning. It is easier to describe what should be as opposed to predicting what will be. However, if we examine the overall development within the field of mental health, for example psychology, we can take some hope. Psychology has expanded exponentially in the past 50 years to address an increasing number of social needs, and although resources may not in all cases be optimal, the societal presence of mental health awareness and services have certainly been enhanced enormously. We have laid out an agenda—perhaps a manifesto—for future directions in geriatric residential care. It seems that although the need for continuing professionalization of general geriatric health care is essential, the situation in a long-term residential care points even more urgently to developing enhanced psychosocial dimensions of care. This dimension of care is not only important in the maintenance of substantive quality of life but also a significant contributor to physical health and well-being.

REFERENCES

Alecxih, L. M. (1997). What is it, who needs it, and who provides it? In B. L. Boyd (Ed.), *Long term care: Knowing the risk, paying the price* (pp. 15–23). Washington DC: Health Insurance Association of America.

Better nursing home care (2000, September 25). *New York Times.*

Binstock, R. H. (1998) Dementia and health care reform. In M. F. Folstein (Ed.) *Neurobiology of Primary Dementia* (pp. 385–408), Washington, DC:

Bishop, C. E. (1999). Where are the missing elders? The decline in nursing home use 1985 and 1995. *Health Affairs, 18*(4), 146–155.

Chambless, D. L., & Hollon, S. D. (1998) Defining empirically supported therapies. *Journal of Consulting and Clinical Psychology, 66,* 7–18.

Crose, R., Duffy, M., Warren, J., & Velasquez, J. (1986). Project OASIS: Volunteer mental health paraprofessionals serving nursing home residents. *The Gerontologist, 27,* 259–362.

Duffy, J. A. and Duffy, M. (1999). The satisfaction mirror. *The Gerontologist, 39*(1), 133.

Duffy, J. A., Duffy, M., & Kilbourne, W. (1997) Crossnational perspectives of service quality in long term health care. *Journal of Aging Studies, 11,* 327–336.

Duffy, M., Bailey, S., Beck, B., & Barker, D. G. (1986). Preferences in nursing home design: A comparison of residents, administrators and designers. *Environment and Behavior, 18,* 246–257.

Duffy, M.(1996) The resident's family: Adversary or advocate in long term care. In R. Crose (Ed.) *Aging is a family affair* (pp. 17–21), Muncie, IN: Ball State University, Center for Gerontology.

Duffy, M. (1999). Reaching the person behind the dementia: Treating comorbid affective disorders through subvocal and non-verbal strategies. In M.Duffy (Ed.) *Handbook of counseling and psychotherapy with older adults* (pp. 577–590). New York: Wiley.

Duffy, M., & Wilson V. L. (1984). The role of design factors of the residential environment in the physical and mental health of the elderly. *Journal of Housing for the Elderly, 2*(3), 37–45.

Feil, N. (1999). Current concepts and techniques in validation therapy. In M. Duffy (Ed.), *Handbook of counseling and psychotherapy with older adults* (pp. 590–613. New York: Wiley.

Friedlob, A. (1993) *The use of physical restraints in nursing homes and the allocation of nursing resources.* Unpublished doctoral dissertation, University of Minnesota, Minneapolis.

Galvin, J. C., & La Buda, D. R. (1991) United States health policy into the next century. *International Journal of Technology and Aging, 4*(2), 115–127.

Hawryluk, M. (1999, June). Quality indicators shift survey focus. *Provider,* 25–29.

Heskett, J. L., Sasser, W. E., & Schlesinger, L. A. (1997). *The service profit chain.* New York: Free Press.

Himes, C. L. (1992). Future caregivers: Projected family structures of older persons. *Journal of Gerontology: Social Sciences, 47*(1), S17–S26.

Hussian, R. A. (1988). Modification of behaviors in dementia via stimulus manipulation. *Clinical Gerontologist, 8,* 37–43.

Lawton, M. P. (1999). Environmental design features and the well-being of older persons. In M.Duffy (Ed.), *Handbook of counseling and psychotherapy with older adults* (pp. 350–363), New York: Wiley.

Lawton, M. P., Van Haitsma, K., & Klapper, J. (1996). Observed affect in nursing home residents with Alzheimer's disease. *Journal of Gerontology: Psychological Sciences, 51B*(1), P3–P14.

Long, M. V., & Martin, P. (2000). Personality, relationship closeness and loneliness of oldest adults and their children. *Journal of Gerontology: Psychological Sciences, 55B*(5), P311–319.

National Institute on Aging (1987) *Personnel for health needs of the elderly.* Washington, DC: Pub. 87–2950.

Omnibus Budget Reconciliation Act (1987). Washington, DC: GAO.

Sanders, K., Brockway, J. A., Ellis, B., Cotton, E. M., & Bredin, J. (1999). Enhancing mental health climate in hospitals and nursing homes: Collaboration strategies for medical and mental health staff. In M. Duffy (Ed.), *Handbook of counseling and psychotherapy for older adults* (pp. 335–349), New York: Wiley.

Schlesinger, L. A. , & Zornitsky, J. (1995). Job satisfaction, service capability and customer satisfaction: An examiniations of linkages and management implications. *Human Resource Planning, 14*(2), 141–149.

Schneider, B. & Bowen, D. E. (1995) New services design development and implementation and the employee. In W. R. George and C. Marshall (Eds.) *New Services* (pp. 217–236), Chicago: The American Marketing Association.

Somers, A. R., & Spears, N. L. (1992) *The continuing care retirement community: A significant option for long-term care.* New York: Springer.

Stone, R. I. (2000). Long-term care for the elderly with disabilities: Current policy, emerging trends, and implications for the twenty-first century. New York: Millbank Memorial Fund.

Tariot, P. N., Podgorske, C. A. and Blazina, L. (1993). Mental disorders in the nursing home: Another perspective. *American Journal of Psychiatry, 150,* 1063–1069.

Author Index

C

Subject Index